Encyclopedia of Wellness

Encyclopedia of Wellness

From Açaí Berry to Yo-Yo Dieting

Volume 1: A–E

Sharon Zoumbaris, Editor

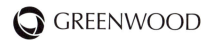 GREENWOOD

AN IMPRINT OF ABC-CLIO, LLC
Santa Barbara, California • Denver, Colorado • Oxford, England

Copyright 2012 by Sharon Zoumbaris

Library of Congress Cataloging-in-Publication Data

Encyclopedia of wellness : from açaí berry to yo-yo dieting / Sharon Zoumbaris,
editor.
    p. cm.
  Includes index.
  ISBN 978-0-313-39333-4 (hardback) — ISBN 978-0-313-39334-1 (ebook)
1. Health—Encyclopedias.   2. Medicine, Preventive—Encyclopedias.
I. Zoumbaris, Sharon, 1955–
  RA776.E524   2012
  613.03—dc23   2011045406

ISBN: 978-0-313-39333-4
EISBN: 978-0-313-39334-1

16 15 14 13 12   1 2 3 4 5

This book is also available on the World Wide Web as an eBook.
Visit www.abc-clio.com for details.

Greenwood
An Imprint of ABC-CLIO, LLC

ABC-CLIO, LLC
130 Cremona Drive, P.O. Box 1911
Santa Barbara, California 93116-1911

This book is printed on acid-free paper (∞)

Manufactured in the United States of America

This book discusses treatments (including types of medication and mental health therapies), diagnostic tests for various symptoms and mental health disorders, and organizations. The authors have made every effort to present accurate and up-to-date information.
However, the information in this book is not intended to recommend or endorse particular treatments or organizations, or substitute for the care or medical advice of a qualified
health professional, or used to alter any medical therapy without a medical doctor's advice.
Specific situations may require specific therapeutic approaches not included in this book.
For those reasons, we recommend that readers follow the advice of qualified health care
professionals directly involved in their care. Readers who suspect they may have specific
medical problems should consult a physician about any suggestions made in this book.

Contents

Alphabetical List of Entries   *vii*

Entries Arranged by Broad Topic   *xv*

Preface   *xxiii*

Introduction: Wellness in the United States   *xxvii*

The Encyclopedia   **1**

Glossary   889

Internet Resources   905

About the Editor and Contributors   937

Index   947

Alphabetical List of Entries

Açaí Berry
Acquired Immune Deficiency Syndrome (AIDS)
Acupuncture
Addiction
Adolescence
Aerobic Exercise
Air Pollution
Alcohol
Allergies
Allergies, Food
Alzheimer's Disease
Amino Acids
Anaerobic Exercise
Anorexia Nervosa
Antibiotics
Antioxidants
Asperger Syndrome
Asthma
Atkins, Robert C.
Attention Deficit Hyperactivity Disorder (ADHD)
Autism
Ayurveda

Back Pain
Bacteria
Bariatric Surgery
Basal Metabolism
Basic Four (Foods)
Biofeedback

Bipolar Disorder
Birth Control
Blood Pressure
Blueberries
Body Image
Body Mass Index (BMI)
Bone Health
Breast-feeding
Bulimia Nervosa

Caffeine
Calcium
Calories
Cancer
Carbohydrates
Cardiopulmonary Resuscitation (CPR)
Cardiovascular Health. *See* Heart Health
Carpal Tunnel Syndrome
Cell Phones
Center for Food Safety and Applied Nutrition (CFSAN)
Centers for Disease Control and Prevention (CDC)
Cheeseburger Bill
Chelation
Cholesterol
Chronic Fatigue Syndrome (CFS)
Cigarettes
Common Cold (Upper Respiratory Viruses)
Comprehensive Smoking Education Act

Daily Value of Nutrients
Dance Therapy
Dental Health
Deoxyribonucleic Acid (DNA)
Depression
Diabetes
Dietary Guidelines for Americans
Dietary Reference Intakes (DRI)
Dietary Supplements
Dieting
Dieting, Online Resources
Diets, Fad
Doctors in the Media
Dream Therapy
Drugs, Recreational

Eating Disorders
E. Coli Infection
Edible Schoolyard Project
Environmental Health
Environmental Protection Agency (EPA)
Ephedra/Ephedrine
Exercise

Fast Food
Fats
Fiber
Fibromyalgia
Flaxseeds
Flexible Spending Account (FSA)
Food Allergies. *See* Allergies, Food
Food and Drug Administration (FDA)
Food-borne Illness
Food Recalls
Food Safety
Free Radicals

Garlic
Gender Identity and Sexual Orientation
Genetically Modified Organisms (GMOs)
Ghrelin
Ginger
Ginseng
Glycemic Index
Graham, Sylvester
Grief
Guided Imagery

Head Start and Healthy Start
Health and Medical Tourism
Health Insurance
Health Savings Account (HSA)
Heart Health
Hepatitis
High-Fructose Corn Syrup
HMO. *See* Managed Care
Homeopathy
Human Chorionic Gonadotropin (HCG)
Human Immunodeficiency Virus (HIV)
Human Papillomavirus (HPV)

Hypertension
Hypnosis

Immune System/Lymphatic System
Immunizations. *See* Vaccinations
Influenza
Inhalants
Insomnia
Institute of Medicine (IOM)
Irradiation

Kava
Kellogg, John Harvey
Ketosis

Lactose Intolerance
Liposuction
Living Wills and Advance Directives
Love Canal
L-Tryptophan
Lupus
Lymphatic System. *See* Immune System/Lymphatic System

Macrobiotics
Malnutrition
Mammography
Managed Care
Manic-Depressive Disorder. *See* Bipolar Disorder
Marijuana. *See* Medical Marijuana; Smoking
Mayo Clinic
Medicaid
Medical Marijuana
Medical Power of Attorney
Medicare
Meditation
Metabolism. *See* Basal Metabolism
Methicillin-Resistant Staphylococcus Aureus (MRSA)
Mind-Body Health. *See* Psychosomatic Health Care
Minerals (Food)
MyPlate

National Cancer Institute
National Center for Complementary and Alternative Medicine (NCCAM)
National Institutes of Health (NIH)

National Organic Program (NOP)
National School Lunch Program (NSLP)
Naturopathic Medicine
Nestle, Marion
Nurse Practitioners
Nutrients
Nutrigenomics
Nutrition
Nutrition Facts Label
Nutritional Diseases

Obesity
Obsessive-Compulsive Disorder (OCD)
Omega 3/6 Fatty Acids. *See* Fats
Online Health Resources
Organic Food
Ornish, Dean
Osteoporosis

Pandemics
Pasteur, Louis
Pauling, Linus
Personal Trainer
Physical Education
Physical Endurance
Pilates
Polycystic Ovary Syndrome (PCOS)
President's Council on Fitness, Sports, and Nutrition
Primary Care Physicians
Pritikin, Nathan
Probiotics
Psychosomatic Health Care
Psychotherapy

Qigong

Recombinant Bovine Growth Hormone (rBGH)
Recommended Dietary Allowance (RDA)
Reflexology
Registered Dietitian
Reiki
Religion and Spirituality
Resting Metabolic Rate
Retail Clinic

Ritalin
Rodale, Jerome

Salmonella
School Meals Initiative
Scoliosis. *See* Bone Health
Seasonal Affective Disorder (SAD)
Secondhand Smoke
Sexually Transmitted Diseases (STDs)
Skin Cancer. *See* Cancer
Sleep
Smoking
Sodium
Soy
Spas, Medical
Staphylococcus
Steroids
Stress
Suicide
Supplements. *See* Dietary Supplements

Tai Chi
Tanning
Target Heart Rate
Therapeutic Touch
Traditional Chinese Medicine
Trans Fats

U.S. Department of Agriculture (USDA)
U.S. Department of Health and Human Services (HHS)

Vaccinations
Vegans. *See* Vegetarians
Vegetables
Vegetarians
Virtual Hospital
Virus
Vitamins

Walking
Water
Waters, Alice
Weight Training
Weight Watchers

White, Ryan
Women's Health Initiative (WHI)
Workplace Wellness
World Health Organization (WHO)

Yoga
Yo-Yo Dieting

Entries Arranged by Broad Topic

Alternative Health Care and Complementary Medicine

Acupuncture
Ayurveda
Biofeedback
Chelation
Dance Therapy
Dietary Supplements
Dream Therapy
Guided Imagery
Homeopathy
Hypnosis
Macrobiotics
Medical Marijuana
Meditation
National Center for Complementary and Alternative Medicine
Naturopathic Medicine
Pauling, Linus
Probiotics
Qigong
Reflexology
Reiki
Rodale, Jerome
Spas, Medical
Tai Chi
Therapeutic Touch
Traditional Chinese Medicine

Diseases and Disorders

Acquired Immune Deficiency Syndrome (AIDS)
Addiction
Alzheimer's Disease
Asperger Syndrome
Asthma
Attention Deficit Hyperactivity Disorder (ADHD)
Autism
Back Pain
Bipolar Disorder
Cancer
Carpal Tunnel Syndrome
Chronic Fatigue Syndrome (CFS)
Common Cold (Upper Respiratory Viruses)
Diabetes
Eating Disorders
Fibromyalgia
Hepatitis
Human Immunodeficiency Virus (HIV)
Human Papillomavirus (HPV)
Influenza
Insomnia
Ketosis
Lupus
Malnutrition
Methicillin-Resistant Staphylococcus Aureus (MRSA)
Nutritional Diseases
Obesity
Obsessive-Compulsive Disorder (OCD)
Osteoporosis
Polycystic Ovary Syndrome (PCOS)
Seasonal Affective Disorder (SAD)
Sexually Transmitted Diseases (STDs)
White, Ryan

Environmental Health

Air Pollution
Cell Phones
Cigarettes
E. Coli Infection
Edible Schoolyard Project
Environmental Health
Ephedra/Ephedrine
Food Safety

Food-borne Illness
Free Radicals
Genetically Modified Organisms (GMOs)
Human Chorionic Gonadotropin (HCG)
Inhalants
Irradiation
Love Canal
L-Tryptophan
Recombinant Bovine Growth Hormone (rBGH)
Salmonella
Secondhand Smoke
Smoking
Staphylococcus
Steroids
Tanning

Exercise and Weight Control

Aerobic Exercise
Anaerobic Exercise
Anorexia Nervosa
Bariatric Surgery
Basal Metabolism
Body Image
Body Mass Index (BMI)
Bulimia Nervosa
Dieting
Dieting, Online Resources
Diets, Fad
Eating Disorders
Exercise
Liposuction
Obesity
Personal Trainer
Physical Endurance
Qigong
Pilates
Resting Metabolic Rate
Tai Chi
Target Heart Rate
Walking
Weight Training
Weight Watchers
Yoga
Yo-Yo Dieting

Government, Legislation, and Public Policy

Center for Food Safety and Applied Nutrition (CFSAN)
Centers for Disease Control and Prevention (CDC)
Cheeseburger Bill
Comprehensive Smoking Education Act
Dietary Guidelines for Americans
Dietary Reference Intakes (DRI)
Environmental Protection Agency (EPA)
Food and Drug Administration (FDA)
Food Recalls
Head Start and Healthy Start
Human Papillomavirus (HPV)
Institute of Medicine (IOM)
Living Wills and Advance Directives
Medicaid
Medical Power of Attorney
Medicare
MyPlate
National Cancer Institute
National Institutes of Health (NIH)
National Organic Program (NOP)
National School Lunch Program (NSLP)
Nutrition Facts Label
Pandemic
Physical Education
President's Council on Fitness, Sports, and Nutrition
Recommended Dietary Allowance (RDA)
School Meals Initiative
U.S. Department of Agriculture (USDA)
U.S. Department of Health and Human Services (HHS)
Vaccinations
Women's Health Initiative (WHI)
Workplace Wellness
World Health Organization (WHO)

Health Care

Antibiotics
Bariatric Surgery
Blood Pressure
Cardiopulmonary Resuscitation (CPR)
Dieting, Online Resources
Doctors in the Media
Health and Medical Tourism

Mammography
Mayo Clinic
Nurse Practitioners
Online Health Resources
Pasteur, Louis
Primary Care Physicians
Psychosomatic Health Care
Registered Dietitians
Retail Clinic
Ritalin
Vaccinations
Virtual Hospital

Insurance and Health Care Costs

Flexible Spending Account (FSA)
Health Insurance
Health Savings Account (HSA)
Managed Care

Mental Health, Social Health, and Addiction

Addiction
Adolescence
Alcohol
Alzheimer's Disease
Anorexia Nervosa
Attention Deficit Hyperactivity Disorder (ADHD)
Bipolar Disorder
Birth Control
Body Image
Bulimia Nervosa
Depression
Drugs, Recreational
Gender Identity and Sexual Orientation
Grief
Obsessive-Compulsive Disorder (OCD)
Psychosomatic Health Care
Psychotherapy
Religion and Spirituality
Seasonal Affective Disorder (SAD)
Sexually Transmitted Diseases (STDs)
Stress
Suicide

Nutritional Health

Açaí Berry
Amino Acids
Atkins, Robert C.
Basic Four (Foods)
Blueberries
Caffeine
Calcium
Calories
Carbohydrates
Cholesterol
Daily Value of Nutrients
Dietary Supplements
Dieting
Diets, Fad
Fast Food
Fats
Fiber
Flaxseeds
Free Radicals
Garlic
Ginger
Ginseng
Glycemic Index
Graham, Sylvester
High-Fructose Corn Syrup
Kava
Kellogg, John Harvey
Lactose Intolerance
Minerals (Food)
Nestle, Marion
Nutrients
Nutrigenomics
Nutrition
Organic Food
Ornish, Dean
Pritikin, Nathan
Sodium
Soy
Trans Fats
Vegetables
Vegetarians
Vitamins
Water

Waters, Alice
Yo-Yo Dieting

Physical Health

Allergies
Allergies, Food
Antioxidants
Back Pain
Bacteria
Basal Metabolism
Bone Health
Common Cold (Upper Respiratory Viruses)
Dental Health
Deoxyribonucleic Acid (DNA)
Ghrelin
Heart Health
Immune System/Lymphatic System
Metabolism
Resting Metabolic Rate
Sleep
Target Heart Rate
Virus
Weight Control. *See* Dieting

Preface

How do individuals achieve wellness in today's busy, stressful world? More important, how does one remain healthy, since wellness and health are not static, and every day can bring new challenges that directly impact an individual's quality of life? While living a long time and not becoming seriously ill or injured may not guarantee anyone a sense of wellness, conversely, being sick may not rob someone of a sense of well-being either.

How is that possible? This three-volume set, the *Encyclopedia of Wellness,* will examine key components that create overall wellness. These include preventive measures such as eating a healthy diet, choosing regular exercise as part of a lifestyle, making self-care decisions that encourage wellness, reducing the risk of chronic diseases, preventing injuries, diminishing safety hazards and environmental issues in the home and workplace, and making the best use of the country's health care system.

A thorough understanding of the changing face of U.S. health care is of growing importance, because the cost of medical care in this country continues to rise rapidly. Knowing what choices to make and how to successfully navigate the medical system frustrates many Americans. These ongoing challenges make information an increasingly valuable component of wellness.

This reference work offers fundamental information about hundreds of topics and methods for examining overall wellness, including health insurance, flexible spending accounts, antioxidants, low-fat versus high-protein diets, smoking, healthy food choices at home as well as in fast food restaurants and schools, vitamins and minerals, diet supplements, drugs and alcohol, and recent changes in national health care legislation and workplace wellness programs that show how corporate America is keeping employees healthy and productive.

The most important aspect of the *Encyclopedia of Wellness* is the wealth of perspectives and information it presents. Leading scholars, well-respected researchers, and up-and-coming professionals have come together to share their wisdom and talents, and readers will be the richer for their efforts. Entries for this encyclopedia have been drawn from all aspects of wellness: physical, mental, emotional, social, and spiritual. The essays have been written in such a way that complex subjects are clear and concise. Even more important, each entry will lead readers to other questions and more information. And they will discover, as I did, just how much there is to learn about living well.

The *Encyclopedia of Wellness* will appeal to students of health and wellness as well as to researchers and laypeople in all different disciplines, including public health, mental health, nutrition, alternative medicine, religious studies, sociology, and philosophy.

The *Encyclopedia of Wellness* offers some 222 entries, from 78 contributors, including notable individuals such as Myrna Chandler Goldstein, Stan Krippner, Reverend Dr. J. Harold Ellens, Harris Friedman, and others. Some of the specially selected material comes from content, updated as appropriate, that has been published in Greenwood's and ABC-CLIO's award-winning encyclopedias and other reference works and from ABC-CLIO's informational databases. Information about the contributors is found in the "About the Editor and Contributors" section at the end of the set.

Each of the essays in this encyclopedia examines an aspect of mental, physical, social, emotional, or spiritual health and looks at current research, its history, and what the future may bring in that subject area. One of the challenges in assembling this encyclopedia was the decision of what to include and what to leave out. There are so many resources available that provide great depth of information on unique aspects of health. This work was not intended to be a comprehensive examination of any single topic. Instead, the goal was to create a resource that covered as many related aspects of health and wellness as possible. The decision was also made not to focus exclusively on disease, although there are entries on specific diseases. The aim instead is to offer readers a well-rounded list of topics that fall under wellness, not just illness, including insurance, exercise, and nutrition.

The volumes are arranged in alphabetical order in standard encyclopedia format. Each entry also provides a list of references and suggestions for related topics. In some entries, short sidebars are intended to provide a personal look into some aspect of health. For example, an article about autism contains a sidebar that describes a very successful summer camp for autistic children. The Internet resource list at the end of the volumes offers a substantial starting point for those wishing to link to other government, nonprofit, and private organizations offering sources of information.

This work is both ambitious and humble. The ambition lies in trying to capture the essence of wellness in just three volumes. The humility, on the other hand, is in realizing that, no matter how much is known, there will always be something new to learn in the quest for a healthy balance in life. As a librarian and researcher, I love books and I love research. My passions joined together in this encyclopedia, a perfect oasis for readers like myself to leisurely browse, roaming from item to item, or to turn directly to whatever information is needed at the moment.

When I was growing up as a child, good nutrition was Wonder Bread with a thick coating of Jiffy peanut butter. The bread was so soft it almost melted before you took your first bite. My rebellious years coincided with the turbulent 1960s and 1970s, when hippies were in vogue and everyone I knew turned vegetarian to help save the planet. I was determined not to be left behind and joined the "granola" crowd, proudly sharing my tofu culinary skills. Once I became a mother of small children, nothing seemed more important than making sure my children were healthy eaters. I did not insist they clean their plates to help starving children in other countries, but I did insist on trying new foods, which helped broaden their taste for fresh fruits and vegetables and the occasional cube of tofu.

Each decade and stage of life brought with it new, sometimes unsettling, information that made me pause, check the latest research, and reevaluate my choices in my quest to create wellness for myself and my family. Each time I looked, I discovered a vast expanse of information available to me, which made me realize just how much I did not know. I hope that the *Encyclopedia of Wellness* provides readers the information they need to live a life of as much well-being as possible.

Introduction: Wellness in the United States

"If you have your health, you have everything." That old adage has been around for a long time because it is true. Health in all its complexities is a necessary foundation for a life well lived. So how do we define health and wellness? One definition comes from the World Health Organization (2009): "Health is a state of complete physical, mental, and social well-being and not merely the absence of disease and infirmity."

This statement recognizes that to be healthy, a person must be more than free of physical problems. He or she must also pay attention to feelings, values, and relationships. In other words, when a healthy person reaches a state of wellness, she or he has demonstrated health in physical, emotional, social, intellectual, and spiritual life.

Even though wellness may be elusive to some Americans, the opportunity to achieve wellness should be available to everyone, no matter their race, gender, or income level. The issue of universal health insurance coverage for Americans took center stage following the passage of a health care reform bill championed by President Barack Obama. However, this is not the first time health care legislation aimed at improving access to insurance coverage for Americans has enjoyed presidential support. In 1912 President Theodore Roosevelt ran on a Progressive Party ticket that endorsed national health insurance. More than two decades later, President Franklin D. Roosevelt created an advisory Committee on Economic Security that called for national health insurance. Their efforts stopped, however, after intense opposition from the American Medical Association and others.

Franklin Roosevelt tried again in 1944 to improve access to insurance for all Americans, and in his State of the Union address he proposed an economic second Bill of Rights that included national health insurance. However, Roosevelt died in office before he could fulfill his goal. His successor, Harry S. Truman, also proposed a national health insurance plan, but his ideas were criticized as big government. Although President John F. Kennedy supported government health coverage for senior citizens in 1962, it was not until 1965 that President Lyndon B.

Johnson was finally able to persuade Congress to approve the creation of the Medicare and Medicaid programs.

Other lawmakers and presidents pushed for health reform in the decades that followed, but it was not until 1993 that another serious attempt was made to offer government health insurance coverage for Americans. President Bill Clinton launched a universal coverage reform effort that was headed by his wife, Hillary Rodham Clinton, and called for private insurers to compete in a regulated market. The Clinton plan died in Congress due to a number of factors, including extensive lobbying against it by insurance interests and strong Republican opposition. One difference in passing the 2010 Affordable Care Act was that the American Medical Association, which had historically opposed all efforts at reform, indicated it would support the Obama legislation. When the bill was brought to the House and Senate, even though each senator and congressperson voted along party lines and the bill received no Republican support, it still passed, thanks to the Democratic super majority in 2010.

The 2010 law was enacted in two parts: The Patient Protection and Affordable Care Act was signed into law on March 23, 2010, and was amended by the Health Care and Reconciliation Act on March 30, 2010. The final version of the law is now referred to as the Affordable Care Act. The reforms in that law apply to all new health plans and many existing health plans, and some benefits have taken effect, such as rebate checks for seniors in the Medicare doughnut hole, and tax credits for small businesses. Still, many effects of the legislation will not be felt for years—some not until 2014—and politicians who are opponents of the law have vowed to stop it, including Republican candidates vying for the presidential nomination to run against President Barack Obama in 2012.

PHYSICAL DIMENSIONS OF WELLNESS

Beyond the dollars and cents of health care, wellness is the responsibility of individuals and their personal choices. Wellness starts with a focus on preventive care and identifying risk factors rather than waiting to treat illness after it occurs. The Affordable Care Act requires new insurance policies to offer preventive services at no additional charge. That means routine immunizations, cancer screenings, and checkups will be paid for and will not be subject to an insurance copayment or a deductible. Children will receive free screenings for conditions such as iron deficiency, sickle cell anemia, and thyroid disease as well as vaccines for hepatitis A and B, tetanus-diphtheria, flu, and human papillomavirus for girls between the ages of 9 and 26. Adult services will include those that the U.S. Preventive Services Task Force, a panel of experts under the Department of Health and Human Services has assigned a top rating. That list includes screenings for HIV, depression, osteoporosis, and breast, colorectal, and cervical cancer.

One of the best ways to practice preventive care is through regular exercise, but anyone not normally active should consult his or her doctor before beginning any exercise program. A good physical workout helps minimize frustrations and stress, and the importance of exercise in improving heart function, lowering blood pressure, and contributing to weight loss is well established. In fact, whether you are 19 or 95, evidence shows exercise can improve your health and well-being. Today, excessive TV watching, computer use, cars, labor-saving appliances, and sedentary hobbies have replaced more active pursuits, which means that millions of Americans simply are not moving enough to burn the calories they eat each day, leading to rapidly growing rates of obesity and other illnesses such as diabetes, heart disease, and stroke.

Just how much exercise is enough? The current government recommendations call for at least 30 minutes of moderate activity each day, but few Americans achieve that goal. In fact, researchers now suggest that to be helpful, the 30 minutes do not need to be all at once; they can be broken into three 10-minute segments and can be accomplished through a variety of activities from walking to biking, strength training, stretching, or cardiovascular workouts. Simply adding 10-minute walks to a daily routine can add up to big health benefits.

Aerobic exercise is vital to any healthy fitness program. Nearly all the research regarding the disease-fighting benefits of exercise focuses on cardiovascular activity such as running or jogging, walking, swimming, and cycling. Strength training or resistance training using weight machines, free weights, or elastic bands is also important as a way to build muscle and protect against bone loss. Although weight training was only popular in the United States with a small number of people in the 1940s, by the 1960s, it began to flourish, and gyms and health clubs that offered a wide range of exercise activities for men and women became common throughout the United States. In recent years, more women have been turning to exercise and weight training to prevent bone diseases and bone density loss. Bones continually lose calcium and can weaken with age; weight and strength training have been shown to slow or reverse the loss and improve bone strength.

Stretching is a third component of a balanced exercise program. Muscles tend to weaken and shorten with age, and many people take that loss for granted. However, deterioration is not inevitable. It is largely a product of inactivity, and older adults with active lifestyles can remain fit and healthy throughout their years. Jack LaLanne, who lived to be 96, had been known for decades as the "godfather of fitness." He was an early fitness pioneer who introduced Americans to television exercise shows. LaLanne, who died in January 2011, was a perfect example of how to stay fit and active throughout life.

Another ingredient in a healthy lifestyle is the proper fuel to keep the human body running like any other piece of machinery. That fuel comes directly from the foods you eat. Proper nutrition is fundamental to every aspect of physical health. The best nutritional program contains a variety of foods that offer proteins, carbohydrates, fiber, fruits and vegetables, and healthy fats.

A focus on nutrition and health reform began in the United States in the 1830s and 1840s thanks to the work of the Reverend Sylvester Graham. Graham first started lecturing on the evils of alcohol and the need for temperance but eventually added the basic U.S. diet to his focus. He criticized the heavy, lard-filled foods most people enjoyed along with white bread and yeasted bread, which he believed produced alcohol. He thought it best to bake bread twice, an idea that led to his invention of a hard cracker, eventually known as the graham cracker.

Then, as well as now, food in the United States symbolizes more than sustenance for many people. For some, food offers comfort and pleasure. Others eat to relieve anxiety or to fill an emotional emptiness. Still others gulp down fast food while they change lanes on the freeway or sit in front of a television set or computer screen. This mindless eating is uniquely American in its reliance on hamburgers, French fries, and other foods high in sodium, fat, and sweeteners and is now being held at least partly responsible for growing numbers of people with illnesses such as heart disease, diabetes, cancer, and hypertension.

People who turn to drugs, alcohol, and tobacco also harm their health with what they put into their bodies. Although the rate of illicit drug use in the United States decreased between 2002 and 2008, the 2009 rate increased, especially among teenagers (Substance Abuse and Mental Health Services Administration, 2010). While the rate of Americans aged 12 years and older who consume alcohol has remained steady, numbers for binge drinking for 2009 showed more than 60 million Americans now binge on alcohol.

The number of Americans who use any kind of tobacco product declined from 30 percent in 2002 to just fewer than 28 percent for 2009; cigarette use was even lower, with a decrease from 26 to 23 percent for those same years. In contrast, the use of smokeless tobacco among youths has increased since 2002, and the popularity of electronic cigarettes is growing, although this use has not yet been surveyed by the Substance Abuse and Mental Health Services Administration (SAMHSA) in its annual National Survey on Drug Use and Health. The SAMHSA survey tracks the use of illicit drugs, alcohol, and tobacco among Americans aged 12 years and older.

Proximity to cigarette smokers remains a physical hazard due to the effects of secondhand smoke, which causes thousands of lung cancer deaths in nonsmokers every year along with hundreds of thousands of lower respiratory infections in children. Secondhand smoke has been shown to increase the chances that children will get asthma and worsens symptoms in those who already have asthma.

Many Americans fail to realize that sleep is another valuable component of preventive health care. How much sleep do we need? Studies show that some people can function well with six hours per night, but others need nine or more hours to feel their best. Experts suggest that individuals find their natural amount of sleep somewhere between seven and nine hours. The way to recognize the correct amount is when an individual can wake up feeling refreshed and is able to stay awake and alert throughout the day without the aid of caffeine or other stimulants.

Sleep helps the brain commit information to memory and can lead to insights and creative problem solving after a restful night's sleep. Scientists continue to study the importance of REM (rapid eye movement) sleep. New studies are also looking at the connection between sleep deprivation and weight gain. Scientists are examining how chronic loss of sleep may alter metabolic function, such as how carbohydrates are processed and stored, and stimulate the release of a stress hormone that has been linked to increased abdominal fat. Health can also be affected by too little sleep when it negatively affects relationships with family and friends and creates problems with job performance.

EMOTIONAL DIMENSIONS OF WELLNESS

In the earliest days, humans lived in caves, and their survival was challenged by three physical factors: predators, the hunt for their own food, and the physical demands of ordinary life. Today's adults rarely face such life-and-death challenges to their survival. However, they are routinely confronted with modern stress, which can cause the fight-or-flight response. Fear and anxiety are important survival mechanisms, but in a modern stress-filled world, they are often triggered inappropriately. People in all walks of life complain about their daily stress, but they are not fighting off a bear; instead, they may be sitting in traffic in the relative safety of their car. Still, the human body acts the same in both situations in which the person experiences fear or anxiety.

Stress has been described as the response of the body to a demand that prompts a needed physical change to meet it. During a stress response, blood flow to the organs and digestion is inhibited so that the arms and legs can work at their greatest capacity. A stressor is the event or trigger that produces stress in people, and, because each person is a unique individual, a stressor for one person might not be a stressor for another. Standing in a long line at a grocery store may be a stressor for one person but not for another.

The ability to deal with stress is important to overall health and wellness, because over time chronic stress can lead to physical or emotional illness. Stress-related disorders include migraine headaches, allergies, ulcers, hypertension, obesity, asthma, anxiety, insomnia, eating disorders, and drug use. Fear, anxiety, excitement, passion, guilt, and remorse are the feelings associated with stress.

Temperament, or the behavioral style that makes up one's day-to-day approach to living, shapes how well someone handles stress and how stress impacts health. An individual's awareness of her or his own temperament can help in dealing with difficult experiences. There are also other ways to prevent and manage stress.

Relaxation is the opposite of stress and is an important tool in relieving stress. The ability to relax can provide a number of physiological changes, including improved blood pressure. There are many ways to relax such as reading, playing a game, taking a hot bath, meditating, or participating in activities with a spiritual component, such as yoga, tai chi, qigong, prayer, and visualization or guided imagery. Once learned, any of these techniques can be practiced regularly, almost anywhere, with no need for expensive equipment.

The relaxation technique of meditation has been shown to have a positive effect on stress and wellness. When people meditate, their bodies' oxygen consumption drops along with their expiration of carbon dioxide. Heartbeat and respiration can slow down, and blood lactate levels, which some scientists believe are a direct link to anxiety, have been known to drop. Meditation can be practiced daily, and many people find that the social support of meditation classes offers an extra positive effect on their health.

Guided imagery or visualization, where practitioners mentally create soothing scenes, is another way to produce a relaxation response to stress. The images—whether they are scenes, places, or experiences—create a feeling of inner calm and are useful in breaking the chain of negative thought that produces stress. Tai chi is a series of slow, fluid circular motions that enhance balance, strengthen muscles, and improve aerobic capacity. Qigong is an ancient Chinese art that resembles tai chi and combines breathing, meditation, flowing movements, and basic exercise. The movements are designed to unblock the chi, or life energy, and return it to a state of equilibrium.

SOCIAL DIMENSIONS OF HEALTH

While surgery, other medical procedures, and medication are important to health, other equally important ingredients for wellness are the ability to connect with others and pursue activities and relationships that add joy to life. This dimension of wellness includes finding meaningful and satisfying work. There is clear evidence that several kinds of social support have a strong impact on health and wellness.

Many people face their biggest problems—problems that engage their defense mechanisms—in spouses, coworkers, children, roommates, friends, and neighbors. The nature of someone's social contacts, the abilities to listen and be empathetic, and the willingness to help others all add to an overall personal sense of wellness. Success in social relationships is an important part of this aspect of health.

Who we are today and how we make sense of the world are products of both genetics and our environment. We are influenced and shaped by our parents, families, and the society around us. Friends, acquaintances, coworkers, relatives, spouses, and partners all add to our social network. Their support may include financial help, emotional support or physical assistance. However, no matter what form the support takes, research has shown that people with a strong social support system do better on everything from exams and job performance to surgery and immune function.

Not surprisingly, the quality of relationships is the key ingredient; a healthy interaction can add to wellness, while negative relationships such as a bitter marriage or draining friendship can be as harmful as a physical illness. Studies show, for example, that women with breast cancer who were involved in an intimate and supportive relationship had more natural killer cells (cells that destroy virus-laden cells) than women who did not have close relationships with family, friends, or caregivers. Physical and emotional health benefits can even come from adopting a pet.

A constellation of work-related factors—from job demands to the related work pressure or overall job satisfaction—all play a role in daily health and longevity according to researchers at the Yale School of Public Health. Workplace satisfaction is closely linked with social support from colleagues, supportive management, and the promotion of wellness by the company. Not only is losing a job bad for individual health, but research in the United States has shown that job insecurity can be as bad for long-term health as a serious illness or an actual job loss (Hobson, 2009). Other studies have shown that people in lower-ranking, lower-paying positions were also more likely to smoke, less likely to be physically active in their leisure time, and less likely to eat fruits and vegetables. Researchers are still trying to understand why public health messages about diet and exercise are heard but not acted on by people who have the least to spend on health care but who would benefit the most from simple lifestyle changes.

Aversion to change may play a role in overall health care decisions. Change requires a great deal of adjustment and brings with it a gamble, a risk. Change also requires problem-solving skills that many people learned early in life. If those skills had a negative focus or were not effective, they remain difficult to unlearn and may influence adult behaviors in key ways. Plus, it is human nature to become accustomed to and comfortable with a point of view, even if it is negative. Still, when ways of dealing with the world are no longer effective or seem self-defeating, a person should consider change as one way to improve her or his health.

INTELLECTUAL DIMENSIONS OF WELLNESS

In an increasingly sedentary world, it may seem that the mind and thinking are the most dependable coping resource for modern life. A book, lecture, sermon, or artistic pursuit may provide refuge from the world. New ideas and new skills can enhance an individual's life and lead to healthy self-questioning. The ability to recognize the nature of personal feelings, interpret their significance, and share those feelings with others is an asset that promotes mental health and physical wellness.

It is also increasingly important to question and understand the changing face of health care and to act as our own personal consumer advocate when it comes to important health care decisions. The new federal health care law will affect almost every American in some way. Unfortunately, confusion remains over important questions, including how Americans can obtain health care, how individuals can improve access to quality medical care, and questions about fairness, efficiency, diagnosis, cost, and the overall effects of medical insurance on quality of care. Interestingly, a 2008 report by the Commonwealth Fund ranked the United States last in the quality of health care among the 19 industrialized countries compared in the study (Roehr, 2008).

Health care in the United States comes primarily from the private sector, and according to the Institute of Medicine (2004) of the National Academy of Sciences, this country is the "only wealthy, industrialized nation that does not ensure that all citizens have (insurance) coverage." That makes health insurance especially important in the United States, because there is no nationwide system of government-owned medical facilities open to the general public. At the same time, U.S. spending on medical care is rising at an unprecedented rate. More money per person is spent on health care in this country than in any other nation in the world, and Americans spend a greater percentage of their income on their health than any other United Nations member state (World Health Organization, 2009).

What little public health care is available comes through Medicaid and Medicare, the military health system, the Federal Employee Health Benefits Program, the Indian Health Service for Native Americans from recognized tribes, the Veterans Health Administration, and the State Children's Health Insurance Program.

For those Americans who have private health insurance coverage, primarily through their employer, participation requires that they select services from a managed care system and choose between health maintenance organizations or preferred provider organizations. They also must evaluate the need for and uses of flexible spending accounts, health reimbursement accounts, health savings accounts, and high-deductible health plans. Although much of this care is paid for in part by employers, each employee may be required to contribute part of the cost of insurance, while the employer chooses the insurance company and tries to use its market power to negotiate price reductions.

Individuals with private insurance are limited to doctors and medical facilities that accept their particular type of insurance. If they choose to visit a provider or medical facility outside of their network, they usually must bear more or all of the cost. Increasingly, doctors and hospitals can refuse to accept a particular insurance, including the federal Medicare and Medicaid programs. However, the Emergency Medical Treatment and Active Labor Act, passed in 1986, requires all hospitals to accept all patients for emergency room care and treatment, regardless of their ability to pay. It does not cover non–emergency room care for anyone who cannot pay.

The result of this law has been a growing national crisis in hospital emergency rooms (ERs), as fewer doctors deal with more patients who come to the emergency room for everything from a sinus infection to a heart attack. The use of the ER for routine medical care bypasses the benefits of preventive care or the importance of seeing a regular primary care doctor. This in turn, fills emergency rooms to over capacity and guarantees long wait times. It is also responsible for running hospitals over budget, because it is generally more expensive to treat a patient in the emergency room than in the primary care physician's office. However, Americans without health insurance routinely turn to ER doctors as their primary care physicians at the same time hospitals are closing or cutting back on their ER staff and facilities.

Access to regular medical care has decreased for some Americans, while advances in medical technology and ongoing improvements in diagnostic and therapeutic procedures have created improved health care standards and improved effectiveness for those who have insurance coverage and access to regular preventive medical care. Unfortunately, these improvements are also the leading driver of rising health care costs. This conflict between cost and access makes it important for U.S. consumers to have a trusted source of information from which they can get up-to-date, objective, and credible information to successfully navigate the various health care choices and obtain services that are most effective and provide the best value.

SPIRITUAL DIMENSIONS OF WELLNESS

The experiences that lead to spiritual growth and the certainty of religious beliefs are an important aspect of individual wellness. Whether those beliefs are part of a mainstream religion or developed through individual events and challenges, the presence of a spiritual focus can lead to a deep sense of personal worth and satisfaction and in that way contribute to wellness. Studies show that people with an active religious life or strong religious beliefs may live longer and be happier, and that religion can reduce anxiety and lower blood pressure. By reinforcing positive emotions, religious beliefs also stimulate healthy responses and encourage better health habits such as avoiding alcohol and tobacco. Religious communities can create several layers of support: emotional support linked to outright assistance as well as a more subtle but equally powerful assistance through prayer and fellowship.

The United States is a land of diversity, and this is true when it comes to religious beliefs and their role in health care issues. Research has found racial differences in prayer and other religious practices among different ethnic groups associated with health concerns. Findings from the Howard University College of Medicine noted that a greater proportion of African Americans and Hispanic Americans used prayer for health reasons. Those same groups were less likely to use other nontraditional spiritual practices such as meditation or tai chi when dealing with health issues (Gillum, 2010).

However, the use of alternative medical practices in general—such as acupuncture, tai chi, and Reiki—is on the rise among many other Americans according to the National Center for Complementary and Alternative Medicine and the National Center for Health Statistics. Their most recent survey found that approximately 38 percent of adults and 12 percent of children in the United States use some form of alternative medicine to supplement their routine care. The most common complementary and alternative therapies mentioned were meditation, massage, yoga, deep breathing, and nonvitamin and nonmineral natural products.

Alternative medicine also encompasses medical techniques that are not considered conventional and are noninvasive and nonpharmaceutical. On one end of the spectrum, some Americans have changed their definition of health care to only include forms of alternative medicine such as homeopathy, botanical remedies, or traditional Chinese medicine and exclude medication or surgical treatments. Still others have embraced a holistic medicine concept, which is a broader approach to life with a focus on how an individual interacts with the environment. It emphasizes the connection of mind, body, and spirit, and it encompasses all forms of treatment, including drugs and surgery.

The pursuit of wellness, like any important goal, needs to be carried out with wisdom and balance. The road to better health is paved with the myriad small decisions made every day. Those who take supplements, avoid traditional medicine, or consume tobacco, alcohol, drugs, or calories in excess must deal with the health effects of those decisions. While most people fall between extremes in choices, many Americans remain passive participants in their health or feel they can do nothing to change their situation. Information is power and can help anyone take control of their health. Take the time to look through the basic information contained in these volumes. It can be the first step toward a life of wellness.

References

Gillum, F. "Prayer and Spiritual Practices for Health Reasons among American Adults: The Role of Race and Ethnicity." *Journal of Religion and Health* 49, no. 3 (2010): 283–95.

Hobson, Katherine. "Is Your Job Killing You? How Work Influences Longevity." *U.S. News and World Report* 147, no. 2 (February 1, 2009): 50.

Institute of Medicine of the National Academies of Science. *Insuring America's Health: Principles and Recommendations* (January 14, 2004), www.iom.edu/Reports/2004/Insuring-Americas-Health-Principles-and-Recommendations.aspx.

Roehr, Bob. "Health Care in US Ranks Lowest among Developed Countries." *British Medical Journal* 337 (July 21, 2008), a889.doi:10.1136/bmj.a889, http://dx.doi.org/10.1136%2Fbmj.a889.

Substance Abuse and Mental Health Services Administration. *Results from the 2009 National Survey on Drug Use and Health:* Vol. 1. *Summary of National Findings.* Office of Applied Studies, NSDUH Series H-38A, HHS Publication No. SMA 10-4586. Rockville, MD: Department of HHS Findings, 2010.

World Health Organization. "World Health Statistics 2009" (November 20, 2010), www.who.int/whosis/whostat/2009/en/index.html.

A

AÇAÍ BERRY

The açaí (pronounced *ah-sah-EE*) berry has joined the ranks of popular super-foods, along with fruits like pomegranate and blueberries. The açaí are the fruit of the South American palm tree known scientifically as *Euterpe oleracea* found in the Amazon rainforests of Brazil and are similar to blueberries and blackberries. The berries are believed to contain antioxidants, which are molecules that may combat cell-damaging free radicals. They also contain amino acids and essential fatty acids in substantial amounts when compared with other foods. The berries were introduced in the United States in 2001, and there are now more than 50 food and drink products containing açaí available to U.S. consumers. Those products include supplements, juices, and vitamins whose manufacturers claim can produce weight loss, improve general health, remove wrinkles, cleanse the body of toxins, and support a healthy immune system. Açaí berries have also been mentioned as having therapeutic value for people with multiple sclerosis (MS). According to the National Multiple Sclerosis Society, however, there is no MS-specific effectiveness information about açaí berry products or their safety for MS patients.

While the açaí has been show to exhibit antioxidant effects in scientific studies, no clinical studies have evaluated the safety of açaí products in general, and high antioxidant scores have not been proven to indicate how effective a food is at preventing disease, according to the Antioxidants Research Laboratory at Tufts University (Colapinto, 2011). As for weight loss, scientists say the fiber content of the berries might suppress the appetite, but drinking expensive bottles of açaí juice is not a magic answer to weight loss. The Center for Science in the Public Interest (CSPI) released a warning to consumers in 2009 cautioning them not to enroll online in supposedly free trials of diet products made with the Brazilian açaí berry. According to the CSPI, despite a lack of evidence that the product works, consumers who took advantage of the free trial also had trouble stopping recurrent charges on their credit cards when they tried to cancel the free trials.

Instead, the CSPI recommends eating a variety of fruits and vegetables that contain natural plant compounds and nutrients that can protect health in many ways.

The berries were virtually unknown outside the Amazon just a decade ago and were not exported in large quantities until 2000. For Brazilian natives, the açaí has long been a staple of their daily diet, and açaí pulp is a filling side dish, especially for poorer families. As international demand for the berries has grown, the price has gone up as well—an increase that benefits those raising açaí but creates problems for poor families in Brazil. The fruit was traditionally collected from wild palms, but açaí plantations have been planted all across the country. Export figures are not exact, but it appears that the region where much of Brazil's açaí is raised has seen a jump in export from 380 metric tons in 2000 to over 9,400 metric tons in 2009 (Kugel, 2010). That amounts to exports totaling some $15 million.

Sharon Zoumbaris

See also Antioxidants.

References

Bowling, Allen C. "Wise Choices in Action: The Example of Açaí." *Momentum* 3, no. 2 (Spring 2010): 46.

Colapinto, John. "Strange Fruit." *New Yorker* (May 30, 2011): 37–43.

Kugel, Seth. "Açaí, a Global Super Fruit Is Dinner in the Amazon." *New York Times* (February 24, 2010): D1.

Moran, Sarah. "Fed up with Diet Myths? Get the Real Skinny on Açaí Berries, Summer Salads and More from Dietitians Who Have the Inside Scoop on How You Can Lose Weight This Season." *Minneapolis Star Tribune* (June 29, 2009): 01E.

ACQUIRED IMMUNE DEFICIENCY SYNDROME (AIDS)

The Centers for Disease Control and Prevention (CDC) defines AIDS as "the late stage of HIV infection, when a person's immune system is severely damaged and has difficulty fighting diseases and certain cancers. HIV is the human immunodeficiency virus, the virus that can lead to acquired immune deficiency syndrome, or AIDS." The CDC (2011) estimates that about 56,000 people in the United States contracted HIV in 2006. AIDS was first recognized in U.S. medical literature in mid-1981. It was named just over a year later to describe the multiple symptoms seen in patients that were the result of an underlying immune deficiency caused by infection with the human immunodeficiency virus (HIV). In the United States, AIDS was discovered in major homosexual communities of large cities and was often initially called gay-related immune deficiency (GRID) or gay cancer. By 1983, medical practitioners and the public came to realize that AIDS could and did affect many others, especially intravenous drug users who shared needles and those who received tainted blood products during medical procedures.

The U.S. Food and Drug Administration (FDA) approved the first successful drug therapy, azidothymidine (AZT), in 1987. While AIDS activist groups

The Death Sentence That Defined My Life

By Mark Trautwein

I haven't died on schedule. Most people don't think death has a schedule, at least a knowable one. But if you were infected early in the AIDS epidemic, you thought otherwise. At 61, I have now lived half my life with AIDS, my constant companion and distant cousin, the inseparable identity I won't let define me, the everyday fact and special circumstance that bent the arc of my life in every way.

As the epidemic grew through the 1980s, all gay men lived with AIDS, whether infected or not. Thirty years ago, the Centers for Disease Control and Prevention reported the first cases of the disease. It was a helpless and terrifying time. Medical information grew. We learned about HIV and sexual transmission, but everything was misty and qualified. Nothing you knew or did mattered. There was no treatment.

Initial medications were eked out of a health care system that had been bashed into compliance by angry activists. They were mere BBs hurled at battleships, but they promised more time, time for better drugs, time for more life.

Then everything changed. Protease inhibitors became available. The "cocktail" was born. You couldn't beat AIDS, but you could fight it to a draw, perhaps indefinitely.

Staying alive was now a full-time job in health management.

My relationship with AIDS is one of my most enduring ones, and has both enriched and beggared my life. It robbed me of friends and loved ones, and with them memories we would have had and repositories of my own history.

What I've gained is precious. Above all, the constant companionship of plague has taught me that life is about living, not cheating death. On that day I walked from the hospital knowing I had "it," I was given a great gift: the realization that we all dangle from that most delicate of threads and that the only way to life a life is to love it. I haven't died on schedule, and I've been learning not to live life on one either.

Excerpt from Mark Trautwein, "The Death Sentence That Defined My Life," *New York Times,* June 4, 2011. Used by permission.

protested the supposed lack of government interest in AIDS and AIDS-related research, laboratories developed multi-drug "cocktails" with varying levels of effectiveness, releasing the first in 1993. In recent years, AIDS has become entrenched in marginalized communities where preventive and therapeutic interventions have been unavailable or have not been adopted.

Recognition of AIDS as a New Disease   Medical research studies indicate that the first, unrecognized cases of AIDS probably occurred in West Africa, where the causative virus mutated from a form that infected monkeys to one that could infect humans. Why, then, was AIDS first recognized as a new disease in the United States? The answer lies in the differences between the ways in which medicine is practiced by physicians and experienced by patients in Africa and in the United States. Individuals in Africa who succumbed to AIDS in the decades before 1981 were most often poor, rural people who rarely consulted physicians practicing Western medicine. Physicians practicing in Africa at the time, upon seeing an African with a fever and wasting, would likely attribute the symptoms to any of a host of diseases present in tropical countries.

The earliest AIDS patients in the United States, in contrast, were largely upper-middle-class whites with health insurance who regularly consulted physicians when they fell ill. Their physicians recognized a disruption in the medical history of their patient populations that led them to question idiosyncratic diagnoses and wonder about the possibility of a novel disease process.

Specifically, in the late 1970s, U.S. dermatologists began seeing young men with rare cancerous lesions (Kaposi's sarcoma) normally found on elderly Mediterranean men. In early 1981, infectious disease physicians encountered patients with infections, especially *Pneumocystis carinii* pneumonia, associated normally with patients whose immune systems had been compromised because of cancer treatments. In June 1981, the cases seen in Los Angeles were described in a short paper in the *Morbidity and Mortality Weekly Reports,* a weekly publication issued by the U.S. Centers for Disease Control and Prevention in Atlanta. Additional papers followed in July and August, all of which observed that the affected patients were previously healthy homosexual men living in gay communities in large cities.

By June 1982, cases of AIDS outside gay communities had been observed, including cases in newborn babies, heterosexual patients who had undergone surgery, Haitian immigrants, and persons who regularly received blood products to treat their hemophilia (a genetic disease characterized by the inability to clot blood). AIDS became known at this time as the "4-H" disease because it had been observed in homosexuals, heroin addicts, Haitians, and hemophiliacs. Epidemiologists understood, however, that these categories of patients also suggested a blood-borne cause.

If AIDS was transmitted by blood, the nation's supply of whole blood and blood products was at risk, a finding that many people, including those who managed blood banks, did not want to believe. Hemophiliacs previously tolerated the possibility of infection with hepatitis B virus because the value of the clotting factor produced from pooling serum outweighed that risk. Hemophiliacs and their families were horrified, however, by the prospect that the lifesaving blood product might harbor a lethal disease agent.

After 1983, when the virus was first isolated in the Paris laboratory of Dr. Luc Montagnier, HIV was demonstrated to be the cause of AIDS. By mid-1984, transfusion-transmitted viruses were no longer considered acceptable risks in reaping the benefits of blood products. An enzyme-linked, immunosorbant assay for antibodies to HIV, developed for use in laboratory research on the etiology of AIDS, was adapted in 1985 as a screening test for blood and blood products. In 1987 the U.S. Food and Drug Administration issued regulations requiring such screening, and in 1988 the FDA began inspecting 100 percent of FDA-regulated blood and plasma donor facilities to enforce screening regulations.

Another consequence of the development of sensitive diagnostic tests for HIV was the transformation of the definition of AIDS. Between 1981 and 1986, the CDC issued successive statements about which opportunistic infections and cancers could be used as the basis for a diagnosis of AIDS. Diseases such as *Pneumocystis carinii* pneumonia, candidiasis (a yeastlike infection) of the esophagus or lungs, toxoplasmosis of the brain, and Kaposi's sarcoma were included early. General wasting symptoms, such as ongoing diarrhea and severe pelvic inflammatory disease in women, were less clearly a part of the syndrome caused by the acquired immunodeficiency.

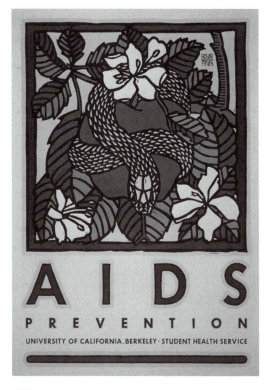

AIDS prevention poster features an image of snake coiled around an apple. (David Lance Goines/LOC)

Details about the various diagnoses mattered, because health insurers and the U.S. federal government based reimbursement payments and access to clinical trials on such information. In August 1987, the CDC revised its definition of AIDS from a list of particular illnesses to any illness that resulted from a long-term infection with HIV. Since that time, the name used for the disease has been HIV/AIDS.

Social, Religious, and Political Reactions to AIDS The social stigma carried by AIDS as a sexually transmitted disease resulted in what some public health leaders called "a second epidemic of fear." From 1983 to 1987, when public fear and panic were at their most destructive, some religious groups proclaimed that AIDS was God's vengeance on the gay community for violating what they viewed as biblical prohibitions against homosexuality. Injecting drug abusers were also viewed as people who made wrong lifestyle choices that led to disease. Hemophiliacs, surgery patients who received infected blood, and women who were infected by their spouses, in contrast, were viewed as innocent victims of AIDS.

This division of people with AIDS into guilty and innocent categories led advocates of conservative views to support research on drugs to treat AIDS but to oppose any public expenditure for condom distribution or needle exchange programs for drug addicts. Teaching personal responsibility—through sexual abstinence and "just say no" to drugs campaigns—was their preferred approach to AIDS prevention efforts. Social and religious reluctance to discuss sexuality in any public setting exacerbated the obstacles to effective public education about AIDS.

Individuals diagnosed with AIDS or as having antibodies to HIV were sometimes fired from their jobs. Police officers, firefighters, ambulance personnel, and other health care workers occasionally refused to take care of AIDS patients. Young Ryan White (1971–1990) in Indiana and three brothers—Ricky (1977–1992), Robert (1978–2000), and Randy (b. 1979) Ray—in Florida, all hemophiliacs who contracted AIDS from contaminated blood products, were denied entrance to schools. Even as medical research demonstrated that AIDS was not transmissible through casual contact, the epidemic of fear moved an arsonist in Arcadia, Florida, to set fire to the Ray brothers' house and the school board in Kokomo, Indiana, to insist that Ryan White take classes over the telephone to avoid accidentally touching his classmates.

The most important tool used by public health leaders to counter this fear was accurate communication about AIDS. Sharing new information as soon as it became available often made the difference between keeping and losing staff at hospitals, firehouses, police departments, and other public service agencies. A concerted education program about AIDS and how it was transmitted helped to defuse fear in school systems.

On the national level, U.S. Surgeon General C. Everett Koop (b. 1916) issued an informational report on AIDS in 1986 and two years later mailed a flier titled "Understanding AIDS" to every household in the United States.

October 2, 1985, marked a turning point in the history of AIDS in the United States. On that date, Hollywood actor Rock Hudson (1925–1985) died of AIDS. Hudson's death seemed to bring home the point to a broad public that anyone, even a movie star, could contract AIDS. The publicity surrounding Hudson's death motivated the U.S. Congress to appropriate significantly more money for AIDS research than it had been willing to commit previously. During the 1990s, other celebrities with AIDS—including tennis player Arthur Ashe (1943–1993) and Elizabeth Glaser (1947–1994), wife of actor Paul Michael Glaser—as well as others without AIDS, such as Elizabeth Taylor (1932–2011), became public spokespersons for raising money to combat AIDS and raising awareness that people with AIDS should be treated fairly and with compassion.

Throughout the 1980s within the gay community, AIDS activists worked from the earliest years of the epidemic to provide care for sick individuals, raise money for foundations, lobby the federal government to increase research, and make possible therapies available more quickly than the traditional drug approval process would allow. To draw attention to their cause, some of the activists staged public demonstrations, or street theater, designed to attract national media attention. In 1987 the organization AIDS Coalition To Unleash Power (ACT UP) was formed by activists in New York City with the initial goal of gaining the release of experimental drugs. Soon ACT UP expanded to advocate for other AIDS issues as well. ACT UP's numerous protests were so successful that they became a model for advocates for other diseases.

Public education programs in the United States about AIDS were strongly split in content according to which group produced them. Those funded by the U.S. government emphasized getting the facts about AIDS. There was virtually no emphasis in government-funded educational campaigns on communicating specifically to the gay community or on discussing safe sex through the campaign's posters. AIDS community action groups and other private-sector groups took the lead in producing stark, graphic messages that communicated the urgent need for condom use and clean needles.

One segment of U.S. society that proved particularly difficult to reach with AIDS prevention messages was the African American community. Traditionally, the black church had been the most effective vehicle for communicating health messages within the African American community, but strong sentiments against homosexuality within the black church made safe gay sex extremely difficult to address. The African American community also had scant trust of health messages from the federal government because of the infamous mid-20th-century Tuskegee syphilis study, in which African American men in Alabama had been left untreated for the disease without their knowledge or consent in order for the effects of syphilis in untreated patients to be observed.

AIDS Doubters and AIDS Quackery In 1987 Peter Duesberg (b. 1936), a distinguished molecular biologist, authority on retroviruses, and member of the U.S. National Academy of Sciences, published a paper asserting that HIV was merely a benign passenger virus and not the cause of AIDS. Leading scientists refuted Duesburg's theory, but his arguments drew adherents from people who wished to believe that AIDS had no link to viral causation and could be cured by living a healthy lifestyle. Questioning the cause of AIDS also fueled the industry of unorthodox treatments for AIDS. From the earliest days of the epidemic, desperate patients had been willing to try almost anything advertised as a cure. Early in the epidemic, promoters of questionable cancer treatments expanded their claims to encompass AIDS because of its link to Kaposi's sarcoma. As the underlying immune deficiency in AIDS became common knowledge, remedies purporting to boost the immune system flowered. The growth of the World Wide Web in the late 1990s allowed the AIDS doubters to spread their message widely and opened the door to multiple quack therapies and urban legends relating to AIDS.

AIDS in the New Millennium In 2001 the world marked 25 years since the earliest recognition of AIDS. By this date, AIDS in the United States had been transformed from a disease identified almost exclusively with affluent homosexual men into a disease of marginalized groups—injecting drug abusers and poor minority populations. Between 2005 and 2008, 50 percent of HIV diagnoses were among African Americans and 17 percent were among Hispanics, even though those groups constituted only 12 percent and 15 percent of the U.S. population, respectively. Men who had sex with other men still accounted for more than 70 percent of AIDS cases in the United States. This was also true in Canada and in Latin America as a whole. Among Caribbean island populations, however, AIDS now strikes men and women equally.

Americans have played a leading role in efforts to halt AIDS in the rest of the world. In poorer regions of the world, AIDS patients cannot afford the cost of antiviral drugs, even those whose prices have been greatly reduced. In 2007 the U.S. government committed $30 billion over five years to fight AIDS in developing countries. Major philanthropic organizations, such as the Bill and Melinda Gates Foundation, have also invested heavily in research on ways to prevent AIDS as well as in helping those already infected.

For the United States, AIDS has become essentially a chronic disease. In 2010, the CDC reported just over 1 million (1,106,400) people living with AIDS in the United States at the end of 2006, the most recent year for which national estimates were available. This represented an 11 percent increase from the previous estimate in 2003. From 2005 through 2007 (the most recent year death data are available), deaths of persons diagnosed with HIV infection has increased 17 percent. Between 1993 and 2003, highly active antiretroviral therapy produced an 80 percent drop in the death rate from AIDS. Since the 1986 release of AZT, new AIDS drugs have been developed that target different points in the life cycle of HIV.

In 1995 a new class of drugs called protease inhibitors was approved, and in 2007 integrase inhibitors were introduced. Even more antiviral drugs are in research and development. None of these drugs, however, can eliminate HIV from an infected person, and the disease requires drug treatment with toxic side effects for the rest of an infected person's life. Because of the rapid mutation of HIV, moreover, a conventional vaccine against AIDS has proved impossible to make, and it may take decades before novel approaches to the vaccine concept produce positive results.

The very success in managing AIDS in the United States has produced worry among public health officials that young people will not understand the serious side effects that accompany antiviral regimens and be lulled into thinking that AIDS is no longer a danger. Among affluent homosexual men—the initial group struck so hard by AIDS—some risky behaviors have reemerged. Many gay bathhouses in major cities, closed in the mid-1980s, reopened quickly with regulations restricting unsafe sexual practices in public areas. Sexual activity in the bathhouses' privately rented rooms was and still is unregulated, illustrating the ongoing tension between personal liberty and the community's right to coerce healthful behavior. Exacerbating the problem has been the widespread use of the drug methamphetamine, which in the 21st century has fueled a return to unsafe sex with multiple partners in bathhouses.

It has been a hard-won truth that AIDS in the United States is best prevented in the 21st century with traditional, 20th-century public health techniques. Educational campaigns about how HIV is transmitted help individuals protect themselves by abstaining from sex or engaging in safe sex practices. Efforts to expand testing for HIV and reduce the stigma of a positive diagnosis likewise help individuals to know their personal status and protect their sexual partners. Before 2005, public health efforts to exchange clean needles for used ones to protect injecting drug users from AIDS had been illegal under most state drug laws, but volunteer programs were often tolerated by law enforcement. In that year, however, needle exchange won official support in California, and since then, other states and municipalities have endorsed this effort.

Joseph P. Byrne

See also Human Immunodeficiency Virus (HIV); Virus; White, Ryan.

References

Baldwin, Peter. *Disease and Democracy: The Industrialized World Faces AIDS.* Berkeley: University of California Press, 2005.

Centers for Disease Control and Prevention. "Basic Information about HIV and AIDS" (July 2011), www.cdc.gov/hiv/topics/basic/index.htm.

Davis, Julia. *Evolution of an Epidemic: 25 Years of HIV/AIDS Media Campaigns in the U.S.* Menlo Park, CA: Henry J. Kaiser Family Foundation, 2006.

Engel, Jonathan. *The Epidemic: A Global History of AIDS.* Washington, DC: Smithsonian Books, 2006.

Feldman, Eric, and Ronald Bayer, eds. *Blood Feuds: AIDS, Blood, and the Politics of Medical Disaster.* New York: Oxford University Press, 1999.

Shilts, Randy. *And the Band Played On: Politics, People, and the AIDS Epidemic.* New York: St. Martin's Press, 1987.

Treichler, Paula. *How to Have Theory in an Epidemic.* Durham, NC: Duke University Press, 1999.

UNAIDS. *AIDS Epidemic Update. Geneva, Switzerland*: World Health Organization/UNAIDS, 2007.

Watney, Simon. *Policing Desire: Pornography, AIDS, and the Media,* 2nd ed. Minneapolis: University of Minnesota Press, 1989.

ACUPUNCTURE

Acupuncture is the procedure of inserting fine needles into specific areas of the body with the purpose of bringing about a therapeutic benefit. Acupuncture is one of the main forms of treatment used in the medical system known as Chinese medicine or traditional Chinese medicine.

Acupuncture was widely believed to have begun in China around 5,000 years ago. However, a recent discovery in Europe opened the possibility that acupuncture has European origins that predate its emergence in the Orient. In 1991 a frozen, mummified human was found emerging from a glacier in Italy. The mummy, named Ötzi, had approximately 57 carbon tattoos consisting of simple dots and lines on his lower spine, behind his left knee, and on his right ankle. Using X-rays, it was determined that the man may have had arthritis in these joints. Some scientists have speculated these marks may be related to an ancient type of acupuncture since they were located at major acupuncture points called meridian lines (Australian Broadcasting Corporation, 2005).

Nonetheless, acupuncture was certainly popularized and refined in China, where its practice has had a long and storied existence. Its beginnings in China have been linked to a legend that told of how ancient Chinese physicians observed surprising effects of puncture wounds in Chinese warriors and used that knowledge to develop acupuncture.

The popularity of acupuncture began to grow in the West in the early 1970s, when President Richard Nixon became the first U.S. president to visit China. Nixon and the journalists traveling with him witnessed major operations being

Acupuncturists

David Teitler, LAc, is a Colorado-based acupuncturist and herbalist. He founded his practice in 1999 to focus on the treatment of respiratory disorders. When he started out, Teitler did not envision his strong affinity for herbal medicine. And he did not anticipate being invited to work in the oncology unit at a nearby hospital. When contacted by the staff of the hospital's integrated medicine department, Teitler brought his knowledge and skills of traditional Chinese medicine and acupuncture to coordinated treatment plans for cancer patients. Despite the gravity of each patient's health situation, Teitler discovered people dedicated to their own care, whether through acupuncture or chemotherapy. He describes his patients as people who are engaged in the moment rather than distracted by everyday stresses.

What that offers him as a practitioner is the opportunity to work with patients who take a strong role in their own physical and emotional health. This often leads to very honest and frank discussions, something Teitler finds extremely rewarding as a health care provider. Looking to the future, Teitler would like to see greater integration between Western medicine and traditional Chinese medicine, looking at each other as partners rather than adversaries. In the treatment of cancer, for instance, it is common practice in China to use Chinese herbal medicine alongside chemotherapy and radiation to help reduce the side effects of the treatment and to strengthen immune function. In time, Teitler thinks this will be acceptable in the United States, just as acupuncture is now used extensively for in vitro fertilization, something which was not practiced or envisioned a decade or two ago. As for Teitler, he plans to keep learning and growing and working with cancer patients, searching for new ways to help individuals achieve wellness.

performed on patients with acupuncture rather than anesthetics. On that trip, *New York Times* journalist James Reston had to undergo an appendectomy and elected to use acupuncture as his only anesthesia. Nixon was impressed, and Reston wrote several stories about its effectiveness. The use of acupuncture gained popularity in the United States and by 2008 had been used by more than 15 million Americans in all 50 states (Dupler, 2009). The chi model remains the best explanation.

The Concept of Chi To understand acupuncture, one must have a basic understanding of the concept of chi. Often translated as energy in the broadest sense, this definition often needs refinement for Westerners. Chi permeates the universe and gives form to the known world. Similar to "the Force" from *Star Wars* lore, chi is an energy that enriches us, protects us, nourishes us, and animates us. The energy behind the process of a seed sprouting into a plant is governed by chi, as is the energy of the spirit within us.

According to the theories of Chinese medicine, acupuncture works by regulating the chi flow in the body. Chi flows through a network of energy pathways called meridians. There are 14 main meridians and many smaller ones throughout the body. Along these meridians are the acupuncture points. By inserting needles into specific points on these meridians, the chi flow of the body is influenced and regulated. When the harmonious flow of chi is interrupted, deficient, or imbalanced, illness ensues. Acupuncture regulates the flow of chi, thereby instilling balance in the body and restoring health.

In Chinese medicine, it is often said that if there is free flow, there is not pain; if there is no free flow, there is pain. This definition refers to the free and unobstructed flow of chi. If the chi flow is blocked, pain ensues. An acupuncture treatment reestablishes the correct flow of chi, resulting in pain relief. Looking at this scenario from a Western science perspective, pain can be seen as a tight muscle. If an acupuncture needle is inserted into the origin of a particularly tight muscle, that muscle will relax, resulting in pain relief.

The exact mechanism, however, of how acupuncture works, has never been thoroughly understood by Western science. Theories abound about an increase in blood circulation, neurotransmitters sending signals to the brain, or stimulating the release of endorphins. Whatever the theory, the fact remains that nobody really knows for sure how acupuncture is able to relieve pain.

Different Points Acupuncture points have different functions. As they relate to chi, some are said to circulate chi and blood, others raise chi, and others strengthen chi. Some points strengthen certain organs. Others are located where muscles and tendons meet, thus being more useful for musculoskeletal conditions such as shoulder pain or tennis elbow.

There are 365 acupuncture points on the 14 main meridians and many others known as extra points. Among these, approximately one hundred are thought of as major points and are more frequently used. Needles are disposable and made from stainless steel. They can be anywhere from one-half inch to two or more inches in length; however, their diameters are very small, usually about the thickness of a dog's whisker.

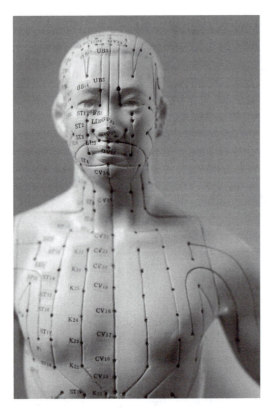

Model displays acupuncture meridian points on head, face, and upper torso. (Orr Zahavi/Dreamstime.com)

During an acupuncture treatment, little sensation is felt when the needle is initially inserted. Once through the skin, a practitioner then manipulates the needle to obtain a sensation called *de chi*. In Chinese, this means the arrival of the chi sensation. This can feel like a dull ache, a sensation of heat, a feeling of prickles or numbness, or a radiating sensation from the acupuncture point.

Acupuncture needles are usually left in for 20 to 30 minutes. An average of 10 to 15 acupuncture points are chosen for an acupuncture treatment. The points are normally chosen bilaterally (the same point on both limbs), but in some cases needling is done on only one side of the body. The points are selected based on the person's ailment and the diagnosis according to the principles of Chinese medicine.

One common experience following an acupuncture treatment is a deep sense of relaxation. Pain relief can be immediate, especially if the condition is acute, such as a recently sprained ankle. If the pain is chronic, such as a bad back, it may take five or more treatments for a patient to begin noticing a difference.

Using a headache as an example, an acupuncturist might place needles in the hands between the thumb and index finger, at the nape of the neck, and along the temple. A couple of extra sets of points in the arms or legs would likely be chosen based on the individual's specific diagnosis.

Some people report feeling the movement of chi during a treatment. However, an equal number do not notice any such sensation, and both of these groups can obtain the same benefit from the acupuncture treatment.

Benefits of Acupuncture   In the United States, some doctors now include treatment with acupuncture for headaches, alcoholism, substance abuse, post-traumatic stress disorder, and arthritis as well as to ease the suffering of cancer and AIDS patients. A study released in 2010 by the Dana-Farber Cancer Institute demonstrated that cancer patients who received a series of 12 acupuncture sessions over eight weeks reported significant improvement in anxiety, fatigue, pain, and depression. Life satisfaction and psychological distress also showed improvement (Dean-Clower, 2010).

Acupuncture performed by a qualified practitioner is very safe. One large study found only 43 minor adverse events associated with over 30,000 acupuncture treatments (MacPherson, 2001). The number of treatments needed varies; anywhere from 2 to 12 or more is a normal series, depending on the condition. For instance, an acute headache may take just a couple of treatments to obtain satisfactory results, while a condition such as chronic fatigue syndrome may take a year or more of treatments to obtain satisfactory results.

The World Health Organization officially recommends acupuncture as an appropriate treatment for a host of medical conditions, including allergies, gastrointestinal disorders, nervous conditions, and chronic pain (Dupler, 2009). In 2002 the National Institutes of Health announced that pain from fibromyalgia could be lessened through acupuncture. Scientists are also continuing to look at acupuncture as a way to improve quality of life for patients with advanced cancer.

Costs for acupuncture treatment vary depending on a number of factors. Insurance reimbursement also varies and is determined by the company and specific state regulations. Some states authorize Medicaid to cover acupuncture for limited health conditions, and some states have mandated that general insurance coverage include acupuncture treatments. Individuals should check with their insurance provider to clarify the specifics of their individual policy regarding acupuncture.

Acupuncture Training The Accreditation Commission for Acupuncture and Oriental Medicine (ACAOM) is the national accrediting agency recognized by the U.S. Department of Education to accredit master-level programs in the acupuncture and Oriental medicine profession. As an independent body, ACAOM accredits a master's degree and master-level acupuncture and Oriental medicine programs. There are currently more than 60 schools and colleges with accredited or candidacy status with the ACAOM.

Information about accredited programs is also available from the Council of Colleges of Acupuncture and Oriental Medicine, which has brochures and catalogs of accredited schools in the United States and in other countries. Requirements vary around the world. For example, in Canada, the provinces of British Columbia, Alberta, and Quebec have licensing requirements. In Australia, the regulations vary by state, and there is no government regulation of acupuncture in the United Kingdom.

When choosing an acupuncturist, it is important to look for the initials LAc, DiplAc, or DOM, which means the practitioner is fully qualified and has passed the national board exam. Licensed acupuncturists (LAc) are required to have a minimum of 1,800 to 2,400 hours or more of educational and clinical training, depending on individual state requirements. In most states, they must also be certified with the NCCAOM. DiplAc signifies completion of a diploma program at schools certified by the ACAOM and usually includes three academic years of study. The DOM is the doctor of Oriental medicine degree, and it indicates additional training beyond state licensure to practice acupuncture.

David S. Teitler

See also Cancer; Health Insurance; Traditional Chinese Medicine.

References

Australian Broadcasting Corporation. *Iceman May Have Been Given the Cold Shoulder* (February 07, 2006), www.abc.net.au/news/2006-02-04/iceman-may-have-been-given-the-cold-shoulder/792734.

Dean-Clower, E. "Acupuncture as Palliative Therapy for Physical Symptoms and Quality of Life for Advanced Cancer Patients." *Integrative Cancer Therapies* 9 (2010): 158–67.

Dupler, Douglas, Teresa Odle, and David Edward Newton. "Acupuncture." *The Gale Encyclopedia of Alternative Medicine,* 3rd ed. 4 vols. Detroit: Gale, 2009.

Focks, Claudia. *Atlas of Acupuncture. Oxford*: Churchill Livingstone, 2008.

Hollifield, M., et al. "Acupuncture for Post-traumatic Stress Disorder: A Randomized Controlled Pilot Trial." *Journal of Nervous Mental Diseases* (June 2007): 504–13.

MacPherson, P., et al. "The York Acupuncture Safety Study: Prospective Survey of 34,000 Treatments by Traditional Acupuncturists." *British Medical Journal* 323 (September 1, 2001): 486–87.

Mayhew, E., and E. Ernst. "Acupuncture for Fibromyalgia: A Systematic Review of Randomized Clinical Trials." *Rheumatology* (May 2007): 801–4.

"Study Results from Dana-Farber Cancer Institute Broaden Understanding of Quality of Life." *Biotech Week* (July 28, 2010): 2122.

ADDICTION

Addiction is a complex disorder whose principal diagnostic feature is a repeated compulsion to take a certain substance or indulge in a certain behavior despite negative consequences. As an addicted person increasingly begins to rely on the object of addiction for physical or emotional gratification, he or she tends to neglect other, healthier aspects of life. It is generally agreed that there are two types of addiction: physical, when people become addicted to substances such as drugs or alcohol, and psychological or behavioral, when people become addicted to activities such as gambling or shopping. A behavioral addiction may also be called a process addiction. Although there is some disagreement over whether behaviors can be addictions in the same sense that drugs can be—some prefer to call such behaviors impulse control disorders or obsessive-compulsive disorders—the addict's need to indulge in them despite adverse consequences has led to their popular identification as addictions.

Both types of addiction initially provide some sort of pleasure, excitement, or gratification—often a combination of these. Addictions may range from mild to severe in degree; mildly addicted people may respond quickly to treatment and have relatively little difficulty refraining from the substance or behavior, whereas severely addicted people may be unable to recover.

Scientific advances over the past 30 to 40 years have revealed that addiction is based on neurochemical changes that take over or hijack a critical chemical pathway in the mesolimbic dopamine system of the brain. Known as the reward pathway, this area is programmed to respond to certain stimuli such as food or sex with feel-good neurotransmitters, primarily dopamine. Scientists believe that the pleasure these stimuli produce is how organisms learn to repeat behaviors important for survival, such as eating and reproduction. In the case of addictive substances, however, this mechanism can backfire.

When someone ingests an addictive drug or engages in addictive behavior, the affected neurons are overstimulated to produce an excess of dopamine that the brain perceives as a significantly more pleasurable experience than that provided by life's natural rewards. With repeated exposure to the psychoactive stimulus, the brain compensates by reducing its neurotransmitter output and producing fewer cellular receptors to receive and transmit dopamine along the reward pathway. As tolerance develops, the individual begins to require more of the drug stimulus to achieve the initial effect. Eventually, his or her use or behavior takes on a compulsive quality as the individual finds him- or herself compelled to indulge more frequently—not to feel good but to avoid feeling bad. In spite of this, the person is likely to deny the problem and claim that usage or behavior falls within normal boundaries. A clear indication that the individual's judgment is impaired, this denial becomes a nearly automatic reflex with which one justifies pathological use or behavior. If the person is unable to indulge, he or she may experience withdrawal, the physical and psychological distress that arises as the brain attempts to adjust to the absence of drugs.

Although behavioral addictions generally do not produce the more severe physical manifestations of withdrawal sometimes seen in substance addictions, individuals suffering from them may experience a certain level of agitation, restlessness, and depression if they cannot satisfy their need. Many drugs, such as certain antidepressants, cause physical dependence in the sense that they rebalance the brain's neurotransmitters, and their abrupt withdrawal can lead to distressing symptoms, but these drugs are not addictive because they do not trigger compulsive use and loss of control.

What Is Addiction? A consensus exists among most scientists that addiction is the process during which the brain's neural pathways—primarily in the mesolimbic dopamine system—are hijacked by the artificial reward of drugs. It is not clear how certain combinations of genetic, biological, and environmental factors allow this to happen in some people and not others; what is known is that, for many, a drug-induced release of dopamine and other neurotransmitters overrides the brain's response to normal rewards that support survival, such as food or sex. This reaction leads to changes in the structure of axons and dendrites and alters synapse formation, a dysregulation that begins to affect the addict's behavior outside of her or his conscious awareness. Although it is not completely understood how this physiological remodeling occurs, the distorted neurochemical messages it transmits affect learning, motivation, and memory. In time, addicts no longer respond to the drug with the same pleasure but find, instead, that they

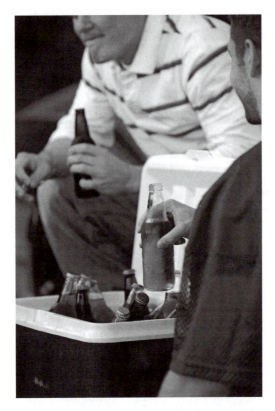

Students drink beer from a cooler. Binge drinking or drinking heavily on weekends or monthly is a form of alcohol abuse. (iStockPhoto)

require the drug to feel normal. As their ability to enjoy other pleasures decreases and their need for the drug increases, many addicts gradually cease to care about families, homes, work, school, or health in their single-minded pursuit of the drug.

Indulging in addictive substances or behaviors does not have to occur on a daily basis for addiction to exist; weekend drinkers or those who go on monthly binges with days of remission between episodes can be addicted, just as heavy drinkers who have several cocktails every night for years are not necessarily addicted if their drinking does not produce negative consequences and if they are able to stop without difficulty.

Recent research on mice has revealed that dopamine-releasing cells in the brain seem to learn and remember their hypersecretion of dopamine in response to addictive drugs. Called long-term potentiation, this cellular memory remains active for some time and may be part of the basis for craving. Researchers also made the intriguing discovery that although psychoactive *nonaddictive* drugs such as antidepressants do not potentiate the cells in the same way, acute stress does. Although stress does not cause addiction, this finding raises questions about how the relationship of drug exposure and stress could affect the brain's chemical threshold for prolonged potentiation and increased vulnerability to addiction. It may also help explain why stress is one of the most powerful threats to abstinence and recovery.

The American Psychiatric Association (APA), in its *Diagnostic and Statistical Manual of Mental Disorders* (*DSM*) published in 2000, presents criteria widely used by mental health experts to diagnose addiction and distinguish it from abuse. Although the *DSM* uses the term *dependence* in an effort to remove the stigma associated with the word *addiction,* this practice has led to considerable confusion, and increasing pressure is on APA editors to revert to the term addiction in the next edition of the *DSM.* Some experts, however, insist that addiction is a vague, clinically inaccurate term that does not properly distinguish between the medical disease that true addiction represents and the overindulgence of drugs or other substances that represents abuse, not addiction. They believe that the term dependence remains appropriate, especially if clear distinctions are made between chemical dependence and drug abuse. Despite this argument, there are indications that the APA will revert to addiction in the fifth edition of the *DSM* due to be published in 2012 rather than continue its use of the term dependence.

Signs of Substance and Behavioral Addictions

- Anticipating the substance or behavior with increased excitement
- Feeling irritable or restless when prevented from indulging in the substance or behavior
- Devoting increasing amounts of time preparing for the substance use or activity or recovering from the effects
- Neglecting responsibilities at home, school, or work
- Indulging in the substance or behavior to manage emotions
- Thinking obsessively about the activity
- Seeking out the substance or activity despite the harm it causes (deterioration of health, complaints from family or coworkers)
- Denying the problem to self and to others despite its obvious negative effects
- Hiding the use or behavior from others
- Suffering blackouts—memory losses while under the influence or an inability when sober to remember behavior that occurred when under the influence
- Becoming depressed; often a contributory factor in the development of an addiction, depression is also a result
- Having a history of anxiety or other mental disorder, psychological or physical abuse, or low self-esteem
- Experiencing some form of sexual dysfunction
- Feeling remorse or shame over use of substance(s) or activities associated with use dependence and physical dependence.

Evidence suggests that behavioral addictions tend to occur later in life and that substance addictions usually have an earlier onset stemming from drug or alcohol use during adolescence. Some studies cite instant-onset addiction, when users report that their initial exposure makes them feel normal for the first time in their lives. Whether this phenomenon represents actual addiction or an unusual reaction to the drug is not yet clear. Late-onset addictions may occur in adulthood, although the National Institute on Drug Abuse (2007) reports that the likelihood of addiction is much greater among adolescents and very young adults due to the plasticity of their developing brains.

The Teen Brain on Drugs   According to the National Institute of Mental Health and other scientists studying the impact that drug abuse has on the brain, adolescents are more vulnerable than adults to the deleterious effects of drugs for three reasons: drugs increase the likelihood of risky behavior; they prime vulnerable areas of the brain for the development of addiction; and, in the long term, they can permanently impair mental capacity.

Once a child reaches puberty, the brain begins to thin out excessive brain-cell connections made when the child was younger and the brain was growing at a rapid rate. This thinning-out process also helps build longer chains of neural networks that are required for the more critical analytical thinking that adults require throughout their lives. The pruning can be likened to how a gardener prunes a bush to remove weaker, ineffective branches to allow the stronger limbs to develop fully so the bush will thrive. A similar process in the brain of someone roughly 11 to 25 years old represents a crucial stage of neurological development.

The final area of the brain to mature is the prefrontal cortex, where higher cognitive functions and judgment reside. With so many structures in the teenage brain set to accelerate, the inhibitory reasoning part of the prefrontal cortex might not engage well enough to adequately guide behavior. Even in their late teens, adolescents are more impulsive, aggressive, and likely to engage in novel or risky activities than people in their mid- to late 20s. By the time adolescents outgrow their impulsive youth and reckless behavior, it may be too late to reverse addictive patterns already laid down in the brain or to undo permanent damage to cognitive abilities.

Addictions for the most part are chronic, progressive, and highly destructive. Long-term drug users develop physical health problems, and interpersonal, social, and occupational relationships break down as well. The ingredients in some drugs that cut or alter the substance can be toxic; snorting—inhaling powdered forms of a drug—can erode nasal tissues; stimulants can cause heart attacks or respiratory arrest; and contaminated needles can transmit HIV and other serious diseases such as malaria, tetanus, blood poisoning, or deadly bacterial infections. Drugs can trigger aberrant or violent behavior, and accidents—particularly automobile accidents—are common. About one-half of all highway fatalities involve alcohol alone.

Behavioral addictions such as eating disorders or sexual addictions that carry a risk of sexually transmitted diseases seriously compromise health. Others, such as pathological gambling, are devastating in other ways. Gambling addicts can squander a lifetime's accumulation of assets as they chase the next win, neglecting eating, sleeping, families, school, and work as their lives unravel.

Although their addictive potential varies widely, legal and illegal addictive substances are generally considered to be narcotics, stimulants, depressants, cannabis, hallucinogens, inhalants, anabolic steroids, nicotine, alcohol, and caffeine. Aside from their inherent chemical properties, factors that affect their addictive liability include the method of administration as well as the addict's genetic and environmental background. Addictive behaviors can arise from normal activities such as gambling, computer usage, sex, shopping and spending, and exercising, or from aberrant practices like kleptomania (stealing), trichotillomania (pulling out of one's hair), self-injury (cutting behaviors), and pyromania (starting fires).

History of Addiction The identification of certain activities as behavioral addictions is a comparatively recent event. Substance addiction has always been recognized, ever since humans began using mind-altering substances. In the fourth century BCE, Aristotle (384–322 BCE) referred to drunkenness as an organic disorder, and discussions of opium addiction appeared in medieval documents. Historical references to addiction focus on its negative aspects, although cultural attitudes about the more controlled use of some addictive drugs have been mixed. At one time, cocaine, marijuana, methamphetamines, and even opium were routinely prescribed for various conditions, and other drugs, such as peyote, are still in legal use among certain religious groups. Today, controlled substances such as codeine are prescribed for pain relief, and Ecstasy is being studied for the treatment of post-traumatic stress disorder.

Until the middle of the 20th century, addicts were usually shunned by the public or incarcerated in prisons or mental institutions. To some degree, modern attitudes have not changed: many people avoid or ignore homeless addicts on the streets of U.S. cities. Others view addiction and the deterioration that accompanies it as behavioral aberrations that should be addressed with cognitive techniques administered through widely available social programs. Still others, increasing numbers of laypeople and professionals alike, have come to regard addiction as an illness. These differing attitudes are reflected in present-day disagreements over whether illegal drug use is best addressed with criminal, behavioral, or medical measures or a combination of all three.

Since the 18th century, three models of addiction have emerged to explain the basis of addiction and to guide treatment strategies to address it: the moral model, the disease model, and the choice model. The disease model has received the most widespread acceptance in modern times, although many continue to support aspects of the moral and choice models.

Today, as accumulating data and brain-imaging studies reveal more about how addictions start and ultimately affect the brain's neurochemistry, the disease model has become widely accepted. The American Medical Association declared addiction a disease in 1956; the National Institute on Drug Abuse defines it as a progressive, chronic, relapsing—and treatable—brain disease; and organizations such as the American Psychiatric Association, the American Psychological Association, the American Society of Addiction Medicine, and the National Council on Alcoholism concur. They agree that although underlying physical or mental illness, genetics, and environmental factors coalesce in complex ways in the development of addiction, almost anyone can become addicted when compulsive behaviors or substance abuse continue long enough. In many people, especially those with a genetic predisposition, brains repeatedly exposed to the addictive substance undergo changes that leave users incapable of making the rational judgments needed to moderate addictive behavior, and so the disease worsens. Fortunately, some of the newer medications that target addiction-related neurochemistry in some cases can help restore the brain to normal functioning and reduce or eliminate craving, a major threat to recovery.

Kathryn H. Hollen

See also Alcohol; Caffeine; Cigarettes; Drugs, Recreational; Stress.

References

American Psychiatric Association. *Diagnostic and Statistical Manual of Mental Disorders,* 4thed., text rev. Washington, DC: American Psychiatric Association, 2000.

Califano, Joseph A., Jr. *High Society: How Substance Abuse Ravages America and What to Do About It.* New York: Perseus Books, 2007.

Erickson, Carlton K. *The Science of Addiction: From Neurobiology to Treatment.* New York: Norton, 2007.

Hanson, Glen R. *Substance Abuse Disorders: Diseases of the Mind.* Utah Addiction Center (July 2007), http://uuhsc.utah.edu/uac.

Hoffman, John, and Susan Froemke, eds. *Addiction: Why Can't They Just Stop?* New York: Rodale, 2007.

Home Box Office. In partnership with the Robert Wood Johnson Foundation, the National Institute on Drug Abuse, and the National Institute on Alcohol Abuse and Alcoholism. *Addiction: Why Can't They Just Stop?* Documentary (March 2007).

Kalivas, Peter, and Nora Volkow. "The Neural Basis of Addiction: A Pathology of Motivation and Choice." *American Journal of Psychiatry* 162, no. 8 (August 2005): 1403–13.

Ketcham, Katherine, and Nicholas A. Pace. *Teens under the Influence: The Truth about Kids, Alcohol, and Other Drugs.* New York: Ballantine Books, 2003.

Lemanski, Michael. *A History of Addiction and Recovery in the United States.* Tucson, AZ: See Sharp Press, 2001.

Miller, Shannon C. "Language and Addiction." *American Journal of Psychiatry* 163 (2006): 2015.

Moyers, William Cope. *Broken: The Story of Addiction and Redemption.* New York: Penguin Group, 2006.

National Institute on Drug Abuse. *The Science of Addiction: Drugs, Brains, and Behavior.* NIH Publication No. 07–5605. Bethesda, MD: NIDA, NIH, DHHS, February 2007.

Nestler, Eric, and Robert Malenka. "The Addicted Brain." *Scientific American* 290, no. 3 (September 2007), www.sciam.com/article.cfm?chanID=sa006&colID=1&articleID=0 001E632978A1019978A83414B7F0101.

Nurnberger, John I., Jr., and Laura Jean Bierut. "Seeking the Connections: Alcoholism and Our Genes." *Scientific American* 296, no. 4 (April 2007): 46–53.

Ozelli, Kristin Leutwyler. "This Is Your Brain on Food." *Scientific American* 297, no. 3 (September 2007): 84–85.

Schaler, Jeffrey A. "Addiction Is a Choice." *Psychiatric Times* 19, no. 10 (October 2002): 54, 62.

Tracy, Sarah, and Caroline Jean Acker, eds. *Altering American Consciousness: The History of Alcohol and Drug Use in the United States, 1800–2000.* Amherst: University of Massachusetts Press, 2004.

U.S. Department of Health and Human Services. *Morbidity and Mortality Weekly Report: Surveillance Summaries.* Centers for Disease Control and Prevention, Youth Risk Behavior Surveillance—United States. Washington, DC: U.S. Government Printing Office, 2009.

U.S. Department of Health and Human Services, National Institute of Dental and Craniofacial Research. *Smokeless Tobacco—A Guide for Quitting.* NIH Publication No. 10-3270. Bethesda, MD: NIDCR, NIH (August 2010), www.nidcr.nih.gov.

U.S. Department of Health and Human Services, National Institute of Mental Health. *Drugs, Brains, and Behavior: The Science of Addiction.* NIH Publication No. 10-5605. Bethesda: MD: NIMH, NIH (August 2010), www.nimh.nih.gov.

U.S. Department of Health and Human Services, National Institute on Alcohol Abuse and Alcoholism. *Reducing Underage and Young Adult Drinking: How to Address Critical Drinking Problems during This Developmental Period.* Volume 33, Number 1 & 2. Bethesda, MD: NIH, NIAAA (July 2010), www.niaaa.nih.gov.

Vaillant, George. *The Natural History of Alcoholism Revisited.* Cambridge, MA: Harvard University Press, 1995.

White, William. "A Disease Concept for the 21st Century." *AddictionInfo.com* (June 2007), www.addictioninfo.org/articles/1051/1/.

Winters, Ken. *Adolescent Brain Development and Drug Abuse.* Philadelphia: Treatment Research Institute, 2008.

ADOLESCENCE

There is much to say about the phase of life known as adolescence. Marked by the beginning of puberty, adolescence is the transition from childhood to adulthood and when a young person experiences physical, mental, and social changes. Within this phase of life are the teenage years.

A relatively recent concept, teenagers became a distinct group when the Great Depression took them out of the workforce and into the classroom. Prior to this, only children of the wealthy received formal education for an extended period of time. Most teens worked on their parents' farms or in factories. Boys left the home as men once they could live on their own and marry. Girls left home as women once a man came along to marry them—some of them married before they turned 18 years of age.

Things would continue to change and evolve for adolescents and teens. In the 1930s, a teenage girl was in a movie theater with friends. She spoke and laughed with them. A man in the theater turned to the girl and asked her to stop. When the girl refused, the man gave her a slap in the face. He was an adult after all, and felt he had the right to administer discipline for what he saw as unruly behavior from a child. The teen girl saw things differently. She sued the man for slapping her. This recorded moment of teen rebellion represented a teenage desire to separate from adults and to take a stand for what she believed to be her rights. Since that time, the rights and lives of teenagers have continued to evolve (Palladino, 1996).

Physical Changes   The most noticeable aspects of adolescence begin at approximately 12 years of age, although girls sometimes begin developing physically into women as young as 8 years of age. Boys tend to begin the journey toward manhood at the age of 9. Girls experience the beginning of breast growth, pubic hair growth, and menstruation. Boys experience the beginning of testicular growth, followed by the lengthening of the penis. Also, their voices begin to deepen.

Most of these physical changes happen in stages known as Tanner Stages, named for the physician who first described the stages of puberty in 1969. There are five stages, each describing the size and appearance of external genitalia, body changes, and breast development in girls. Stage 1 is considered prepubertal. Stage 5 is considered to be a mature adult level (medicinenet.com/puberty/page2.htm).

Tanner Stages for Girls

Stage 1: Preadolescent; elevation of papilla only.

Stage 2: Breast bud stage; elevation of breast and papilla as a small mound, enlargement of areola diameter.

Stage 3: Further enlargement of breast and areola, with no separation of their contours.

Stage 4: Projection of areola and papilla to form a secondary mound above the level of the breast.

Stage 5: Mature stage; projection of papilla only, due to recession of the areola to the general contour of the breast. (Marshall & Tanner, 1969)

Tanner Stages for Boys

Stage 1: Preadolescent; testes, scrotum, and penis about same size and proportion as in early childhood.

Stage 2: Scrotum and testes enlarge, and change in the texture of the scrotal skin; some reddening of the scrotal skin.

Stage 3: Growth of the penis, at first mainly in length but with some increase in breadth; further growth of testes and scrotum.

Stage 4: Penis further enlarged in length and breadth with development of glands; testes and scrotum further enlarged; further darkening of the scrotal skin.

Stage 5: Genitalia adult in size and shape. (Marshall & Tanner, 1970)

The Teenage Brain Adolescents and teens are works in progress, and so are their brains. In fact, researchers suggest that brain development is not complete until a person reaches his or her mid-20s. According to medical literature, the prefrontal cortex—which is one of the last areas of the brain to fully mature—controls a person's ability to make sound and reasonable judgments, controls impulses, and enables a person to take a long view of one's circumstances. These are important abilities for a person to have when navigating the world. To begin meeting these challenges, the adolescent brain develops a more complex wiring and improves in efficiency, particularly in the prefrontal cortex.

Over time, the maturing brain grows neural connections that can perform several tasks at once. Dopamine is an important chemical for the adolescent brain; it sends signals to the prefrontal cortex to help an individual focus when there are competing options. Throughout adolescence, these signals increase.

With the help of this information, researchers understand that loving parents, other adults, and institutions can help teens learn specific adult skills and behaviors. Also, teens themselves can have a hand in their own brain development by participating in positive experiences to grow more complex and adaptive brains (Weinberger, Elvevåg, & Giedd, 2005).

During adolescence a greater understanding of the world and its people emerges. Adolescents begin to grasp abstract concepts in areas such as math, philosophy, and law. They also gain a greater understanding of morals and develop a sense of right and wrong. They learn to establish and maintain relationships and move gradually toward a more mature sense of identity and purpose. Also, adolescents may begin to question old values.

In early adolescence, friends and relationships become very important. Adolescents' peer groups often consist of platonic friendships, including cliques, gangs, or clubs. Members of the peer group often attempt to behave alike, dress alike, have secret codes or rituals, and participate in the same activities. As young people move into mid-adolescence, also known as the teenage years, their peer groups expand to include romantic relationships.

This is also a time when adolescents begin to separate from their parents in an attempt to establish their own identity. In some cases, this social transition is uneventful. In other cases, conflicts can arise. As adolescents pull away from parents in a search for identity, their peer groups take on a special significance. These peer groups may become a safe haven, in which the adolescent can test new ideas and compare physical and psychological growth.

As they continue to grow, adolescents face safety concerns that stem and from the development of increased strength and agility and from increased mobility as a result of being able to drive. These concerns sometimes arise before a teen or adolescent has developed good decision-making skills. Armed with feelings of invincibility, teens may participate in a variety of risk-taking behaviors. Adolescents and teens are also affected by a strong need for approval from their peer groups—also known as peer pressure—which also can lead to risky behaviors.

Adolescents involved in sports and other recreational activities should always follow the safety rules and recommendations associated with the activity. Appropriate motor vehicle safety should be emphasized with teens as well. These lessons include the responsibilities of drivers, passengers, and pedestrians. They should understand the legal and accidental consequences of driving under the influence of drugs and alcohol. Teens also need to be reminded of the importance of wearing seat belts.

Mental and Emotional Issues The transition from childhood to adulthood can be smooth and uneventful or tumultuous, and how individual youth handle the experience can vary. The rapid physical, mental, and emotional developments that occur can lead to feelings of self-consciousness and concern over body changes. Adolescents and teens frequently compare themselves to their peers.

One myth of adolescence that is typically responsible for the angst demonstrated by so many teens and preteens is the belief that all eyes are on them all of the time. In reality, peers are typically too preoccupied with their own situations to pay to close attention to others. While it can be off-putting to adults, this behavior is perfectly normal.

However, if the angst does not pass or change as the adolescent or teen ages, parents and other adults should pay special attention to the young person's behaviors. Many teens who develop depression also can be at risk for suicide. If adolescents appear to be isolated from peers and family, uninterested in school or typical teen activities, or are deteriorating in school or sports performance, a psychological evaluation may be needed. Parents should seek advice from their adolescent's pediatrician (MedlinePlus, 2011a).

Depression in adolescents and teens can be a temporary response to many things, including normal maturation, fluctuation of sex hormones, parental conflict, a breakup with a boyfriend or girlfriend, or failure at school. Adolescents with low self-esteem and who feel they have no control over negative events are especially at risk for depression.

Girls are twice as likely as boys to suffer from depression. A family history of depression increases the chances of an adolescent or teen experiencing the disorder. Where there is depression, there also may be anxiety disorders, attention deficit hyperactivity disorder, bipolar disorder, or eating disorders such as bulimia and anorexia.

Signs of depression in teens include agitation, appetite changes, difficulty concentrating, difficulty making decisions, fatigue, feelings of worthlessness, loss of interest in activities, or trouble sleeping. In some cases, depression exists where there are no signs of sadness. Instead, depression can manifest itself through acting-out behaviors, criminal behavior, a drop in grades, irresponsible behavior, or substance abuse.

It may seem as if the signs of depression mimic the typical emotions and behaviors of adolescence. However, there are ways that parents and other adults can tell the difference. If signs and symptoms persist longer than two weeks without any periods of the adolescent experiencing joy and if they cause a significant inability to function, parents should seek treatment. Also, a worsening of symptoms or side effects from medications should be reported to a health care provider. If the adolescent starts giving away cherished possessions, his or her personality changes, or she or he threatens suicide, these are major causes for alarm, and parents should seek treatment. A suicide attempt should never be ignored.

To test for depression, a physical examination is performed and blood tests are ordered to rule out medical causes for the symptoms. The patient is also tested for signs of substance abuse, which can cause depression. A psychiatric evaluation will seek the patient's history of sadness, irritability, and loss of interest and pleasure in normal activities. The patient will be evaluated for other psychiatric disorders as well.

Treatment for youth with depression includes supportive parents, care from a medical provider, and talk therapy. Antidepressant medications may be an option as well. The good news is that depression in adolescents typically responds to treatment. The bad news is that teens with depression usually battle depression as adults.

While periods of having a depressed mood are normal in teens, it is still important for them to develop healthy coping skills and to have supportive relationships. When there is open communication in the home, parents may be able to identify their child's depression early. Early identification and a prompt response can stave off further episodes of depression.

In homes with children and adolescents, it is a good idea to make sure that alcohol, guns and ammunition, and prescription medications are locked away or in some way inaccessible.

Adolescent Rituals   Entering the world of adolescence is not all negative. In many ways and throughout many cultures, adolescence is celebrated with rites of passage. These are ceremonies or practices that mark changes in an individual's social status. They occur around events such as childbirth, puberty, marriage, and death. When practiced, these events symbolize the separation of an individual from one group or phase of life to another. At the end of the ritual, the individual is presented to society in his or her new role.

There are many categories under which rites of passage are celebrated. Life cycle events are acknowledged in just about every culture in the world. For adolescents and teens, these rituals are most often connected to coming of age, religion, and education attainment.

In the United States, certain groups select debutantes (girls in their late teens) to participate in coming-out parties or ceremonies where they are presented to society as young women ready to work toward adult goals. Coming-of-age celebrations in the United States are also connected to birthday milestones such as turning 16 or "sweet sixteen." The Hispanic tradition of celebrating a daughter's 15th birthday is called a *quinceañera* and is similar to a sweet sixteen party. In other cultures, coming-of-age customs can be serious and painful, such as scarification, killing a wild animal, or enduring physical pain. Australian Aborigines, for example, send youths into the wilderness to spend a period of time alone ("Rite of Passage," 2008).

Religious celebrations may also be connected with age. In the Jewish tradition, 12-year-old girls receive a bat mitzvah, and 13-year-old boys receive a bar mitzvah. These celebrations acknowledge the honoree's receiving of full adult rights. Poy Sang Long is a ceremony held for boys in Burma and in Thailand and requires them to become novice monks. Young children in some Hindu castes celebrate the sacred thread ceremony, which marks the beginning of their education. In Amish communities, adolescents sometimes participate in a rite called *rumspringa,* where they spend time living outside of the community before deciding whether to join the Amish church and be baptized as an adult. Some Native American youths participate in vision quests, where they undergo sensory deprivation in order to make contact with the spirits.

Education rituals are important in Western cultures. In the United States, many schools hold graduation ceremonies and farewell programs for elementary and middle school students. High school graduation is a big event involving a ceremony where students receive diplomas and listen to speeches. Sometimes these events are followed by graduation parties. The prom, an event where seniors dress formally and attend a dance, is another important rite of passage associated with graduation from high school. Graduations held in other parts of the world happen a bit differently. In Scandinavia, for example, students celebrate during the entire month when they graduate from high school.

Abena Foreman-Trice

See also Anorexia Nervosa; Depression; Eating Disorders.

References

Conrad Stöppler, Melissa. "Puberty." MedicineNet.com, http://medicinenet.com/puberty/page2.htm.

Marshall, W.A., and J.M. Tanner. "Variations in Pattern of Pubertal Changes in Girls." From the Department of Growth and Development, Institute of Child Health, University of London, *Archives of Disease in Childhood* 44 (1969): 291.

Marshall, W.A., and J.M. Tanner. "Variations in the Pattern of Pubertal Changes in Boys." From the Department of Growth and Development, Institute of Child Health, University of London, *Archives of Disease in Childhood* 45 (1970): 13.

MedlinePlus. "Adolescent Depression" (January 17, 2011a), nlm.nih.gov/medlineplus/ency/article/001518.htm.

MedlinePlus. "Adolescent Development" (January 17, 2011b), nlm.nih.gov/medlineplus/ency/article/002003.htm.

Palladino, Grace. *Teenagers: An American History.* Basic Books, 1996.

"Rite of Passage." *New World Encyclopedia* (2008), newworldencyclopedia.org/entry/Rite_of_passage.

Weinberger, Daniel R., Brita Elvevåg, & Jay N. Giedd. "The Adolescent Brain: A Work in Progress." National Campaign to Prevent Teen Pregnancy (June 2005), www.thenationalcampaign.org/resources/pdf/BRAIN.pdf.

AEROBIC EXERCISE

From Olivia Newton John's song, "Let's Get Physical" to Jane Fonda's workout tapes, by the 1980s, aerobic exercise had permeated U.S. life and culture. However, its origins go back to 1968, when Dr. Kenneth H. Cooper, a flight surgeon who was also a director of the U.S. Air Force Aerospace Medical Laboratory in San Antonio, Texas, published a book on the benefits of aerobic activity for cardiovascular health. The effort was prompted by a health scare that highlighted his own need to get into shape and his subsequent development of physical conditioning programs for U.S. astronauts.

His book, called, simply, *Aerobics,* launched a new devotion to physical fitness that grew by leaps and bounds and continues today. Decades later, Cooper still devotes his time to helping people improve their physical fitness. He leads the Cooper Institute, which he founded in 1970. The institute is devoted to research, training, and educating the public—including youth—on the benefits of exercise for health and wellness (Cooper Aerobics, 2011).

Aerobic exercise is any exercise done while the body uses oxygen to sustain activities for a long period of time. Almost any activity can be aerobic and can fall into categories such as running, water aerobics, dance aerobics, low-impact aerobics, and sport aerobics. Studies show that aerobic exercise brings many health benefits. It is nearly the opposite of anaerobic exercise, which is short-lasting, high-intensity exercise requiring almost more oxygen than the body has to give.

After Cooper, who was a runner, popularized aerobic exercise, others soon followed to spur the aerobics movement. Jackie Sorensen is credited with developing aerobic dance routines. Howard and Karen Schwartz were credited with bringing the world aerobic championships, turning the exercise into a sport in

1984. Gin Miller, a former gymnast who suffered from overuse injuries to her muscles, has been credited with developing step aerobics—a popular form of exercise where participants step up onto small, portable platforms and conduct a series of movements to music. Initially, stepping up and down on a milk crate and then her porch steps was a form of therapy for Miller, who needed to rehabilitate her knee muscles (Aerobic.org, n.d.).

An aerobics program or routine usually begins with a warm-up session to get the body ready to engage in significant activity. Once engaged in aerobic activity, the goal is to progressively move into a rigorous level of intensity that raises the heart rate and that typically lasts from 15 to 25 minutes. A cool-down period ends the exercise session, allowing individuals to stretch, improve flexibility, and lower the heart rate.

Other behaviors can make aerobic exercise more effective. For example, weights can provide the added benefit of strengthening muscles. However, it is important to give muscles time to recuperate. Therefore, the same muscles should not perform weight-bearing exercise two or more days in a row. Personal trainers and exercise physiologists are in positions to advise individuals on appropriate aerobic regimens. Also, the U.S. government offers exercise recommendations for children and adults. According to the Centers for Disease Control and Prevention (CDC), adults need 150 minutes of moderate aerobic activity each week or 75 minutes of vigorous aerobic activity each week (CDC, 2011a).

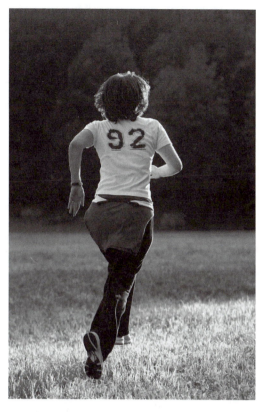

Female jogger crosses an open field. Millions of Americans became part of the jogging craze that swept the country in the early 1970s. Jogging continues to be a popular form of aerobic exercise. (iStockPhoto)

How can individuals know if they are engaging in true aerobic activity? According to the experts, true aerobic activity will not leave one breathing easy. If a person has to take more breaths at a faster pace and his or her heart rate increases, then the activity is bringing aerobic benefits. Everyday activities such as pushing a lawn mower, taking a dance class, or biking to the store all count toward daily aerobic activity if done correctly. Running and jogging provide excellent aerobic exercise. The activity has to last for at least 10 minutes at a certain level of intensity. That benefit of aerobic exercise means that while recommendations call for 30 minutes per day at a minimum, those minutes do not have to be all at once (CDC, 2011b).

The intensity level of physical activities is important, because it requires the body to work hard, increasing the body's heart rate. This heart-healthy effect is another reason aerobic workouts are also referred to as cardio workouts. Light activities that do not require much physical exertion such as shopping, cooking, doing laundry, and running errands do not qualify as aerobic activity. Activities that range from moderate to vigorous levels of intensity and cause individuals to perspire, prevent conversations (or require a person to take breaths every few moments in order to carry a conversation), and raise the heart rate significantly are aerobic activity. The most intense of these exercises are running, swimming laps, fast-paced bike riding, and playing tennis or basketball (CDC, 2011b).

For those who need more ways to tell if activities are vigorous enough, many types of measurements exist. Two types of aerobic intensity levels—relative intensity and absolute intensity—describe an individual's level of exertion physical activity.

Relative intensity is the basic level of effort required to perform an activity. Relative intensity calls on people to pay attention to how their heart rate and breathing are affected by what they are doing. An easy way to tell whether an activity is of relative intensity is to take the talk test. If a person engaged in aerobic activity can talk but is unable to sing, then he or she is exercising at a moderate level of intensity.

At a more vigorous level of intensity known as absolute intensity, a person cannot speak freely without frequently stopping to take a breath. Absolute intensity indicates how much energy the body uses per minute to conduct activity.

There also is a more scientific or mathematical way to figure out the body's level of exertion when doing exercises. A person can measure his or her heart rate to determine the intensity of the physical activity. Each person has a target zone and a maximum heart rate, depending upon age. During moderate exercise, a person's heart rate should fall between 50 and 70 percent of their maximum heart rate. The traditional calculation for maximum heart rate has been to subtract a person's age from the number 220, but that method has been cited as erroneous. A slightly more accurate calculation may be $205.8 - (0.685 \times age)$, but it too has been cited as prone to error (Robergs & Landwehr, 2002).

For example, for a 20-year-old, , 205.8 minus (0.685×20), would be 205.8 minus 13.7, which is 192.1 beats per minute (bpm) for *maximum heart rate*. For the traditional method, the maximum heart rate would be 200 bpm (220 minus age of 20). For moderate exercise, 50 percent of 200 $(200 \times .50)$, would be 100. This means that at a moderate level of exercise intensity, the heart rate for a 20-year-old should equal at least 100 beats per minute. To determine more vigorous levels of physical intensity, the heart's target zone should be 70 percent to 85 percent of a person's maximum heart rate. So, for example, the same 20-year-old conducting more rigorous exercise would have a target heart rate of 140 $(200 \times .70)$ beats per minute.

Another way to measure target heart rate is to pause during exercise and measure one's pulse at the neck, chest, or wrist. Experts at the CDC recommend that people use their wrists for this measurement. This is done by taking the index finger and the two middle fingers and applying gentle pressure on the wrist's artery. A person can either count heart beats for 60 seconds (or for 30 seconds and then multiply that number by two). Again, for the 20-year-old, more than 100 beats per minute indicates moderate exercise, and more than 140 beats per minute indicates a more rigorous level of exercise (CDC, 2011a).

Inactive individuals planning to begin an aerobic exercise regimen should first consult their primary care physicians. Once they have discussed plans with their doctor, they may begin at a moderate level, but they should feel at ease before gradually increasing to a more intense level of activity. By following government and medical guidelines in addition to consulting a physician, individuals can develop an appropriate aerobic exercise regimen and improve their overall health and wellness.

Abena Foreman-Trice

See also Anaerobic Exercise; Exercise; Heart Health; Physical Endurance; Target Heart Rate.

References

Aerobic.org. "Aerobic History" (n.d.),www.aerobic.org/aerobic/aerobic-history.asp.

Aerobic.org. "Types of Aerobics" (n.d.), www.aerobic.org/aerobic/types/.

Centers for Disease Control and Prevention. *Physical Activity for Everyone* (March 2011a), www.cdc.gov/physicalactivity/everyone/guidelines/adults.html.

Centers for Disease Control and Prevention. *Physical Activity for Everyone:* Measuring Intensity (March 2011b), www.cdc.gov/physicalactivity/everyone/measuring/index.html.

Cooper, Kenneth H. *The Aerobics Way: New Data on the World's Most Popular Exercise Program.* New York: Bantam Books, 1978.

Cooper Aerobics. "Dr. Kenneth Cooper" (2011), www.cooperaerobics.com/About-Cooper/Dr--Kenneth Cooper.aspx.

Robergs, Robert A., and Roberto Landwehr. "The Surprising History of the 'HRmax= 220–age' Equation." *Journal of Exercise Physiology* 5, no. 2 (2002): 1–10.

Sharkey, Brain J., and Steven E. Gaskill. *Fitness and Health,* 6th ed. Champaign, IL: Human Kinetics, 2007.

Sutton, Amy L. *Fitness and Exercise Sourcebook,* 3rd ed. Detroit: Omnigraphics, 2007.

Wright, Vonda, and Ruth Winter. *Fitness after 40: How to Stay Strong at Any Age.* New York: AMACOM, 2009.

AIR POLLUTION

Taking a walk outdoors may seem like one of the healthiest things a person can do. However, such may not always be the case. The World Health Organization estimates that about 3 million people die worldwide each year as a result of breathing polluted air. In the United States, air pollution is responsible for about 70,000 deaths annually. By comparison, vehicle-related accidents kill about 40,000 people.

Even sitting at home in your own living room can be a hazard to your health. Many homes, offices, and other buildings are poorly ventilated. Breathing the air in such buildings can expose a person to a variety of harmful substances, such as radon, carbon monoxide, and secondhand tobacco smoke. The American Lung Association estimates that radon trapped inside buildings is responsible for 15,000 to 21,000 lung cancer deaths in the United States each year.

Air pollution has been a problem for human societies for hundreds of years. As far back as the 14th century, air pollution was so bad in England that King Edward I banned the use of coal for making fires, declaring, "whosoever shall be found guilty of burning coal shall suffer the loss of his head." The problem became much worse with the rise of the Industrial Revolution in the early 19th century. The combustion of coal became the primary means of operating factories, running railroad engines, and heating homes and offices. This practice produced huge amounts of waste products, such as soot and ash, which filled the skies over most urban areas with clouds of smoke. People continued to complain about the inconvenience of polluted air, but governments usually accepted the problem as an unfortunate side effect of a growing prosperity. As industrial development continued through the 19th and 20th centuries, air pollution became a more severe and more widespread problem. By the 1950s, parts of the Earth that had once been pristine—like the skies over the Arctic—had also started to become polluted.

The term *air pollution* refers to the presence of substances in the air at a level that can harm the health and survival of humans, other animals, and plants. The most common substances present in polluted air are carbon monoxide, oxides of nitrogen, sulfur dioxide, ozone, particulate matter, volatile organic compounds (VOCs), and lead. By far the most important source of these pollutants is the combustion of fossil fuels: coal, oil, and natural gas. Each pollutant has specific harmful effects on living organisms that vary depending on the amount of pollutant present and the time one is exposed to the pollutant. Carbon monoxide in small doses over short periods can cause headache, nausea, and disorientation; in larger doses, it can cause loss of consciousness and death. Long-term exposure to oxides of nitrogen or sulfur dioxide can produce bronchitis, pneumonia, emphysema, and other respiratory disorders. VOCs and ozone also act as irritants to the lungs and can cause respiratory disorders as well as make the lungs more sensitive to other irritants. Particulate matter consists of tiny particles of unburned carbon and other solids that lodge in lung tissue, causing a variety of respiratory problems. Lead is a toxic material that can cause various physical and mental disorders, including reproductive and digestive problems and mental retardation.

Air pollutants can produce other harmful effects. Smog—a form of air pollution produced when sunlight acts on pollutants to form a smoky fog—is responsible for reduced visibility that may result in automobile or airplane accidents. Oxides of nitrogen and sulfur dioxide can attack plants, destroying leaves, flowers, and fruits. Most air pollutants also have health effects on domestic animals similar to the effects on humans. Mercury in the air dissolves in water, where it is ingested by aquatic plants and animals and becomes part of the food chain.

The earliest legislation in the United States dealing with air pollution was the Air Pollution Control Act of 1955, allocating $5 million to the states to carry out research on air pollution. That act was followed by a series of Clean Air Acts and amendments in the 1960s, none of which was very effective in reducing air pollution. The first successful piece of legislation concerned with air pollution was the Clean Air Act of 1970. The act established National Ambient Air Quality Standards and New Source Performance Standards that form the bases of air pollution reduction programs even today. It also created standards for automobile emissions. The 1970 act has been amended and revised a number of times, most importantly in 1977 and 1990.

Efforts to combat air pollution in the United States have been quite successful. The Environmental Protection Agency reported in 2005 that total emissions from six major air pollutants—nitrogen dioxide, ozone, sulfur dioxide, particulate matter, carbon monoxide, and lead—had dropped by 54 percent between 1970 and 2004. The worldwide situation was not as promising. While developed nations were finally getting air pollution problems under control, developing nations were only beginning to realize the magnitude of the challenge they face. China was perhaps the most troublesome example. In the early 21st century, 16 of the world's 20 most polluted cities were in China. As the nation continues to burn coal at a voracious rate to drive its burgeoning economy, air pollution is certain to become an even more serious problem for the giant, as it will for many other growing economies throughout the world.

David E. Newton

See also Environmental Health; Environmental Protection Agency (EPA); World Health Association (WHO).

References

Elsom, Derek M. *Atmospheric Pollution: A Global Problem.* Oxford: Blackwell, 1992.

Graham, Ian. *Air: A Resource Our World Depends On.* Chicago: Heinemann Library, 2005.

Kidd, J.S., and Renee A. Kidd. *Into Thin Air: The Problem of Air Pollution.* New York: Facts on File, 1998.

Rapp, Valerie. *Protecting Earth's Air Quality.* Minneapolis: Lerner Publications, 2009.

Turco, Richard P. *Earth under Siege: From Air Pollution to Global Change.* New York: Oxford University Press, 2002.

ALCOHOL

Alcohol has been associated with health problems—and also wellness—since prehistory. It has been used for medicine, as part of the diet, for religious rituals, and as a social lubricant. Alcohol (ethanol, ethyl alcohol) comes in three basic beverage forms: wines, beers, and distilled liquors or spirits. Alcoholic beverages were likely discovered by early humans when mixtures of crushed fruits or honey mixed with water were left exposed to airborne yeasts in a warm atmosphere.

The yeast converts the natural sugars into alcohol and carbon dioxide by fermentation.

Wines are made from the fermentation of fruits, honey, and simple grains such as rice (mead is made from honey; ciders are made from fruit but have less alcohol content than wine). Beers and ales are made by fermenting more complex sugars such as grains, hops, corn, and potatoes after the starch has been broken down by such substances as malts. Distilled spirits such as gin, rum, whiskey, and brandy are made by distilling the alcohol from crude wines or beers. Fortified wines such as sherry and port are wines to which distilled alcohol has been added. Liqueurs (cordials) are made in a similar way; the addition of sugar and spices gives them a thick and syrupy consistency.

Most beers in North America contain 3 to 6 percent, wines 12 to 21 percent, and distilled spirits 40 to 50 percent alcohol by volume. Proof is designated as twice the percentage of alcohol by volume. A 12-ounce bottle, glass, or can of beer is one drink; a 4- to 5-ounce glass of wine is a drink; and a 1.5-ounce jigger of spirits is one drink. Each gram of alcohol contains 7 calories. Beers range from light to stout and contain 95 to 200 calories; white and red table wines range from 85 to 105 calories; distilled spirits range from 90 to 150 calories.

History and Cultural Use of Alcoholic Beverages Today most cultures around the world, with the exception of Islamic societies and some Protestant religious groups, consume alcohol. Moreover, alcoholic beverages have been drunk throughout human history. Residues of wines and beers have been identified in archeological finds from numerous preliterate societies. Although alcohol has been widely used, many cultures gave warning of the harmful effects of excessive drinking. For this entry, the terms *drink* and *drinking* refer to the consumption of an alcoholic beverage and not other liquids.

References to wine making are found in abundance in Judeo-Christian scriptures and in other ancient writings. Alcohol was used in the Greek and Roman civilizations, by the gods in myth and legend, as well as by the people of all social classes. Wines fermented from rice were widely used by Asian cultures; the Middle Eastern Arabs first distilled alcohol around 500 CE.

In Europe, the northern and the southern regions have traditionally been seen as having different drinking patterns and attitudes toward drinking. Moreover, these preferences appear to have persisted from a more distant past. It is hypothesized that from antiquity, different drinking cultures concerning alcohol developed in the northern and in the Mediterranean areas of Western Europe. During the expansion of the Roman Empire, rural areas of west central Europe became Romanized (urbanized). As a part of this process, indigenous inhabitants adopted some customs from urban Roman culture, including moderate wine drinking with meals.

When Rome's influence declined in the West, Engs (1995) suggests that former provinces that retained Roman culture also retained drinking patterns characterized by moderation. The northern Celtic and Germanic cultures, untouched by direct Roman influence, continued their traditional, heavy, feast drinking patterns and developed an ambiguous attitude toward alcohol. Malt liquor, mead, and later spirits, but not wine, were the preferred alcoholic beverages. Southern Britain and a few areas of continental Europe integrated some aspects of the northern drinking into its predominantly southern pattern. These patterns congealed during the early Middle Ages and became the underlying drinking cultures for the regions overlaying these areas into modern times.

In Europe during the Middle Ages, when the water supplies were often polluted, beer, wine, and cider were commonly drunk in place of water. Although many church leaders denounced drunkenness, they seldom criticized the daily use of alcoholic beverages, as they were considered a necessity for maintaining good health. This attitude was brought to North America by the early settlers. However, severe penalties were imposed for drunkenness. In New England the production of rum became an important business, and the trade of rum, molasses, and slaves flourished for many years in the colonies.

As early American settlers pushed farther west, whiskey making became common inasmuch as the pioneers found it easier to transport whiskey made from corn rather than bulky containers of wine and beer. However, during the frontier days, a number of people became concerned about the heavy drinking of the pioneers and began to question the health-giving qualities of rum, gin, and whiskey. Church leaders pleaded for temperance (moderate and responsible use of alcohol). But later these leaders urged people not to drink at all and started lobbying for laws against drinking, as they felt that alcohol caused too many social and health problems.

In the United States, these concerns resulted in three waves of prohibition emerging out of clean living movements. In these health and social reform movements, reformers attempted to "clean up" society. This included the elimination of tobacco, drugs, and alcohol and the promotion of exercise, better diet, and pure food and water for better health of the population. State prohibition in all states north of the Mason-Dixon Line and east of the Mississippi River was legislated in the early 1850s. These laws were repealed during the Civil War. National Prohibition began in 1920 with the 18th Amendment to the Constitution and was repealed in 1933. The National Minimum Drinking Age Act of 1984 required all states to raise their minimum purchase and public possession of alcohol to age 21. States that did not comply faced a reduction in highway funds under the Federal Highway Aid Act.

The United States has one of the highest legal drinking ages in the world. In most countries, 18 years is the legal drinking age, and many nations do not even enforce this age. Canada, which has a drinking age of 19, has a lower alcohol consumption rate compared to the United States. In the United States, the per capita consumption of alcohol reached a peak in 1980 and declined through 2002. However, after 2003 it began to rise again. English-speaking countries have lower consumption rates compared to other nations.

Alcohol and Its Unhealthy Use   Alcohol is a classic depressant of the central nervous system. In increasing amounts, it causes uncoordination, slurred speech, sleepiness, stupor, and even death from alcohol intoxication. In small amounts, alcohol can cause an apparent stimulation in some people. This results from

Table 1. Ranking of English-Speaking Countries among 30 Nations in Terms of Per Capita Consumption of Absolute Alcohol

Rank	Nation	Liters Consumed per Capita
9	United Kingdom	11.2
14	Australia	9.8
19	New Zealand	8.9
20	United States	8.3
23	Canada	7.8

Adapted from: Organisation for Economic Co-operation and Development. *Health Data 2010,* http://stats.oecd.org/index.aspx.

unrestrained activity on various parts of the brain that have been freed from inhibition as a result of the depression of inhibitory control mechanisms. The consumption of too much alcohol over time can result in serious health and social problems.

Approximately 10 percent to 15 percent of adults who drink have mental, physical, or social problems resulting from its consumption. *Alcohol abuse* is generally defined as alcohol consumption that results in occasional problems such as drunkenness, being arrested for driving while intoxicated, or missing work due to a hangover. *Alcoholism,* or *chronic alcohol dependence,* is drinking over a long period of time that results in social, physical, or psychological problems. These can include loss of employment, financial problems, serious health problems, domestic abuse, or repeated arrests.

Alcohol abuse and alcoholism are found in all age groups, ranging from teenagers to the elderly. Youth in the United States tend to have more problems with drunkenness and alcohol abuse compared to older individuals. One of the most serious results of alcohol misuse is that approximately 32 percent of all U.S. traffic deaths are caused by alcohol-impaired driving.

Research suggests that more than one drink per day in some individuals, in particular women, can cause an increase in blood pressure. Heavy drinkers are more likely to have strokes, heart disease, obesity, cancer, and a host of other physical problems. Some medical authorities advise against pregnant women consuming alcoholic beverages due to the risk of fetal alcohol syndrome.

Common signs of problem drinking can become obvious to friends and family members, especially if the individual becomes *obsessed* with drinking. Other symptoms of problem drinking include if the individual constantly talks about drinking or partying. He or she continues to drink even though the drinking behavior *causes harm* to himself or herself or others. When the individual cannot obtain alcohol, *withdrawal* symptoms can occur. These symptoms include irritability, longing for a drink, restlessness, or more serious problems such as *delirium tremens* and convulsions. Some people experience *loss of control.* The person drinks six beers when he or she only wanted to drink one. The individual often *denies problems apparent to others* resulting from his or her drinking and often blames others for all his or her problems. The individual may *hide his or her drinking* after family or close friends have mentioned their concern, experiences a *blackout* after drinking (do not remember what happened at a party).

There is no consensus as to the etiology (cause), prevention, and treatment of alcoholism or problem drinking. A U.S. government publication titled "Theories on Drug Abuse: Selected Contemporary Perspectives" came up with no less than 43 theories of chemical (alcohol and drug) addiction and at least 15 methods of treatment (Lettieri, 1980).

To add to the confusion, some people consider alcoholism a disease, but others consider it a learned behavior in response to the complex interplay between heredity and environmental factors. Still others argue for a genetic cause. Some researchers point out that, unlike most common diseases such as tuberculosis, which has a definite cause (a microbe) and a definite treatment model upon which everyone agrees, there is no conclusive cause or definite prevention or treatment method upon which everyone agrees for chronic alcohol dependence.

This lack of agreement among experts causes problems with prevention and treatment approaches. Professionals debate whether total abstinence, such as is followed by Alcoholics Anonymous or professional 12-step programs, or controlled drinking, such as proposed by Moderation Management, is effective. Others debate whether medication, such as antabuse, is a desirable treatment method.

Help for Problem Drinking and Alcoholism   Although the theories for the causes of alcoholism, and its prevention and treatment are numerous, various types of therapy can help a person who has this potentially life-threatening condition. It is suggested that a family physician, clergyperson, counselor, or support or educational group be contacted for help and referral. Some sources of help include:

- Al-Anon for family and friends (www.al-anon.alateen.org/)
- Alcoholics Anonymous (www.aa.org/)
- Moderation Management (www.moderation.org/)
- Women for Sobriety (www.womenforsobriety.org/)

Alcohol Consumption and Wellness   Over the past 30 years, numerous research studies have suggested that moderate alcohol consumption—in particular, wine—is associated with longevity. This longevity is reflected in a decrease in heart disease, strokes, some cancers, diabetes, dementia, and many other chronic diseases. Regular moderate drinkers are more likely to get more sleep, to exercise, be happier, and have fewer gall bladder and heartburn problems.

The National Institute on Alcohol Abuse and Alcoholism (1999), for example, conducted a review of research on drinking and health from about 20 countries. The results of almost all of the studies suggested a 20 percent to 40 percent lower incidence of heart disease among drinkers compared to nondrinkers. Moderate drinkers had the lowest rate of mortality compared to either heavy drinkers or abstainers for heart disease.

Two major health problems in Western society include Type 2 diabetes and obesity, which are often associated with each other. Some research suggests that moderate drinking may reduce the risk for Type 2 diabetes and even obesity. However, heavy alcohol intake increases the risk for both of these conditions.

Several studies have suggested a decreased risk of cognitive decline, dementia, and Alzheimer's disease among older individuals who drink moderately. Some studies have found that those who consume beer, wine, or spirits in moderation several times a week are less likely to develop dementia than nondrinkers. On the other hand, other studies have found that either heavy drinking or abstinence increases the risk of cognitive decline and dementia in later life.

Drinking, like eating or any social activity, has guidelines to help the participant get more enjoyment out of the activity. Many are related to health. Gobbling down a whole chocolate cake at a party would not be considered responsible eating or even polite behavior in most cultures. In addition, you would probably get sick. If you did this several times per week, you could become obese or develop other serious health problems. The same is true for drinking.

Guidelines for what constitutes moderate and safe drinking differ slightly between cultures. In general, moderate and safe drinking levels for women are no more than one or two drinks per day and for men no more than two or three drinks per day.

The following are some tips for healthy choices concerning alcohol consumption that can enhance health and a healthy lifestyle.

- *Drink no more than one drink per hour.* Consuming one drink or less over an hour allows the liver to detoxify the alcohol and avoid drunkenness.
- *Eat food while drinking.* Many cultures consume alcohol only with food to enhance a meal and to avoid intoxication.
- *Sip, don't gulp, the beverage.* Taste and smell the various flavors. This is particularly true for wine.
- *Cultivate taste.* Choose quality rather than quantity. Learn the names of fine wines, whiskeys, and beers. Learn what beverages go with what foods.
- *Avoid drinking when taking medications.* This includes over-the-counter drugs such as sleeping pills and cold or cough medicines. Alcohol should not be used while taking certain antibiotics, antidepressant, and many other prescription medications. Check with your physician or pharmacy before you drink while on any prescription drug.
- *Appoint a designated driver.* If you do not have one and you must drive home, consume no more than one drink with a meal.
- *If you have close relatives who have had drinking problem, be careful of your own alcohol consumption.*
- When hosting a party, *serve alcohol adjunct to an activity* rather than as the primary focus. Have plenty of nonalcoholic beverages and snacks on hand.

In summary, alcoholic beverages have been used throughout human history. Alcohol consumption can lead to both psychological and physiological social and health problems. However, alcohol used in moderation can enhance health and a healthy lifestyle.

Ruth C. Engs

See also Addiction; Heart Health; Obesity.

References

Centers for Disease Control and Prevention. "Alcohol and Public Health: Frequently Asked Questions" (July 10, 2010), www.cdc.gov/alcohol/faqs.htm.

Engs, Ruth C. *Clean Living Movements: American Cycles of Health Reform.* Westport, CT: Praeger, 2000.

Engs, Ruth C. "Do Traditional Western European Drinking Practices Have Origins in Antiquity?" *Addiction Research* 2, no. 3 (1995): 227–39, www.indiana.edu/~engs/articles/ar1096.htm.

Hendrick, Bill. "Moderate Drinking Linked to Better Health: Study Shows Moderate Drinkers of Alcohol Are Healthier Than Nondrinkers." *WebMD Health News* (May 19, 2010), www.webmd.com/food-recipes/news/20100519/moderate-drinking-linked-to-better-health.

Lettieri, Dan J., Sayers, Mollie, Pearson, Helen Wallenstein. *Theories on Drug Abuse: Selected Contemporary Perspectives.* NIDA Research Monograph 30, March 1980. Rockville, MD: NIDA. http://archives.drugabuse.gov/pdf/monographs/30.pdf.

National Institute on Alcohol Abuse and Alcoholism. *Alcohol Epidemiologic Data Directory* (June 2008), http://pubs.niaaa.nih.gov/publications/datasys.htm.

National Institute on Alcohol Abuse and Alcoholism. *Alcohol Alert,* no. 45 (October 1999).

Organisation for Economic Co-operation and Development. *Health Data 2010,* http://stats.oecd.org/index.aspx.

Peck, Garrett. *The Prohibition Hangover: Alcohol in America from Demon Rum to Cult Cabernet.* Piscataway, NJ: Rutgers University Press, 2009.

U.S. Department of Agriculture. "Chapter 9: Alcoholic Beverages." *Dietary Guidelines for Americans 2005* (July 2008), www.health.gov/DIETARYGUIDELINES/dga2005/document/html/chapter9.htm.

World Health Organization. "Core Health Indicators" (May 2008), http://apps.who.int/whosis/database/core/core_select_process.cfm?strISO3_select=ALL&strIndicator_select=AlcoholConsumption&intYear_select=latest&language=English.

ALLERGIES

Allergic reactions are an immune response against a harmless substance. While scientists know how they occur and when, they still puzzle over why some people have allergies and others do not. The substance that stimulates the allergic reaction is called an allergen. Allergens come in the form of drugs or food, insect venom, pollen, mold, pollutants, and poisonous plants. In other words, they are all around us. That may explain why allergies are so common. According to the Centers for Disease Control and Prevention, one in five Americans, more than 50 million people, have some type of allergy that creates symptoms and affects their lives (Castells, 2007).

There are two main reasons individuals develop allergies: genetics and the environment. A child with one allergic parent has a 30 percent chance of developing allergies, and the likelihood grows to 70 percent if both parents have allergies (Asthma and Allergy Foundation of America, 2011). A genetic predisposition to allergies is called atopic, and children with this genetic predisposition often experience eczema or dermatitis, rhinitis or sinus symptoms, and atopic asthma or breathing symptoms. Some children outgrow allergies to certain foods, but scientists say children who are atopic rarely outgrow allergies and may face one or more allergies as adults.

However, atopy and allergy are not the same thing. Atopy means a genetic predisposition to be allergic, but allergy simply describes an individual hypersensitivity to something after exposure. In some cases, children with atopy do not develop allergies, but some people with no genetic link do develop allergies. Some people with allergies also have asthma, and allergens are a very common trigger for asthma. Asthma is a disease that involves a chronic inflammation of the lungs and their passages and it can develop at any age.

Some research shows that environment and birth order may play a role in influencing allergy development. Children who have three or more older siblings have been shown to be less likely to develop allergies than children born earlier. Scientists suspect this may be linked to germ exposure and that exposure may help temper the immune system's response (Castells, 2007). In fact, the first year of life is seen as very important in the development or lack of allergies in children. Research shows that children living with a pet in their first year of life may be less likely to develop allergies (Gordon, 2011).

Allergic reactions appear to be growing in Western industrialized countries but not in other, less developed areas of the world. Scientists suggest this may be related to the introduction of antibiotics and vaccines, which, while reducing the number of diseases, also exposes children to fewer germs during their formative years. With little exposure, researchers theorize that the developing immune system lacks training as it matures. The theory, known as the hygiene hypotheses, came largely from research on young children living on farms in part of Europe. Those studies showed the children who grew surrounded by farm animals and barns had fewer allergies than non-farm children from the same region (Castells, 2007).

There are no cures for allergies, but there are three basic categories of treatment: avoidance, medications, and desensitization or immunotherapy allergy shots. To avoid contact with known allergens, individuals can stop eating certain foods, use air filters, and eliminate pets or remove problem fabrics or chemicals from their immediate surroundings. Standard medications for allergies include antihistamines, decongestants, and nasal sprays. These medicines may be obtained with or without a prescription, depending on the individual's degree of allergic reaction.

The third form of treatment is allergy shots that gradually expose the person to increasing amounts of specific allergens. In this situation, an allergist will inject a small amount of allergen into a patient, and this signals to body to make natural antibodies, which are supposed to increase immunity to that allergen. The benefit is that an allergist mixes the shot according to each individual's needs, and the treatment aims to eventually eliminate the symptoms, sometimes after only

18 months (Konrad, 2010). A study released in early 2010 found that shots were especially effective in reducing symptoms in children.

When symptoms first appear, there are several ways to diagnose allergies. Physicians suggest the first step is to create a detailed log of symptoms and situations that trigger those symptoms. This should include both home and work or school environments along with a list of any additional medications and prescription or over-the-counter and alternative medicines, herbs, or vitamins. The most routine form of testing is a skin test that is designed to detect immunoglobulin E (IgE) antibodies. When a person has an allergic response, the body produces IgE antibodies. The IgE then signals the body to produce histamine and to release a chain reaction of allergy symptoms, including red or runny eyes, congestion, itchy nose, coughing, wheezing, clogged ears, nausea, diarrhea, or itching on the roof of the mouth or in the throat.

In rare cases, a person can experience a very severe allergic reaction known as anaphylaxis or anaphylactic shock, which includes swelling shut of airways and a serious drop in blood pressure. If that occurs, the individual needs an emergency injection of epinephrine and immediate emergency medical care.

The skin test places the possible allergen on a superficial layer of the skin and provides quick results, often within 10 to 15 minutes. If the spot turns red, swells, or begins to itch, that shows the IgE was released to attack the offending area. The prick test is another skin test for allergies; the skin is punctured on the back or inside of the arm, and a small amount of allergen is introduced. The response of redness, swelling, or itching can be almost instantaneous if there is sensitivity.

The intracutaneous test also calls for an injection and usually follows a prick test to confirm sensitivity to a specific allergen. The patch test involves no injection; instead, the allergen is placed on the skin under a bandage and left for 48 hours. When the patch is removed, any sign of redness, swelling, or blisters confirms an allergic reaction. Of course, tests can provide false positives, and sometimes an individual shows sensitivity but never exhibits allergy symptoms.

Allergists are also turning to blood tests in increasing numbers. One test, called RAST (which stands for radioallergosorbent test), looks for the IgE antibodies in the blood. Blood tests are helpful for individuals who cannot interrupt medications, such as antidepressants. The original RAST used an antibody that included a radioactive element, but modern tests now use chemical labels.

Sharon Zoumbaris

See also Allergies, Food; Asthma; Vaccinations.

References

Asthma and Allergy Foundation of America. "Allergy Facts and Figures," www.aafa.org.

Castells, Mariana C. "What to Do about Allergies." *Harvard Special Health Report Annual 2007*: 5.

Gordon, Serena. "Early Exposure to Pets Won't Up Kids' Allergy Risk." *Consumer Health News* (June 13, 2011), http://consumer.healthday.com/Article.asp?AID=653836.

Hicks, Rob. *Beat Your Allergies: Simple, Effective Ways to Stop Sneezing and Scratching.* New York: Perigee, 2007.

Konrad, Walecia. "A Child's Allergies Are Serious but Can Be Treated Effectively." *New York Times* (March 5, 2010), www.nytimes.com.

Wegienka C., C. Johnson, S. Havstad, D.R. Ownby, C. Nicholas, & E.M. Zoratti. "Lifetime Dog and Cat Exposure and Dog- and Cat-Specific Sensitization at Age 18 years." *Clinical and Experimental Allergy*, 41, no. 7 (July 2011): 979–86.

ALLERGIES, FOOD

Food plays a significant and important role in our lives, for both good health and social well-being. Religious holidays, family celebrations, and social gatherings often include special dishes made just for the occasion. Then there are birthdays, sporting events, ice cream socials, movies, weddings, ad infinitum, where food is an integral part of the event. But for those living with a food allergy, special occasions or a visit to a friend's house can turn into a deadly experience.

While it would be nice to eat anything and everything without a care in the world, it is just not realistic for anyone who experiences a food allergy or hypersensitivity. For reasons still not fully understood, the human immune system reacts abnormally to some foods. So is it even possible to eat safely, enjoy social gatherings, and stay healthy when living with adverse food reactions? No matter what food a person struggles with, there is a way to stay safe, consume all the nutrients necessary for good health, and still enjoy life.

Are Food Allergies on the Rise?   The Centers for Disease Control and Prevention (CDC) estimates that approximately 12 million Americans (2 million of whom are children) experience some type of adverse reaction to a food. An estimated 30,000 Americans are rushed to emergency rooms for severe food reactions, and between 100 and 200 die from food-related anaphylaxis annually (CDC, 2007). Food allergies are not, however, restricted to just the United States. In Europe and most developed countries, an estimated 1 to 2 percent of adults and 5 to 7 percent of children have reported food allergies, making them a worldwide concern.

More than 200 foods are reported to cause adverse reactions, and most people assume they are allergic to a food after experiencing an adverse reaction. However, only eight foods—eggs, fish, milk, peanuts, shellfish, soy, tree nuts (almonds, cashews, pecans, pistachios, walnuts), and wheat—are responsible for over 90 percent of true food allergy reactions worldwide (Food Allergy & Anaphylaxis Network, 2008). Other medical conditions or food hypersensitivities can mimic symptoms similar to those of a food allergy.

Prevalence of adverse food reactions varies regionally and is largely influenced by a country's dietary habits and food preparation methods. In the United States, eggs, milk, and peanut allergies are the most prevalent food allergies affecting children. Fish, peanuts, tree nuts, and shellfish commonly affect U.S. adults. In Australia, Denmark, and Sweden, cow's milk allergy is quite common in infants and children under the age of two. In Southeast Asian countries, such as Japan and South Korea, buckwheat allergies are prevalent. In China, where peanut consumption (in the form of boiled or fried peanuts) is the same as in the United States (in the form of dry roasted peanuts, which makes the protein allergens stronger), peanut allergies are negligible. In Israel, where peanuts are also a staple of the daily diet, sesame seed allergies are far more common than peanut allergies.

Many experts believe food allergies associated with life-threatening anaphylaxis are on the rise worldwide. Although studies have yet to prove this beyond a shadow of a doubt, some data do suggest that these types of allergies are on the increase. Pediatric peanut allergies doubled from 1997 to 2002 in the United States. Since 1990, food allergy reactions increased hospital admissions by 500 percent in the United Kingdom. Asthma cases, a reliable predictor of food allergy susceptibility, increased 100 percent over the past 30 years (although other factors, such as air pollution, may play a role) (Wood, 2007). Increasing global travel and the importation of food products from other countries also expose populations to new foods. For example, in the United States, kiwi allergies were uncommon until this fruit (which is indigenous to China) became increasingly popular in the United States. Increasing concerns about food hypersensitivities prompted the European Union in 2005 to begin a multidisciplinary project, known as EuroPrevall, to study the problem and develop diagnostic tools and databases.

Although theories abound, there are still no clear-cut reasons for these increases. Family genetics appear to play a key role in food allergy susceptibility. Research studies performed with twins found that when one twin has a peanut allergy, an identical twin will have a 64 percent chance of having a peanut allergy as well. However, a nonidentical twin only has a 7 percent chance of sharing the same peanut allergy (Wood, 2007).

Although this confirms a strong genetic link to food allergy susceptibility, experts in the field believe a combination of genetics and environmental factors are the cause of many food allergies and hypersensitivities. Certainly, increased awareness about food allergies today has led to improved detection and diagnosis, yet better detection does not totally account for the dramatic increases being seen. Some theories point to ingredients and food additives used in commercially prepared foods, increased use of vitamin supplements and antacids, exposure to tobacco smoke, living in a "too clean" environment with lack of exposure to germs that build up immunity, introducing food at too young an age, and use of bioengineered foods as culprits. Much more research still needs to be done.

When U.S. scientists first began to bioengineer food, the first food they selected to modify was the soy plant, a relatively inexpensive source of protein. Scientists wanted to develop a disease-resistant plant that would increase the yield of soy nuts. To do this, they took genetic material from Brazil nuts and inserted it into soy plants. However, the Brazil nut is a tree nut and one of a group of nuts that often trigger severe allergic reactions. Thus, the potential for widespread life-threatening allergic reactions was astronomical.

Fortunately, scientists realized the potential hazard and removed this plant from production. Industry safeguards against a similar modification in the future were implemented, and bioengineered foods must now be labeled. But this one example highlights the potential danger to consumers when foods are modified from their natural state and the need for consumers to be vigilant about what they eat.

Living with a food allergy or hypersensitivity can be difficult, frustrating, and sometimes deadly. Preventing exposure to food allergens is the only way to avoid symptoms, but just avoiding an allergen is not as simple as it might seem. Many processed foods and restaurant meals contain hidden allergens. Safe foods sometimes become cross-contaminated when accidentally exposed to allergens via cooking methods, contaminated work surfaces and utensils, or during processing. Convenience foods occasionally have ingredient substitutions or changes that are not declared on the label. Food labels can be misleading; for instance, coffee creamers and margarines may be labeled nondairy, yet still contain milk proteins. Even walking through a supermarket or fish market can elicit a reaction if airborne food allergens are present and inhaled. So how can anyone with food allergies or hypersensitivities live a normal life?

Living with Food Allergies and Hypersensitivities Symptoms of most nonallergic food hypersensitivities are mostly inconvenient, disruptive, and annoying. But as a rule they are not usually life-threatening. However, true food allergies and some hypersensitivities (anaphylactoid reactions and some food-related medical disorders) can be deadly. Treatment of true food allergies and nonallergic food hypersensitivities are similar in many ways, but also different. Obtaining an accurate diagnosis from a qualified health care professional is extremely important when planning correct treatment options.

In addition to the previously mentioned eight foods that account for most food allergies worldwide, foods that are naturally high in histamine content or foods and medications with food preservatives or additives that trigger histamine release from mast cells can also trigger severe reactions. Medical disorders, oral allergy syndrome, food-dependent exercise-induced anaphylaxis, and some cross-reactivity reactions are also capable of producing severe, life-threatening reactions.

Strictly avoiding a food allergen or trigger is the only proven treatment currently available. Strict vigilance of food is critical, and an effective food allergy treatment plan should always include the following components:

- Avoidance diet
- Emergency and nonemergency treatment plans
- Extra caution when eating away from home
- Label-reading skills
- Medical alert information

Avoidance diets are eating plans specifically designed to avoid the food or compound that triggers a reaction while also balancing daily nutrients necessary to maintain good health. But eating the right balance of nutrients when it is necessary to eliminate one or more food groups can be a challenge. Working with a registered dietitian is well worth the investment of time and money to ensure a nutritionally balanced and safe diet plan specifically tailored to the individual.

Treatment plans save lives. In general, anyone who has experienced or has the potential to experience a severe reaction, such as anaphylaxis, will be given a prescription for an epinephrine autoinjector. This medication comes in two strengths:

junior (for children or anyone weighing between 33 and 66 pounds) and regular (for adults or those weighing over 66 pounds). The best known brands of epinephrine autoinjectors are EpiPenJr., EpiPen Twinjet, and Ana Guard. Additional medications, such as antihistamines (diphenhydramine [Benadryl]; histamine-2 receptor antagonists blockers [Zantac or Tagamet]); inhalant asthma medications (albuterol); and corticosteroids (prednisone) may also be prescribed and combined with epinephrine when symptoms are life-threatening.

Carrying the right medications at all times and in all circumstances is extremely important, even if severe reactions are rare or circumstances appear nonthreatening. A 2008 study at the University of Michigan found that only 50 percent of college students with food allergies avoided eating the food they were allergic to. Twenty percent carried an epinephrine autoinjector with them at all times, and 43 percent had some other emergency medication with them at all times (University of Michigan Health System, 2008).

These study results highlight the tragic case of 19-year-old James, who had a peanut allergy. James ate a chocolate chip cookie at his girlfriend's house and immediately experienced itching in his mouth and throat, alerting him to the fact that a severe reaction was imminent. But he had never had a severe reaction before and had not filled his EpiPen prescription. By the time paramedics arrived to provide emergency treatment 10 minutes later, his heart had stopped, and it was too late to save him (Sicherer, 2006). *Life-threatening reactions can occur at any time and from foods that appear safe.* It is also important to know that not all states allow paramedics to carry epinephrine.

Besides carrying medications at all times, it is equally important to become familiar with and practice how to use a prescribed epinephrine autoinjector and educate family, friends, coworkers, and teachers about how to manage an anaphylactic emergency. The University of Michigan study also found less than half of elementary school staff recognized and knew how to respond to a food allergy emergency, and less than one-third of reactions were treated with epinephrine immediately. This lifesaving treatment was often delayed for 15 minutes or longer.

For anyone with food allergies or life-threatening hypersensitivities and their caregivers, it is critically important to recognize symptoms early, give immediate treatment with the right medications, and seek medical care quickly to minimize the chance of severe reactions such as anaphylaxis. Most fatal anaphylactic reactions follow a clear pattern. They usually involve young adults or teenagers who have asthma and peanut or tree nut allergies, who ate away from home, and who did not carry epinephrine medications with them.

Even after symptoms appear to be under control, the individual must continue to be monitored for at least four hours for signs of delayed reactions (known as biphasic reactions). In anaphylactic reactions, both the respiratory and cardiovascular systems are involved. Individuals with asthma and food allergies or a prior history of anaphylactic reactions are at high risk for severe and potentially fatal reactions.

Extra caution is always needed when living with food allergies. Unfortunately, many people do not think food allergies are a serious threat to life. Take the case of Irene, who had a severe allergy to nuts and was dining out at an Italian restaurant. Irene carefully questioned the server about a menu item, checking to be sure it was not made with nuts. The server, who unfortunately did not take Irene's allergy seriously, assured her that the food did not contain nuts, even though she never checked with the kitchen staff. But the meal included a sauce that was nut based and Irene suffered a reaction, later dying at the hospital. As a rule of thumb, when eating away from home, always ask to speak directly to whoever is preparing the meal or the manager and explain the severity of a reaction to a particular food allergen. Don't be afraid to ask; it can mean the difference between life and death.

Contamination of safe foods by unsafe foods, called cross-contamination, is another key concern for those living with food allergies. Food-processing equipment is often shared with different food products. If cleaning between different food batches is not thorough enough, traces of potential allergens may still remain on processing equipment, contaminating the next food product that is processed. Take the case of Stephen, who has an allergy to milk. Stephen drank an apple juice pack with his lunch. After he experienced a severe reaction, which had never occurred before, an investigation revealed that the equipment used to fill the apple juice containers in the processing facility was also used to fill milk containers. Apparently, the cleaning process between foods had accidentally left milk allergens on the equipment, thus contaminating the apple juice. But contamination can occur even in processing plants that have separate processing lines for their food products via airborne allergens. Cross-contamination can occur anywhere—in the home, in restaurants, in supermarkets, and anywhere foods are kept or served. Being aware of this potential risk and asking questions helps to decrease risk.

Fortunately, many restaurants are beginning to take food allergies more seriously and are increasingly willing to work with their patrons to ensure an allergen-free meal. The New Jersey Department of Health and Senior Services, Rutgers University, and the New Jersey Restaurant Association partnered to develop the Ask Before You Eat Program (www.foodallergy.rutgers.edu), implementing Public Law 2005, c.026 (A303 ACS 2R) that targets New Jersey residents who have food allergies. Sloane Miller, a psychotherapeutic social worker with food allergies living in New York, also developed an Internet blog to help those with food allergies dine out safely. Worry-Free Dinners (http://worryfreedinners.blogspot.com) is a website that provides information about restaurants and chefs who offer allergy-safe meals for members of a food allergy group in the New York City area.

The Food Allergy and Anaphylaxis Network implemented a restaurant training program for the National Restaurant Association and is currently planning a food allergy training program for managers and employees. Restaurants in Sweden are receiving allergy-free certificates if their staff undergo a special training course that teaches them about food allergies and how to meet the needs of their patrons to help them avoid allergic reactions. But even with this increased attention to food allergies, caution is still advised when eating out.

Label reading is also extremely important. In the United States, the Food Allergen Labeling and Consumer Protection Act of 2004 (FALCPA) became effective January 1, 2006. Gluten must also be listed as of August 2008. FALCPA requires the top eight food allergens (eggs, fish, milk, peanuts, shellfish, soybeans, tree nuts, and wheat) to be listed on food labels by their common name if used as a food ingredient. If cross-contamination is possible where the food is processed, the food label must list a warning about this potential danger.

Prior to this law, although inclusion of all ingredients was required on the food label, loopholes in food laws allowed the "2 percent rule." This rule did not require ingredients to be listed in order by weight if 2 percent or less of the ingredient was added. Exemptions also allowed additives to be listed as "flavors" or "spices," putting individuals at risk for unknown food allergens. Soy, a common ingredient added to cans of tuna, is one example that many consumers with soy allergies were unaware of prior to the new law.

The Food Allergy and Anaphylaxis Network provides a timely "Special Allergy Alert" page, which can be accessed at www.foodallergy.org/alerts.html. Health agencies of many countries and most food manufacturers also issue food alerts when food safety is in question.

Medical alert information can mean the difference between life and death. Wearing a medical identification bracelet or necklace can be lifesaving when an exposure occurs unexpectedly. If a reaction renders an individual unable to communicate, this easily identifiable accessory can allow rapid and accurate treatment before it is too late. MedicAlert jewelry is available at a number of medical identification websites. Allergy Cards, a business card that lists food allergies and prohibited foods, can also be carried and given to restaurant chefs and waitstaff. One website, www.allergycards.com, offers them at no charge. If traveling oversees, Allergy Translation (www.allergytranslation.com) and Select Wisely (www.selectwisely.com) offer cards translated into different languages for a fee. The Food Allergy Initiative offers free food allergy restaurant cards translated into 10 languages, and these can be accessed at its website www.faiusa.org under the "Downloads" tab.

Alice C. Richer

See also Allergies; Asthma; Vaccinations.

References

American Academy of Allergy, Asthma and Immunology. "Food Allergy Statistics" (May 2008), www.aaaai.org.

Broussard, M. "Everyone's Gone Nuts: The Exaggerated Threat of Food Allergies." *Harper's Magazine* (January 2008): annotation 64–65.

Food Allergy and Anaphylaxis Network. "Food Allergy Facts and Statistics" (May 2008), www.foodallergy.org.

Food and Agriculture Organization of the United Nations and the World Health Organization. "Safety Aspects of Genetically Modified Foods of Plant Origin." *Report of a Joint FAO/WHO Expert Consultation on Foods Derived from Biotechnology* (2000): 20–23.

Sicherer, Scott H. *Understanding and Managing Your Child's Food Allergies. Baltimore*: Johns Hopkins University Press, 2006.

University of Michigan Health System. "Students with Food Allergies Often Not Prepared." *ScienceDaily* (August 2008), www.sciencedaily.com/releases/2008/08/080806081451.

U.S. Food and Drug Administration. "Food Allergen Labeling and Consumer Protection Act of 2004" (September 2008), www.cfsan.fda.gov/dms/alrgact.

Wood, Robert A. *Food Allergies for Dummies.* Indianapolis, Indiana: Wiley, 2007.

ALZHEIMER'S DISEASE

Alzheimer's disease is a type of dementia that causes problems with memory, thinking, and behavior. Dementia is "a general term for memory loss and other intellectual abilities serious enough to interfere with daily life" (Alzheimer's Association, 2010). Alzheimer's is just one form of dementia, but it is the most common one, accounting for 50 to 80 percent of all dementia cases (Alzheimer's Association, 2010). Other types of dementias include Parkinson's disease, Creutzfeldt-Jakob disease, and Huntington's disease. Furthermore, there are many causes of memory loss. Thus, just because a person is suffering from memory loss, it does not necessarily mean they have Alzheimer's disease.

Currently, more than 5 million Americans are afflicted with Alzheimer's disease, but by 2050 this number is expected to rise to 13.4 million (Park, 2010). This rise will be observed because overall people are living longer and the greatest known risk factor for this illness is increasing age. Americans over the age of 65 have a one in eight chance of developing Alzheimer's disease, while those over the age of 85 have a 50 percent chance of having it (Alzheimer's Association, 2010). However, this disease is *not* just a disease of old age. Approximately 5 percent of those with the disease have early-onset Alzheimer's, which typically manifests when someone is in their 40s or 50s. Furthermore, the disease afflicts women more often than men. Two-thirds of those with Alzheimer's, 3.4 million people, are women (Alzheimer's Association, 2010).

Alzheimer's disease is currently the sixth leading cause of death in the United States (Alzheimer's Association, 2010). However, unlike the other major causes of death, Alzheimer's is the only illness without treatment available to prevent or cure it. Moreover, while mortality rates declined for most major diseases between 2000 and 2008, deaths from Alzheimer's increased 66 percent during this time period (Alzheimer's Association, 2010). Those who are diagnosed with the disease typically survive an average of 4 to 8 years after their diagnosis, but some can live for up to 20 years.

Symptoms   Experts have identified 10 warning signs of Alzheimer's disease:

1. Memory loss that disrupts daily life and that is marked by forgetting recently learned information, forgetting important dates or events, and asking for the same information over and over.
2. Challenges in planning or solving problems, including changes in the ability to develop and follow a plan, difficulty concentrating, and trouble following a familiar recipe or working with numbers.

3. Driving to a familiar place, remembering the rules to a favorite game, and other daily tasks are often difficult to complete.
4. Confusion with time or place.
5. Trouble understanding visual images and spatial relationships.
6. The development of new problems with words in speaking or writing; difficulty having a conversation.
7. Misplacing things and losing the ability to retrace steps.
8. Decreased or poor judgment in decision making.
9. Withdrawal from work or social activities.
10. Changes in mood and personality; the person may become confused, suspicious, depressed, fearful, or anxious.

People who have already begun to experience memory loss or to exhibit other signs of Alzheimer's disease may have difficulty recognizing a worsening in their condition and the development of other symptoms. Thus, it may be more apparent to friends and family that a person is exhibiting signs of dementia and should see a doctor.

Alzheimer's is a progressively degenerative disease where symptoms gradually get worse over time. Early on, symptoms include the loss of cognitive skills and memories. As the disease advances through the brain, symptoms become more severe and include disorientation, mood and behavior changes, and difficulty with speaking and abstract thinking. The progression of the disease occurs in seven stages, which provide a general guideline as to how a person's abilities change from normal function to advanced Alzheimer's (Alzheimer's Association, 2010).

In Stage 1, there is no impairment and no evidence of dementia at all. Stage 2 is marked by mild cognitive decline, which could be normal changes due to aging or the earliest signs of Alzheimer's. Mild cognitive decline could include having memory lapses or forgetting words. However, at this stage, a medical exam does not indicate any signs of dementia. Stage 3 is early-stage Alzheimer's disease, which can be diagnosed in some, but not all, individuals. Often family members, friends, or physicians may begin to notice a person struggling. Common problems experienced in this stage include difficulty coming up with the right word or name, struggles with functioning in social settings, misplacing important objects, an inability to concentrate, and trouble making plans.

In Stage 4, a medical interview will reveal problems with forgetting recent events or personal history and an impaired ability to perform mental math. This stage is indicative of mild or early-stage Alzheimer's and may also be marked by mood swings and difficulty performing complex tasks such as paying bills. Stage 5 is moderate or mid-stage dementia. Gaps in memory and thinking become very noticeable. A person may be unable to recall his or her own address or telephone number and may be confused about his or her location and what day it is. The person may need assistance completing daily activities such as selecting appropriate clothing, but not with activities such as eating and toileting. At this stage, an individual can still recall significant information about him- or herself and about his or her family.

In Stage 6, moderately severe or mid-stage Alzheimer's, the disease reaches a point such that a person can no longer remember his or her own personal history. In addition, personality changes may take place; an individual may become suspicious of others or experience delusions. Memory continues to fail and wandering may begin. By Stage 6, a person with Alzheimer's disease typically needs extensive help with daily activities. The seventh and final stage is severe or late-stage Alzheimer's. Symptoms of this stage include losing the ability to respond to one's environment, carry on conversation, and control movement. Reflexes may become abnormal and swallowing impaired. Often 40 percent of a person's years with Alzheimer's disease are spent in the Stage 7.

Biology of Alzheimer's Disease The brain has a highwaylike network of more than 100 billion nerve cells called neurons that communicate with each other through electrical signals. These electrical signals regulate thoughts, memories, sensory perception, and movement. The changes in memory, thinking, and behavior associated with Alzheimer's disease are thought to occur because of disruptions in electrical signaling due to damaged or dead nerve cells. Two abnormal structures implicated in the damaging and death of nerve cells and thus in Alzheimer's disease are plaques, which are made from beta-amyloid protein, and tangles, which are made from tau, a protein that stabilizes the structure of nerve cells (Alzheimer's Association, 2010).

Beta-amyloid protein is made from a larger molecule called the amyloid-precursor protein (APP). APP is a normal protein. While it performs its duties in and around the cell, it typically gets chopped up by an enzyme called alpha-secretase (Bloom, 2010). Being chopped or cleaved by this enzyme leaves fragments that dissolve in the watery environment of the brain. However, beta-amyloid protein is produced when APP is cleaved by the enzymes beta-secretase or gamma-secretase as opposed to alpha-secretase. Beta- and gamma-secretase cut the APP in the wrong places, leaving behind beta-amyloid fragments that cannot be dissolved. Certain mutations in APP make the APP more prone to cleavage by beta-secretase, which results in a greater production of beta-amyloid protein (Bloom, 2010).

As they accumulate, beta-amyloid proteins lose their helical shape and flatten out to form beta-sheet structures. These sheets bind together to form tough, stringy fibrils, which then clump together to create masses of plaque. As Alzheimer's progresses, more and more healthy brain tissue is displaced by tough, insoluble plaque. As plaque builds up, tau begins to breakdown. Without tau present, the structure of neurons begins to deteriorate. This leaves gaps such that electrical signals get broken up and the flow of communication is interrupted. The neurons then shrivel and die, leaving their tangled debris behind.

It is this destruction of nerve cells that causes memory failure, personality change, and other symptoms of Alzheimer's disease. The presence of cellular debris also activates the immune system's inflammatory response, which attempts to remove debris. Ultimately, the result of this cascade of events is a brain full of dead and dying neurons and the shutdown of neural connections. At the time of death, an patient with Alzheimer's disease will have lost one-third of all neurons in the brain.

The precise role of plaques and tangles in the development of Alzheimer's is still unknown and remains a source of controversy (Cowley, 2002). To begin, most people, even those without Alzheimer's, develop plaques and tangles as they age. However, researchers are still trying to figure out the threshold between a healthy and a diseased brain. In addition, the severity of cognitive decline has been shown to "correlate more closely with the burden of tangles" than with the amount of plaque (Cowley, 2002). Studies in genetically engineered mice also suggest that it is mutant tau proteins rather than the actual tangles that are the primary entity of toxicity. If this is the case, the plaques and tangles may not be causative agents in Alzheimer's symptoms, but rather simply serve as visible markers of the ailment (Bloom, 2010).

The development of Alzheimer's also involves several genes. Some of these are risk genes, which increase the likelihood of developing a disease but do not guarantee it will happen, and others are deterministic genes, whose presence means the individual definitively will develop the disease. Apolipoprotein E-e4 (APOE-e4) is a risk gene with the greatest known impact on Alzheimer's. On the other hand, genes coding the proteins amyloid precursor protein (APP), presenilin-1 (PS-1) and presenilin-2 (PS-2) are deterministic genes. APP mutations have been found to cause an inherited form of Alzheimer's, while PS-1 and PS-2 mutations have been seen to cause early-onset Alzheimer's (Alzheimer's Association, 2010).

Diagnosis While it is relatively easy to determine if a person has dementia, establishing whether it is Alzheimer's disease specifically is much more difficult to do. There is no single, standard test used to diagnose the disease (Park, 2010). Typically, it is diagnosed through a complete medical assessment, including a thorough medical history, mental status testing involving memory and recall

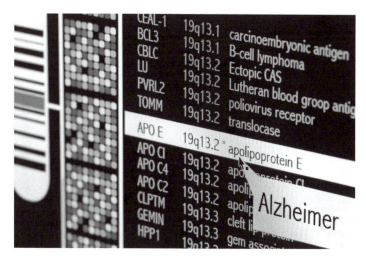

Computer screen displays genomic mapping of APO E, one of the markers for Alzheimer's disease. (iStockPhoto)

exercises, a physical and neurological exam, reports from family members, and diagnostic tests such as blood tests, spinal taps (which reveal the presence of amyloid protein), and brain imaging. Again, just because an individual experiences dementialike symptoms does not automatically mean that he or she has Alzheimer's. Other potential causes of memory and thinking problems—such as depression, thyroid issues, and certain vitamin deficiencies—must be ruled out as possible causes.

Although Alzheimer's cannot be stopped or reversed, early detection of this disease is still key. Early detection allows an individual to get the maximum benefit from available treatments, which can provide relief from symptoms and extend independence (Alzheimer's Association, 2010). Early detection also gives the person more time to plan for the future and allows him or her to have a greater role in that planning process while mental capacity is greater. Finally, as Alzheimer's patient Mary Ann Becklenberg commented in a *Time* magazine article in the fall of 2010, it is also "terribly important to know that you have the disease. If you know, then you don't feel that you're crazy, falling apart, inadequate and terrified" (Park, 2010). Understanding the cause of problems being experienced can provide comfort and reduce anxiety about the unknown.

A complete medical evaluation is sufficient for diagnosing Alzheimer's and is the best diagnostic available, but a truly absolute diagnosis of the disease is only possible postmortem (Park, 2010). At this point, an autopsy of the brain can be conducted, which can reveal signature lesions associated with Alzheimer's disease.

As previously mentioned, there are no current treatments to stop the disease or to reverse the damage it has caused. Many attempts have been made to develop such drugs, but they have largely failed and have been associated with very negative side effects (Park, 2010). However, every day researchers are making progress. Therapies do exist that can temporarily slow the worsening of dementia symptoms and improve the quality of life of those with Alzheimer's. Furthermore, it has been determined that it is important to start treating Alzheimer's patients as early as possible and that a multipronged approach that addresses as many of the disease's complex abnormalities as possible has the greatest potential to improve an individual's condition (Park, 2010).

At present the drug treatments available for Alzheimer's disease are largely made up of cholinesterase inhibitors. These treatments do benefit some patients, but researchers recognize the urgent need for other therapies. One area of study is in the use of autoantibodies, which are antibodies that target an individual's own proteins. Scientists have discovered the presence of autoantibodies in Alzheimer's patients and are working to uncover new treatments based on their findings. There are some 35 new candidate treatments for Alzheimer's in the development pipeline in various stages of research ("Alzheimer's Disease Autoantibodies," 2011).

Risk Factors   The primary risk factors for Alzheimer's disease are age, family history, and genetics, with age having the most well-known influence (Alzheimer's Association, 2010). As previously mentioned, most people with Alzheimer's are over age 65, and once an individual reaches 85 years of age, there is a 50 percent chance of developing the disease. People with a parent or sibling with Alzheimer's also are at greater risk of having the disease. Furthermore, this risk increases with the number of family members who have suffered from it. Because of the role risk genes such as APOE-e4 and deterministic genes such as APP play in the development of Alzheimer's, one's genetic makeup can put a person at a greater risk for having the disease. Finally, it is important to note that aluminum is not a risk factor. This is a myth that emerged in the 1960s and 1970s.

While Alzheimer's major risk factors—age, family history, and genetics—cannot be controlled, there are steps that individuals can take to mitigate other risk factors and decrease their chance of developing the disease (Alzheimer's Association, 2010). For instance, there may be a link between head trauma and Alzheimer's, so a person can lower the risk of developing the disease by exercising caution with one's head with practices such as wearing helmets and seat belts. Evidence also suggests a link between heart health and the health of the brain. Because the brain uses an extensive network of blood vessels to receive essential blood from the heart, any condition that damages the heart or blood vessels—such as high blood pressure, diabetes, and heart disease—seems to increase the likelihood of having Alzheimer's. In light of this, those who have higher rates of vascular disease—such as African Americans and Latinos—may be at greater risk for Alzheimer's. Finally, generally healthy lifestyle choices such as refraining from tobacco use, exercising both the body and the mind regularly, and engaging socially may provide some protection against developing the disease.

Cost of Care   The impact of Alzheimer's disease reaches far beyond the afflicted individual. A person with Alzheimer's will, at some point, require assistance with daily activities. In many instances, this care is provided by family members or friends. "In 2010, 14.9 million Alzheimer's and dementia caregivers provided 17 billion hours of unpaid care valued at $202.6 billion" (Alzheimer's Association, 2010). A study conducted by the Alzheimer's Association revealed that providing this care is both physically and mentally taxing. Alzheimer's and dementia caregivers had "$7.9 billion in additional health care costs in 2010 and more than 60 percent of them rated the emotional stress of providing care as high or very high" (Alzheimer's Association, 2010).

Beyond the family unit, Alzheimer's is also costly to society in general. It is projected that in 2011 the cost of caring for those with Alzheimer's to the American society will be $183 billion; this is $11 billion more than was spent in 2010 (Alzheimer's Association, 2010). By 2050, this number is expected to be $1.1 trillion. A person with Alzheimer's or another dementia typically uses three times as many Medicare dollars as a person without. In addition, the baby boomers are now beginning to reach the age where the disease typically manifests itself. This group coming of age, so to speak, is anticipated to add $627 billion in Alzheimer's-related health care costs to Medicare (Park, 2010).

Research   Alzheimer's is an incredibly complex disease which has mystified doctors and researchers for quite some time. Ninety percent of what is known about the disease has been discovered in the last 15 years (Park, 2010). However, while it has been slow, progress has been made. Today, there is a much better understanding of how Alzheimer's disease impacts the brain and the pathology of the disease. Furthermore, there is a community that is extraordinarily committed to the cause of the disease, and a worldwide effort is underway to find new treatments to delay its onset, reverse its damage, and even prevent it from developing in the first place.

Laura McLaughlin

See also Depression; Diabetes; Medicare.

References

Alzheimer's Association. "Alzheimer's Disease" (November 2010), www.alz.org/alzheimers_disease_alzheimers_disease.asp.

"Alzheimer's Disease Autoantibodies, Vaccines and Therapeutic Antibodies Pipeline—2011 Report." *Biotech Week* (April 13, 2011): 309.

Bloom, George. "Alzheimer's Disease." Lecture, University of Virginia (March 2010).

Cowley, Geoffrey. "The Disappearing Mind." *Newsweek,* June 24, 2002.

Hoblitzelle, Olivia Ames. *Ten Thousand Joys and Ten Thousand Sorrows: A Couple's Journey through Alzheimer's.* New York: Jeremy P. Tarcher/Penguin, 2010.

London, Judith L. *Connecting the Dots: Breakthroughs in Communication as Alzheimer's Advances.* Oakland, CA: New Harbinger, 2009.

Masoumi, A., B. Goldenson, and S. Ghirmai. "J Alzheimers Dis: 1 alpha, 25-dihydroxyvitamin D Interacts with Curcuminoids to Stimulate Amyloid-beta Clearance by Macro-phages of Alzheimer's Disease Patients." *Alternative Medicine Review* 14, no. 3 (2009): 314.

Park, Alice. "New Research on Understanding Alzheimer's." *Time,* October 25, 2010.

Reiswig, Gary. *The Thousand Mile Stare: One Family's Journey through the Struggle and Science of Alzheimer's.* Boston: Nicholas Brealey, 2010.

Turkington, Carol, and Deborah Mitchell. *The Encyclopedia of Alzheimer's Disease.* New York: Facts on File, 2010.

AMINO ACIDS

The main components of the human body are proteins, fats, and carbohydrates. While fats and carbohydrates play important roles in fuel production and metabolism, the proteins perform a consortium of important physiological functions. The building blocks of proteins are amino acids (AAs), and the human body must have some 20 in the right amounts to function properly.

The name *amino acid* describes their composition with an amine group and an acidic group (carboxylic acid) in their structure. Depending on individual chemical structure, AAs can be classified as linear-chain or branched-chain. There are four elements that compose the AAs: carbon, oxygen, hydrogen, and nitrogen. When they combine to form proteins, amino acids join their amine groups with their acid groups to form bonds known as peptide bonds. The creation of peptide bonds by the body is not a simple, direct chemical reaction. Rather, it involves several pathways leading to the formation of the bond. Nevertheless, the end result is a chain of AAs lined up together to form the final structure known as a peptide or protein. If the chain has fewer than 50 AAs, the product is called a peptide; if it has more than 50, it is a protein.

Among the celebrated proteins in the human body is insulin. This important protein is composed of 51 AAs forming two chains held together with bridges containing sulfur known as the disulfide bonds. Insulin is a small protein, but it has a huge job. It regulates how the body utilizes glucose as a fuel for cells, especially muscle cells and brain cells. If the human body does not produce enough insulin, then Type 1 diabetes develops. If it cannot utilize the insulin produced by the pancreas, then Type 2 diabetes develops. Diabetic patients are commonly prescribed insulin to regain control of their glucose utilization. Insulin has normally been given by injection because the digestive system contains enzymes that will degrade insulin given orally. Research is ongoing globally to create an injectionless insulin for Type 1 diabetics (Madhumathi, 2011). Other routes of insulin administration being investigated include an aerosol via the lungs, nasally, or as an oral spray.

Enzymes are also made of amino acids. Enzymes perform a colossal number of activities within the body, including digestion, building, storage, and transportation. Other examples of biological materials that are made of AAs include chemicals involved in brain signaling known as neurotransmitters, the building components of the genetic material known as the nucleotides, and the protein essential for carrying oxygen in the blood known as hemoglobin.

An individual is capable of making the majority of the amino acids needed to sustain life. However, a few are not synthesized by the body and must be supplied by diet. They are labeled essential amino acids (EAAs) because they must be obtained from an outside source. The eight EAAs are isoleucine, leucine, lysine, methionine, phenylalanine, threonine, tryptophan, and valine.

The other amino acids, known as nonessential, are alanine, arginine, asparagine, aspartic acid, cysteine, glutamic acid, glutamine, glycine, histidine, ornithine, proline, taurine, selenocysteine, serine, and tyrosine. Five other amino acids are sometimes listed as conditionally essential because they may be essential under special circumstances, such as in the case of infants, children, or those suffering from certain diseases. All amino acids can be easily obtained from a balanced diet, including vegetarian diets. The important point to remember is the word *balanced,* because some sources may be lacking or may contain only a small amount of the needed AAs. This is especially important with special diets such as vegan and vegetarian diets.

In addition, the amino acids arginine, cysteine, glutamine, leucine, proline, and tryptophan are known as functional AAs. The term *functional* signifies their role in regulating key metabolic processes important for immunity, reproduction, growth, and overall maintenance. Some food products are considered complete sources of amino acids (such as animal meats and soy products), and others may be incomplete (such as vegetables).

In 1994, the United States Congress passed the Dietary Supplement Health and Education Act. This act classified and distinguished products containing herbs/botanicals, vitamins, minerals, amino acids, enzymes, glandular, organ tissues, metabolites, or a combination as dietary supplements. The supplements became popular for a variety of uses, including fitness training, weight loss, and certain chronic diseases. Although many of these supplements continue to be used by the public as medications to help manage different diseases, the manufacturers cannot legally claim a medical or clinical effect for its content. The U.S. Food and Drug Administration (FDA) only allows a structure/function claim to be placed on the label. For example, a label for the supplement containing the amino acid arginine may state, "Amino acids are the building blocks of protein and help fuel skeletal muscles."

The FDA also requires the manufacturer to place a statement on the same label to indicate the product is not intended for medical use: "The label claims have not been evaluated by the Food and Drug Administration. This product is not intended to diagnose, treat, cure or prevent any disease. Consult your healthcare professional before taking any dietary supplements." It is extremely important for anyone thinking of using dietary supplements, including products containing amino acids, to consult first with his or her health care provider as many of these supplements can adversely interact with prescription or over-the-counter medications, which can lead to life-threatening conditions. Advertising on television and radio has led to a greater public demand for a number of supplements.

Research studies conducted on the use of amino acids in the treatment of diseases are constantly emerging in medical literature. In the case of arginine, several clinical effects have been suggested for its use. As an amino acid, arginine plays an important role in the cellular synthesis of many compounds, including nitric oxide, polyamines, creatine, and the amino acid ornithine. Being a substrate for nitric oxide synthases, the family of enzymes that produce nitric oxide, arginine consumption suggests a potential benefit from this amino acid in the management of asthma and high blood pressure. Due to the vasodilation potential of arginine use, many patients with erectile dysfunction have promoted this supplement for the purpose of overcoming this condition. Also, clinical studies of arginine oral administration have demonstrated a reduction in the inflammatory markers in the blood of angina pectoris patients, a beneficial effect for heart failure patients.

The essential amino acid lysine has its own therapeutic claims as well. Lysine is found in meat products, beans (including lentils and soybeans), and wheat germ (although wheat itself is a poor source for lysine). This amino acid plays a significant role in the synthesis of carnitine (important for generating energy from fats) and collagen (important for healthy skin, bones, tendons, and cartilages). Clinical studies have shown lysine improves the absorption of calcium from the gastrointestinal tract and at the same time reduces the amount of calcium excreted in urine. Together these two effects may help maintain bone health and prevent osteoporosis. In clinical trials, lysine was shown to be effective in reducing the rate of infection with herpes simplex virus, in particular when the diet was high in lysine and low in arginine. Another possible application of lysine comes from limited observational data that suggest that a high daily dose of lysine (6 g) may help in relieving the painful symptoms of angina pectoris. However, no controlled clinical trials are available to support the pain relief action of lysine in angina pectoris patients.

Another amino acid with a positive effect on health is the essential amino acid tryptophan. It is abundant in meat products, especially in turkey. Tryptophan is widely used for sleep or insomnia and for anxiety and depression. Scientific and medical research on tryptophan supports the anecdotal folklore use of this amino acid, at least to a certain extent. Tryptophan gets converted in the body to serotonin, which is a neurotransmitter that affects mood. In turn, serotonin is converted to melatonin, the sleep hormone that is secreted from the pineal gland. There is an added benefit to tryptophan's mood and sleep normalizing effects: Any portion of tryptophan that gets absorbed from the intestine undergoes conversion to niacin by the liver, and niacin, or vitamin B3, is important in the control of cholesterol and triglycerides in the blood.

The best sources of the amino acid tyrosine are meat products, oat, and wheat. The human body is also capable of converting the amino acid phenylalanine to tyrosine. However, in the case of phenylketonuria, a genetic disease, patients are not able to convert phenylalanine to tyrosine due to a deficient amount of the converting enzyme in their liver. Patients who suffer from this disease are placed on natural protein restriction and given a protein substitute enriched with tyrosine without any added phenylalanine. For these patients, tyrosine is considered an essential amino acid. Tyrosine is also used to make several important neurotransmitters, including dopamine, epinephrine, and norepinephrine, which regulate mood. Low levels of these neurotransmitters cause sadness and irritability.

Exposure to cold temperatures produces a drop in cognitive, physical, and psychomotor functions; tyrosine supplementation was shown to reverse this reduction to normal levels (O'Brien, 2007). Researchers suggest tyrosine overcomes the effect of cold by suppressing the depletion of epinephrine and norepinephrine during exposure to environmental stress. While there is some support for using tyrosine in the management of attention deficit hyperactivity disorder, there are no clinical trials that show a strong enough connection at this time.

Another popular use of protein or amino acid supplements is by professional athletes to enhance their physical performance. For example, use of beta-alanine is growing among athletes because it is the precursor of carnosine, a dipeptide or two amino-acid peptides found in high concentration in the skeletal muscles. Studies have shown that athletes trained in different sports such as sailing, resistance training, heavy-load training programs, cycling, and others have all experienced, to some extent, a degree of enhanced endurance performance while taking mixtures of amino acids (Sharp, 2010). In general, athletes should rely more on a high-quality balanced protein diet to support their exercise training programs rather than supplements.

What does a well balanced protein diet look like? For protein consumption, this translates into 25 to 30 grams of high-quality protein for each meal, the equivalent to two average-size hamburger meat patties. These nutrients along with micronutrients of minerals and vitamins should come from as many natural unprocessed foods as possible.

When Americans try to lose weight, they often adopt different fad diets, some of which advocate the elimination of whole groups of nutrients. For example, the

Atkins diet consists of low-carbohydrate and high-protein food choices. The diet became popular after Robert Atkins published *Dr. Atkins' Diet Revolution* in 1972. While the Atkins diet can deliver what it promises regarding weight loss for some dieters, it has been plagued by numerous reports of potentially harmful cardiovascular effects. In addition, high-protein unbalanced diets can cause a significant loss in calcium, which promotes bone loss and the development of osteoporosis and can lower citric acid secretion in urine. This can lead to the development of kidney stones.

Amino acid supplements, while considered relatively safe beyond the possible development of osteoporosis and kidney stones, have been shown at higher doses to cause rapid heart rate, anxiety, and restlessness. Nonprotein amino acids from plant sources can result in toxicity if ingested by humans in the diet. Examples of AAs that are *not* harmful are canavanine from alfalfa and homoarginine from lentil. Neurotoxicity can come from ingesting some of the seeds of the *Lathyrus* species.

Beyond the naturally occurring amino acids, synthetic AAs also play a growing role in science and medicine. More importantly, biotechnology is now a major player in the production of therapeutic proteins, also known as recombinant proteins, which are produced by the recombinant DNA technology. Human insulin production and its use in the management of diabetes is an example of this progress. The insulin is produced from microorganisms specifically engineered to synthesize it. Following its production, the hormone is extracted, purified, and then packaged into sterile products. The obvious advantage of human insulin is that it is a human form of the hormone. Older forms of insulin were from animal sources. Other new proteins and peptides biotechnology products include Aranesp (Amgen, California), which is used as an erythropoiesis-stimulating protein, and Avonex (Biogen Idec, Massachusetts), which is a form of beta-inteferon employed in the treatment of multiple sclerosis.

Antoine Al-Achi

See also Atkins, Robert C.; Calcium; Diabetes; Insomnia; Osteoporosis.

References

Braverman, Eric R. *The Healing Nutrients Within: Facts, Findings, and New Research on Amino Acids.* Laguna Beach, CA: Basic Health, 2003.

Cordes, Eugene H. *The Tao of Chemistry and Life: A Scientific Journey.* Oxford and New York: Oxford University Press, 2009.

Emsley, John. *Molecules at an Exhibition: Portraits of Intriguing Materials in Everyday Life.* Oxford and New York: Oxford University Press, 1998.

Hoffer, Abram. *Putting It All Together: The New Orthomolecular Nutrition.* New York: McGraw-Hill, 1998.

Madhumathi, D. S. "Biocon to Go for Fresh Oral Insulin Trials with New Partner." *Business Line* (January 24, 2011).

O'Brien, C., C. Mahoney, W.J. Tharion, I.V. Sils, and J.W. Castellani. "Dietary Tyrosine Benefits Cognitive and Psychomotor Performance during Body Cooling." *Physiology & Behavior* 90, nos. 2–3 (February 28, 2007): 301–7.

Sharp C.P., and D.R. Pearson. "Amino Acid Supplements and Recovery from High-Intensity Resistance Training." *Journal of Strength & Conditioning Research* 24, no. 4 (2010): 1125–30.

ANAEROBIC EXERCISE

Slow and steady wins the race, as the saying goes. However, sometimes, fast and flexible have benefits just as great. Much is known about the benefits of aerobic exercise, a form of cardiovascular fitness that relies on oxygen for endurance. The lesser known opposite of aerobic exercise, anaerobic, is short-lasting, high-intensity exercise that requires more oxygen than the body has to give (Nichols & Mueller, 2011). An example is interval training, where a runner, for example, sprints very fast, with sudden bursts of energy.

While aerobic and anaerobic exercises are needed to be physically fit, anaerobic exercise uses muscles to allow the body to move at a level of high intensity for a short period of time. It also helps people to increase muscle strength and always be ready and capable of quick bursts of speed (McKesson Health Solutions, 1998).

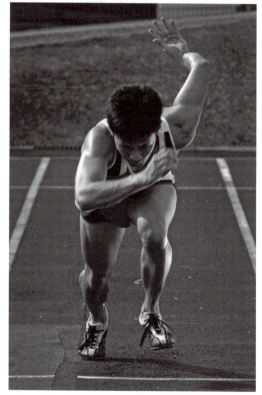

When people exercise for fitness or to lose weight, they may find that they hit plateau. This means their efforts either do not allow them to move beyond their current level of activity intensity, or their exercise regimen will not allow them to lose those last few pounds to reach a weight goal. With the use of anaerobic exercise, according to some experts, people who reach a plateau can surpass it and get to their next level of weight loss, physical ability, and endurance (Nitti & Nitti, 2001).

Anaerobic exercise works by creating a buildup of lactic acid in muscles during exercise. Lactic acid results from the creation of energy without the presence of oxygen. When too much lactic acid accumulates in the blood stream, muscles grow weary. This is why anaerobic exercise cannot be sustained for long periods of time (Nichols & Mueller, 2011).

Lactic acid helps to tire muscles and is burned during periods of

A sprinter powers off the starting line. Anaerobic exercises, like sprinting, are short-lasting, high-intensity exercises. (Koh Sze Kia/Dreamstime.com)

rest when muscles are recuperating. This prepares the body for another possible attempt at anaerobic exercise and gives muscles the chance to replace the energy used during the just-completed high-impact bout of extreme physical activity (McKesson Health Solutions, 1998).

While a doctor should always be consulted before a person adds anaerobic activity to his or her regimen, the good news is that the body can become accustomed to anaerobic activity with training. Over time, an individual can improve the ability to deal with lactic acid and even will produce less of it. An individual in training can even reduce the time it takes to grow tired during anaerobic exercise. In fact, there is some evidence that the ability of muscles to protect themselves against the effects of lactic acid can increase anywhere from 12 percent to 50 percent (Nichols & Mueller, 2011). This allows those with good conditioning to continue to perform high-intensity exercises without becoming tired too quickly.

Anaerobic exercise also utilizes small and large muscle fibers. Small fibers use oxygen for sustained physical activity. Larger muscle fibers do not. They pack more power than small muscle fibers, however, and are mainly used for strenuous, anaerobic activities. If these large muscles are underutilized, they may become diminished and weak. Anaerobic exercise helps large muscle fibers stay strong (Nitti & Nitti, 2001).

Anaerobic training is usually the province of seasoned athletes or individuals who are in top physical condition and want to enhance their abilities. Beginners can start with low-intensity aerobic exercise and slowly work their way up to the high-intensity activities. Anaerobic exercise is also known as interval training. An example of interval training is a jogger speeding up the pace to a fast sprint for perhaps a minute, then returning to a slower, sustainable pace. Interval training can be performed during almost any type of exercise or activity; the key is doing the activity at such a high pace that brief breathlessness occurs. Exercises and activities such as swimming, biking, hiking, dancing, kick-boxing and even climbing stairs can all be accomplished anaerobically. Experts recommend always warming up before anaerobic exercise and cooling down afterward (Nichols & Mueller, 2011).

For some athletes, anaerobic exercise can alter the effects of certain ergogenic aids. Ergogenic aids are compounds or substances that enhance performance or increase one's ability to participate in physically or mentally strenuous activity. In addition to helping people with heartburn and acid indigestion, sodium bicarbonate, is a common ergogenic aid. Research has shown that at 10- and 30-minute intervals, compared to longer intervals of exercise, sodium bicarbonate has little to no benefit in terms of increased performance or ability. The results were measured within groups of men using an ergometer, a device that measures the effectiveness of ergogenic aids (McNaughton, 1992)

Anaerobic exercise can also improve the level at which aerobic activity is sustained. The anaerobic threshold is the point at which the body's manufacture of lactic acid is higher than the rate at which the body can remove it from the bloodstream. Anaerobic threshold training is activity that occurs at a pace just below an individual's anaerobic threshold. At this point, breathing becomes only slightly elevated and a conversation can still take place. This form of training is said to enhance performance and improve the body's aerobic energy mechanisms (Kent, 2011).

Anaerobic exercise provides many health benefits. Individuals who improve their muscle mass due to anaerobic exercise tend to be leaner and able to more effectively manage their weight in part because more calories are burned (Nichols & Mueller, 2011). A healthy weight is associated with a reduced risk of heart disease, diabetes, and high blood pressure. Anaerobic exercise has also been shown to create growth hormone. The body creates human growth hormone (HGH) naturally, especially in response to intense, high-impact exercise and activity. This act stimulates muscle growth and increases fat's usefulness as fuel.

For this reason, anaerobic exercise has been called a fountain of youth of sorts. In children, HGH contributes to growth in height; as adults—especially those middle-aged and older—HGH helps lower body fat and girth and promote physical fitness. Sprinting, for example, could raise a person's HGH up to 530 percent above normal, according to one study (Campbell, 2005). Additional health benefits from HGH for older adults include help for patients with chronic heart failure (CHF). In patients with CHF, the anaerobic threshold by gas exchange, achieved through anaerobic activity, reportedly has the capacity to determine the level at which a person cannot perform physical activities. It also can tell medical practitioners how well a patient with CHF might respond to techniques meant to improve physical ability (Sullivan & Cobb, 1990)

Anaerobic exercise is not without its risks. Research has shown that repetitive anaerobic cycling sessions, for instance, create something called an acute phase response. An acute phase response is a series of physiological reactions to tissue damage. The damage can be pronounced after just one session. During an acute phase response, the liver releases physiologically active proteins in response to cytokines that promote healing. This can cause inflammation, something that is evident, according to scientists, even a day after stopping the exercise session. Inflammation is of concern because once it has done its job to promote healing, too much inflammation can lead to extraneous tissue damage. Researchers caution that athletes should be mindful of participating in too much anaerobic exercise in the course of one week (Meyer, 2001).

From high-performance athletes to older adults seeking to improve or maintain good health, everyone can experience some benefit from implementing anaerobic exercise into their routine. Users should consult their primary care physician before starting any rigorous exercise program.

Abena Foreman-Trice

See also Aerobic Exercise; Calories.

References

Campbell, Phil. *How Seniors Can Benefit from Anaerobic Exercise* (2005), www.eldercarezone.com/2590.php.

Kent, Linda Tarr. *Aerobic and Anaerobic Speed Training* (2011), www.livestrong.com/article/413896-aerobic-anaerobic-speed-training/.

Lewis, Carl. "Foreword." In *The Interval Training Workout: Build Muscle and Burn Fat with Anaerobic Exercise,* by Joseph T. Nitti and Kimberly Nitti, 1–6. Alameda, CA: Hunter House, 2001.

McKesson Health Solutions. *Anaerobic Exercise: Energy without Oxygen.* University of Iowa Health Care (1998), www.uihealthcare.com/topics/exercisefitness/exer3098.html.

McNaughton, L. R. "Sodium Bicarbonate Ingestion and Its Effects on Anaerobic Exercise of Various Durations." *Journal of Sports Science and Medicine* 10, no. 5 (October 1992): 425–35.

Meyer, T., H.H.W. Gabriel, M. Ratz, H.J. Muller, and W. Kindermann. "Anaerobic Exercise Induces Moderate Acute Phase Response." *Medicine & Science in Sports & Exercise* 33 (2001): 549–55.

Nichols, Jen, and Nicole Mueller. *Reference Guide to Anaerobic Exercise* (2011), www.sparkpeople.com/resource/fitness_articles.asp?id=1035.

SportsMed Web. "Anaerobic Threshold" (1997), www.rice.edu/~jenky/sports/anaerobic.threshold.html.

Sullivan, M.J., and F.R. Cobb. *The Anaerobic Threshold in Chronic Heart Failure: Relation to Blood Lactate, Ventilatory Basis, Reproducibility, and Response to Exercise Training* (January 1990), www.ncbi.nlm.nih.gov/pubmed/2295152.

Weil, Richard, and Melissa Conrad Stoppler. *Aerobic Exercise Health and Fitness Benefits: Types, Programs and Routines by Medicine Net,* www.medicinenet.com/aerobic_exercise/article.htm.

ANOREXIA NERVOSA

Anorexia nervosa (sometimes referred to simply as anorexia) is an eating disorder—a pathological fear of weight gain. The National Association of Anorexia and Associated Disorders estimates that more than 8 million Americans suffer from full-blown eating disorders—including anorexia nervosa and bulimia nervosa—and 86 percent of them develop the problem before age 20. Intentional starving often begins around the time of puberty and involves extreme weight loss, defined as at least 15 percent below one's normal body weight (National Alliance on Mental Illness, 2010). For regularly menstruating adolescent girls and women, skipping three menstrual cycles (except pregnancy) is another medical indicator of a serious problem. Even though someone with anorexia may look emaciated, she may still be convinced that she's too heavy.

The vast majority of people affected by eating disorders are adolescent and young adult women. Males and older women can also develop eating disorders, but young women are often most influenced by idealistic—and generally unachievable—standards of beauty. In a survey by the Centers for Disease Control and Prevention, more than one-third of the high school girls surveyed thought they were overweight. That compares to 15 percent of the boys who answered the same way (Austin et al., 2008). However, the National Association for Males with Eating Disorders (NAMED) refers on its website to statistics that suggest up to 25 percent of the estimated 8 million Americans with eating disorders are now male (NAMED, 2007).

According to the National Institute of Mental Health (NIMH), results from a national survey released in 2007 suggest that binge-eating disorder is now more

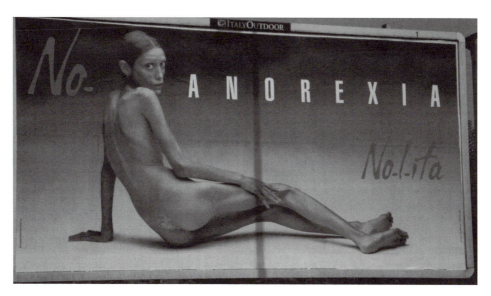

This Italian billboard features an anorexic young woman. The disease affects people all over the world. (AP/Wide World Photos)

prevalent than both anorexia nervosa and bulimia nervosa. The study (Austin et al., 2008) was based on data gleaned from the NIMH-funded National Comorbidity Survey Replication. Statistics indicated that approximately 1 percent of adolescent girls develop anorexia nervosa and another 2 to 3 percent develop bulimia nervosa. As girls approach adulthood, the numbers increase; according to the latest data, 9 percent of women and 3 percent of men reported having anorexia at some time in their lives. They also found that people with eating disorders, regardless of the type, often have other disorders, including mood, anxiety, impulse control, or substance abuse.

All eating disorders are destructive conditions and can lead to serious damage, even death. One in 10 cases of anorexia nervosa leads to death from starvation, cardiac arrest, other medical complications, or suicide. About 1,000 women die of anorexia each year, according to the National Alliance on Mental Illness (NAMI, 2010). The NIMH (2008) calls anorexia the eating disorder with the highest mortality rate among eating disorders. A study published in the *International Journal of Eating Disorders* (Button et al., 2010) looked at mortality among the various eating disorders and agreed with this earlier assessment. The researchers wrote that their work "confirmed previous evidence of a markedly increased mortality risk for anorexia nervosa" ("Findings from Leicester General Hospital," 2010). However, the study also suggested the risk of death for those suffering from other eating disorders had increased as well.

Marjolijn Bijlefeld and Sharon Zoumbaris

See also Bulimia Nervosa; Diets, Fad; Eating Disorders.

References

"Anorexia and Bulimia: What You Should Know." *American Family Physician* 77, no. 2 (January 15, 2008): 196.

Austin, S.B., N.J. Ziyadeh, S. Forman, L.A. Prokop, A. Keliher, and D. Jacobs. "Screening High School Students for Eating Disorders: Results of a National Initiative." *Preventing Chronic Disease* 5, no. 4 (2008), www.cdc.gov/pcd/issues/2008/?oct/07_0164.htm.

Bennett, Jessica. "It's Not Just White Girls." *Newsweek,* September 15, 2008, 96.

Bulik, Cynthia M. *Crave: Why You Binge Eat and How to Stop.* New York: Walker, 2009.

Button, E.J., et al. "Mortality and Predictors of Death in a Cohort of Patients Presenting to an Eating Disorder Service." *International Journal of Eating Disorders* 43, no. 5 (2010): 387–92.

"Eating Disorders." *The Columbia Encyclopedia,* 6th ed. Farmington Hills, MI: Gale Group, 2000: 11949.

"Findings from Leicester General Hospital Advance Knowledge in Eating Disorders." *Mental Health Weekly Digest* (June 28, 2010).

Fowells, Asha. "Understanding Eating Disorders." *Chemist and Druggist* (June 27, 2009): 16.

Hudson, J.I., E. Hiripi, H.G. Pope, and R.C. Kessler. "The Prevalence and Correlates of Eating Disorders in the National Comorbidity Survey Replication." *Biological Psychiatry* 61 (2007): 348–58.

Latner, Janet D. "Self-Help for Obesity and Binge Eating." *Nutrition Today* 42, no. 2 (March–April 2007): 81–86.

Mazek, Melissa. "Eating Disorders Are a Campus Problem." *America's Intelligence Wire* (April 20, 2009). General Reference Center Gold. Web.

National Alliance on Mental Illness. "What Is Anorexia Nervosa?" (August 27, 2010), www.nami.org.

National Association for Males with Eating Disorders, "Statistics" (August 22, 2010), www.namedinc.org/statistics.asp..

National Institute of Mental Health. "Eating Disorders" (2008), www.nimh.nih.gov/health/publications/eating-disorders.

Tomaselli, Kathleen Phalen. "Starving for Perfection: The Changing Face of Anorexia." *American Medical News* 51, no. 17 (May 5, 2008): 27.

University of Maryland Medical Center. "Eating Disorders: Complications of Anorexia" (January 2009), www.umm.edu/patiented/articles/how_serious_anorexia_nervosa_000049_5.htm

ANTIBIOTICS

The term *antibiotic* was adopted to refer to a category of drugs—compounds produced by microorganisms that inhibit the growth of other microorganisms. Most antibiotics are the products of filamentous fungi, like penicillin from *Penicillium notatum,* but some soil bacteria of the actinomycete group also produce important antibiotics. Antibiotics kill or inhibit pathogens by inhibiting nucleic acid or protein synthesis, damaging the plasma membrane, preventing cell wall synthesis, or interfering with cell metabolism.

Bacteria and other microorganisms that cause infections are resilient and even as scientists continue to search for new antibiotics, the bacteria are also developing ways to survive these new drugs. Antibiotic resistance is now considered a pressing public health concern in the United States and other nations. The overuse of antibiotics has promoted the emergence of more strains of resistant bacteria. In fact, some health officials worry that if overuse of antibiotics is not slowed, there could be a return to the days before antibiotics, when common diseases were often lethal.

Development History   By the 1870s, several scientists had called attention to the implications of what was called antibiosis (the struggle for existence between different microorganisms). The transformation of this vague idea into a new source of powerful therapeutic agents was the result of Alexander Fleming's study of the antibacterial effects of the mold *P. notatum.*

Fleming became interested in antibacterial agents while serving as a military physician during World War I, but his experience in treating infected wounds convinced him that chemical antiseptics were generally more harmful to human tissues than to bacteria. After the war, Fleming devoted himself to bacteriological research.

In 1928, while conducting a study of staphylococci, Fleming discovered the remarkable effect of the mold *P. notatum* on these bacteria. The mold was apparently killing staphylococci on one of Fleming's discarded petri dishes.

Penicillin   Mold contamination of bacteriological preparations is a common laboratory accident, generally considered a sign of poor technique. Acknowledging

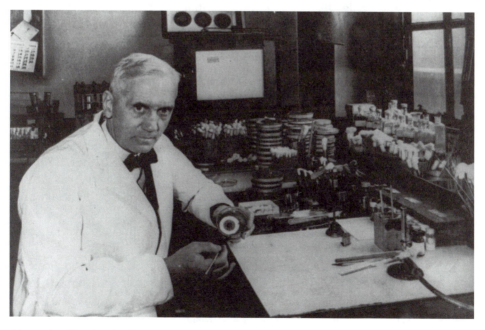

Alexander Fleming holds a Petri dish in his laboratory. Fleming was awarded the Nobel Prize in medicine in 1945 for his discovery of penicillin more than 15 years earlier. (Library of Congress)

this correlation, Fleming often said that he would have made no discoveries if his laboratory bench had always been uncluttered and overly tidy. When he went on vacation, Fleming left behind stacks of dirty petri dishes from old experiments. On his return to the laboratory, Fleming noticed that staphylococci growing on one of these petri dishes had been destroyed in the vicinity of a certain mold colony, which was identified as *P. notatum*. Fleming assumed that the fungal colony was the product of a spore that had contaminated the bacterial culture and that something produced by the growing fungus had inhibited or killed the bacteria. Scientists who have attempted to recreate Fleming's discovery of the antibacterial properties of penicillin have called it the luckiest, greatest, and most improbable accidental discovery in the history of science. Very few species of mold actually produce useful therapeutic agents, and *P. notatum* is fairly uncommon. Because penicillin cannot dissolve fully grown colonies of staphylococci, the mold must have been growing and releasing penicillin into the medium before the bacteria began growing.

Intrigued by the antibacterial properties of the mold that had killed his staphylococci, Fleming began a series of experiments, including some attempts to identify the active agent. Although his attempts to purify penicillin were unsuccessful, even in crude, dilute preparations, penicillin inhibited the growth of many different bacteria. Although penicillin was powerful enough to kill bacteria, Fleming noted that it was harmless to white blood cells in the test tube and to experimental animals.

The story of Fleming's accidental discovery of penicillin in 1928 is well known, but the fact that penicillin's therapeutic potential was not realized until World War II is often forgotten. Both aspects of the penicillin story were recognized in 1945 when the Nobel Prize for Physiology or Medicine was awarded to Alexander Fleming, Howard Walter Florey, and Ernst Boris Chain for the discovery of penicillin and for demonstrating its effectiveness in the treatment of infectious diseases.

Penicillin was effective against a host of gram-positive bacteria, including pneumococci, staphylococci, and streptococci. By 1950, penicillin was widely available for use in the treatment of syphilis, gonorrhea, pneumonia, diphtheria, meningitis, strep throat, tonsillitis, rheumatic fever, boils, and abscesses. Although it was not effective against all pathogens, penicillin was generally seen as a revolutionary new therapeutic agent. Moreover, the successful use of penicillin provided proof of the concept that the microbial world itself might be the source of many valuable compounds that were too complex for chemists to synthesize in the laboratory.

Streptomycin, which is produced by *Streptomyces griseus*, was discovered by Selman A. Waksman and his colleagues Elizabeth Bugie and Albert Schatz in 1944. Because it was effective against tuberculosis, streptomycin was especially valuable, but neomycin, chloramphenicol, aureomycin, erythromycin, and nystatin also expanded the range of pathogens that could be treated with antibiotics.

In his systematic studies of soil microbes, Waksman, a pioneer in soil microbiology, discovered more than 20 antibiotics, but most were too weak or too toxic for human use. Streptomycin was toxic to many species of bacteria, including *Mycobacterium tuberculosis* and the bacteria that cause typhoid, tularemia, and plague. Evaluating remedies for tuberculosis was very difficult because the disease is unpredictable, develops slowly, and is affected by nonspecific factors such as diet and rest. The failure of Robert Koch's tuberculin led to considerable skepticism about other alleged miracle cures. Koch was among the first scientists to identify the organism that causes tuberculosis. William H. Feldman and Horton Corwin Hinshaw were conducting tests of various possible therapeutic agents, using guinea pigs as an experimental model for tuberculosis, when they learned about streptomycin's effect on *M. tuberculosis*. After experiments with guinea pigs demonstrated that streptomycin was effective against tuberculous infections, tests were conducted on patients with pulmonary tuberculosis as well as deadly meningeal and miliary tuberculosis. Despite popular references to streptomycin as a miracle drug, early, impure preparations raised doubts about its safety and efficacy. Some patients suffered adverse effects, including nerve damage and deafness, but pharmaceutical companies were able to produce and market improved preparations of the drug by 1948. Waksman was awarded the Nobel Prize for the discovery of streptomycin in 1952, two years after the legal settlement of a complex royalty dispute initiated by his former associate, Albert Schatz. In 1994, Schatz, who insisted that he had not received sufficient credit for the discovery of streptomycin, received the Rutgers University Medal.

Golden Age of Antibiotics   The success of penicillin and streptomycin stimulated the growth of the pharmaceutical industry and encouraged unprecedented support for biomedical research. Reflecting the optimism of the 1940s and 1950s, a period that has been called the golden age of antibiotics, Waksman predicted that future research would lead to the discovery of more powerful and less toxic antibacterial agents. By the 1960s, however, hopes that an ever-accelerating pace of discovery would continue seemed overly optimistic. Moreover, the overuse and misuse of antibiotics resulted in unanticipated adverse side effects and promoted the development of drug-resistant strains of bacteria. The prolonged course of treatment required to cure tuberculosis creates ideal conditions for the evolution of drug-resistant bacteria. Combination therapy using streptomycin, para-amino-salicylic acid, isoniazid, and rifampin transformed the management and treatment of tuberculosis. Clinical trials proved that combination therapies were more effective in the treatment of tuberculosis than individual drugs. Multidrug therapy helped avoid the proliferation and survival of drug-resistant bacteria. Although even with a combination of antibiotics, a complete cure took many months, a partial course of treatment generally arrested active tuberculosis infections, thus preventing the transmission of the disease.

Streptomycin and other antibiotics so revolutionized the treatment of tuberculosis that by the 1960s, infectious disease experts were optimistic about the prospects for controlling, or even eradicating, the disease. The major obstacles, as observed by 19th-century reformers, were associated with poverty and the consequent lack of medical and public health resources in areas where the burden of disease was greatest. As with any infectious disease, the persistence of the pathogen, even in isolated, impoverished populations, meant that the disease could still be a threat to wealthy countries where the incidence of tuberculosis had been drastically reduced.

During the 1980s, public health authorities detected increases in the incidence of tuberculosis, especially in areas where poverty and the spread of HIV/AIDS facilitated the transmission of opportunistic infections. Despite improvements in the control of tuberculosis in some regions, significant increases in the incidence of the disease occurred in Africa and especially Eastern Europe during the 1990s, when the World Health Organization (WHO) declared tuberculosis a global health emergency. Tuberculosis remains a serious problem in India, China, Indonesia, and Africa, especially South Africa and Nigeria. The emergence of drug-resistant bacteria is particularly likely to occur where treatment is inadequate, public health programs have been neglected, and antibiotics are widely available without prescriptions or medical supervision. Antibiotics generally affect a limited spectrum of bacteria, and they are all ineffective against viruses. Some antibiotics are quite toxic and are only prescribed when no other alternatives are available.

At the 2002 World Congress on Tuberculosis, experts estimated that about 2 billion people—about one-third of the global population—were infected with tuberculosis. Most tuberculosis infections are asymptomatic or latent, but about 10 million people become clinically ill each year, and about 2 million people die of the disease. Globally, in 2006, about 700,000 tuberculosis cases and 200,000 deaths caused by tuberculosis occurred among people with HIV/AIDS. Tuberculosis experts predict that unless all parts of the world cooperate in a coordinated global control plan, or establish a safe and effective vaccine, tuberculosis will infect an additional 1 billion people by 2020, raising the death toll to 70 million per year.

Drug-resistant strains of *M. tuberculosis*—multidrug-resistant tuberculosis (MDR-TB) strains and extremely drug-resistant strains (XDR-TB)—are considered a growing threat to tuberculosis control programs throughout the world. Many of the drug-resistant microbes are resistant to at least three of the four first-line drugs recommended by the WHO: streptomycin, isoniazid, rifampicin, and ethambutol. XDR-TB cases were most commonly found in Russia, India, Asia, and Africa. In 2008, when the WHO released its fourth global report on tuberculosis and drug resistance, XDR-TB had been reported in 45 countries.

Ordinary tuberculosis can be cured in about 95 percent of patients, but the cure rate is less than 70 percent for MDR-TB and falls below 30 percent for XDR-TB. Treating patients who are coinfected with tuberculosis and HIV/AIDS is particularly difficult. In an outbreak of XDR-TB in South Africa in 2005, 52 out of 53 HIV/AIDS patients with XDR-TB died. Like medieval lepers, patients with XDR-TB are often confined to institutions that are more like prisons than hospitals in an attempt to prevent the spread of XDR-TB. Protecting the public and respecting the rights of those already infected is a difficult balancing act for public health officials. Most countries rely on voluntary cooperation and outpatient treatment, but many health officials argue that it is sometimes necessary to isolate the sick to protect society. Because detecting drug resistance can take many months, patients may be taking useless drugs and infecting others before the extent of drug resistance is finally identified. If antibiotics fail because of drug resistance, traditional public health measures might provide the only useful approach to controlling the disease. International travel makes drug resistance a global threat. Guidelines issued in 2006 by the WHO say that patients with MDR-TB should not travel by public air transportation until they have proved that they are noninfectious, but compliance and enforcement options are negligible. Tuberculosis is not considered highly contagious, but the lack of a serious, global response to XDR-TB suggests that international boundaries would not stop a highly contagious disease like influenza or severe acute respiratory syndrome.

Still, health organizations continue to blame antibiotic resistance on the overuse of antibiotic drugs and the practice of putting antibiotics into the feed of healthy domestic farm animals to promote faster growth and move them more quickly to market. According to the U.S. Food and Drug Administration, meat, poultry, and dairy producers used almost 29 million pounds of antibiotics for livestock in 2009 ("Revisiting the Use of Antibiotics," 2011). Organizations including the World Health Organization, the Centers for Disease Control and Prevention, and the American Medical Association continue to call for the U.S. Congress to enact legislation that would require a review of previously approved antibiotics for animal use to see if they are unsafe from a resistance standpoint.

Lois N. Magner

See also Bacteria; Influenza; World Health Organization (WHO).

References

Allen, A. *Vaccine: The Controversial Story of Medicine's Greatest Lifesaver.* New York: W.W. Norton, 2007.

Behrman, G. *The Invisible People: How the U.S. Has Slept through the Global AIDS Pandemic, the Greatest Humanitarian Catastrophe of Our Time.* New York: Free Press, 2004.

Gandy, M., and A. Zumla, eds. *The Return of the White Plague: Global Poverty and the "New" Tuberculosis.* London: Verso, 2003.

Glynn, I., and J. Glynn. *The Life and Death of Smallpox.* Cambridge: Cambridge University Press, 2004.

Häusler, T. *Viruses vs. Superbugs: A Solution to the Antibiotics Crisis?* Translated by K. Leube. New York: Macmillan, 2006.

Lesch, J.E. *The First Miracle Drugs: How the Sulfa Drugs Transformed Medicine.* New York: Oxford University Press, 2007.

Moberg, C.L., and Z.A. Cohn, eds. *Launching the Antibiotic Era: Personal Accounts of the Discovery and Use of the First Antibiotics.* New York: Rockefeller University Press, 1990.

Ryan, F. *The Forgotten Plague: How the Battle against Tuberculosis Was Won—And Lost.* Boston: Little, Brown, 1993.

Sachs, J.S. *Good Germs, Bad Germs: Health and Survival in a Bacterial World.* New York: Hill and Wang, 2007.

Thomas, A. *Twenty-first Century Plague: The Story of SARS.* Baltimore: Johns Hopkins University Press, 2005.

World Health Organization. *The Global Eradication of Smallpox: Final Report of the Global Commission for the Certification of Smallpox Eradication, Geneva, December 1979.* Geneva: World Health Organization, 1980.

ANTIOXIDANTS

Many claims have been made about the health benefits of antioxidants. These are substances that counteract the harmful free radicals created by oxidation. Oxidation, for example, can rust cars. Some oxidation in the body is good because it produces energy and kills bacterial invaders. But, in excess, it can damage tissues. Antioxidants are found naturally in many foods, primarily fruits and vegetables. They are also available as supplements, but whether they are helpful is still a matter of debate. There are claims that antioxidants in large quantities can help prevent or reduce the effects of a variety of diseases, including cardiovascular disease, diabetes, Alzheimer's disease, and various forms of cancer.

An eight-year study, led by researchers at the University of Oslo, Norway, and published in January 2010 created a comprehensive antioxidant food database aimed at identifying the total antioxidant capacity of fruits, vegetables, beverages, spices, and herbs in addition to nonplant foods (Carlsen et al., 2010). According to the published results, the study clearly demonstrated that plant-based foods introduce significantly more antioxidants into the human diet than nonplant foods. The results also suggested that individual antioxidants may increase their health benefits in combination with other foods, especially those rich in antioxidants. The database is available online to other researchers through the university's website. Scientists are also studying the effects of a diet rich in natural antioxidants on diabetics after an Italian study released in June 2010 and presented at that time to the Endocrine Society's 92nd Annual Meeting in San Diego showed that a diet high in antioxidant foods can improve insulin resistance.

Vitamins with antioxidant properties include vitamins E, C, and A as well as beta-carotene. Some minerals, such as selenium, are also considered to have antioxidant properties. Earlier research had cast some doubt on the health effects of antioxidants. A 2000 report by a panel at the Institute of Medicine of the National Academies of Science reported that megadoses of antioxidants have not yet been proven to be helpful and might in fact be dangerous. According to the press release announcing the findings, "A direct connection between the intake of antioxidants and the prevention of chronic disease has yet to be adequately established," said Norman I. Krinsky, chair of the study's Panel on Dietary Antioxidants and Related Compounds, and a professor of biochemistry at Tufts University School of Medicine, Boston. "We do know, however, that dietary antioxidants can in some cases prevent or counteract cell damage that stems from exposure to oxidants, which are agents that affect a cell's molecular composition. But much more research is needed to determine whether dietary antioxidants can actually stave off chronic disease" (National Academy of Sciences, 2000).

The panel established the following recommendations for dietary supplementation of antioxidants. It increased recommended intake levels of vitamin C to

75 milligrams per day for women and 90 milligrams per day for men. Smokers, who are more likely to be impacted from the cell-damaging biological processes and deplete more vitamin C, need an additional 35 milligrams per day. The report set the upper intake level for vitamin C, from both food and supplements, at 2,000 milligrams per day for adults, adding that intakes above this amount may cause diarrhea. Food sources for vitamin C include citrus fruit, potatoes, strawberries, broccoli, and leafy green vegetables.

Vitamin E recommendations were also increased, and men and women are now advised to consume 15 milligrams of vitamin E from food. Food sources for this vitamin are vegetable oils, nuts, seeds, liver, and leafy green vegetables. Synthetic vitamin E from vitamin supplements should not exceed 1,000 milligrams of alpha-tocopherol per day for adults. Alpha-tocopherol is the only type of vitamin E that human blood can maintain and transfer to cells when needed. People who consume more than this amount place themselves at greater risk of hemorrhagic damage because the nutrient can act as an anticoagulant, according to the report.

The report also recommended that men and women need 55 micrograms of selenium per day. Food sources include seafood, liver, meat, and grains. The upper level of selenium, including natural and supplement sources, should be less than 400 micrograms per day. More could result in selenosis, a toxic reaction that can cause hair loss and nail sloughing. The report did not set a recommended daily intake or upper intake level for beta-carotene and other carotenoids, which are found naturally in dark green and deep yellow vegetables. However, it cautioned against high doses, recommending supplementation only for the prevention and control of vitamin A deficiency.

The report also stressed that a balanced and varied diet will provide adequate amounts of these vitamins and minerals without requiring supplements. The American Heart Association concurred in a February 1999 Science Advisory, "Antioxidant Consumption and Risk of Coronary Heart Disease: Emphasis on Vitamin C, Vitamin E, and Beta-Carotene," which concluded,

> The most prudent and scientifically supportable recommendation for the general population is to consume a balanced diet with emphasis on antioxidant-rich fruits and vegetables and whole grains.
>
> This advice, which is consistent with the current dietary guidelines of the American Heart Association, considers the role of the total diet in influencing disease risk. Although diet alone may not provide the levels of vitamin E intake that have been associated with the lowest risk in a few observational studies, the absence of efficacy and safety data from randomized trials precludes the establishment of population-wide recommendations regarding vitamin E supplementation.

The role of antioxidants is complex, but basically scientists say that antioxidants combine with free radicals to prevent them from oxidizing other molecules and in this way are thought to help prevent diseases—specifically heart disease, some forms of cancer, macular degeneration, Parkinson's disease, rheumatoid arthritis, and Alzheimer's disease. Free radicals do some good in the body by improving basic immune function, but they begin to oxidize when they are present in large numbers and the oxidization then damages healthy cells. While research has not proven the direct relationship between antioxidant intake and disease prevention, research has shown that antioxidant supplements do not provide the same health benefits as dietary antioxidants found in fresh foods.

The several classes of antioxidants include carotenoids, isothiocyanates, flavonoids, phenols, sulfides, and whole grains. Carotenoids include beta-carotene found in vegetables such as carrots; lutein found in collards, kale, and some citrus fruits; and lycopene found in tomatoes. Different categories of flavonoids can be found in berries, red grapes, dark red fruits such as cherries, apples, citrus fruits, strawberries, and cinnamon. Sulfides include diallyl sulfide found in garlic, leeks, and scallions and dithiolthiones from broccoli and collard greens.

The antioxidants thought most important to human health include vitamins A, C, and E as well as beta-carotene flavonoids and selenium. Researchers have found that foods can contain thousands of different antioxidants, which is a better choice than a supplement containing only a single type of antioxidant. The medical community has theorized that antioxidants from food are able to form strong chemical networks; the end result of those networks is then individualized by each person's unique genetic profile.

In terms of antioxidant intake, the best choice is to include a large variety of fresh fruits and vegetables as part of a healthy diet. The foods with the highest per-serving content of antioxidants are dark-colored berries such as blueberries, blackberries, raspberries, cranberries, and strawberries. Beans are also a rich source of antioxidants, especially red beans, kidney, pinto, and black beans. Apples with the peel are a good source of antioxidants. Other strong antioxidant fruit choices include cherries, pears, plums, pineapple, kiwi, and avocados.

Many vegetables contain a high antioxidant count; the highest are

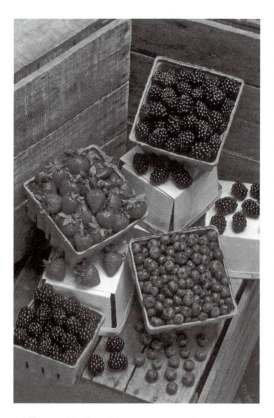

Different kinds of berries are rich in antioxidants, the disease-fighting compounds thought to prevent or repair cell damage. (U.S. Department of Agriculture)

artichokes, spinach, red cabbage, sweet potatoes, and broccoli. While cooking can increase antioxidant levels in some foods, it can decrease antioxidant levels in other foods. Nuts such as walnuts, almonds, and pistachios are antioxidant-rich foods, as are some herbs and spices, including cinnamon, ginger, ground cloves, and oregano leaf. Whole grains are important sources of antioxidants; however, oat-based foods are higher than other grain sources. There is increasing interest in beverages as antioxidant sources, such as green tea, fruit juices such as pomegranate and açaí, plus coffee and red wine.

As researchers work to unravel the connection between an antioxidant-rich diet and health, the added benefit is that foods high in antioxidants are also loaded with vitamins and minerals, high in fiber, and low in fat and cholesterol. In other words, they are all healthy foods that are good for you.

Marjolijn Bijlefeld and Sharon Zoumbaris

See also Açaí Berry; Fiber; Vegetables; Vitamins.

References

Balch, James F. *The Super Antioxidants: Why They Will Change the Face of Healthcare in the 21st Century.* New York: M. Evans, 1998.

Carlsen, Monica H., et al. "The Total Antioxidant Content of More Than 3100 Foods, Beverages, Spices, Herbs and Supplements Used Worldwide." *Nutrition Journal* 9 (January 22, 2010): 3.

Ellin, Abby. "Food Claims Raise Questions." *New York Times* (March 12, 2009): E3.

Fabricant, Florence. "To Your Health, from the Amazon." *New York Times* (July 13, 2005): F6.

Hensrud, Donald. "Food Sources the Best Choices for Antioxidants." Mayo Clinic (June 5, 2009), www.mayoclinic.org/medical-edge-newspaper-2009/jun-05b.html.

Kris-Etherton, Penny M., Alice H. Lichtenstein, Barbara V. Howard, Daniel Steinberg, and Joseph L. Witztum. "Antioxidant Vitamin Supplements and Cardiovascular Disease." *Circulation* 110 (2004): 637–41.

National Academy of Sciences. "Antioxidants' Role in Chronic Disease Prevention Still Uncertain: Huge Doses Considered Risky" (April 10, 2000), www.nationalacademies.org.

Schwartz, Joseph A. *An Apple a Day: The Myths, Misconceptions and Truths about the Foods We Eat.* New York: Other Press, 2009.

"Well-Defined Quantity of Antioxidants in Diet Can Improve Insulin Resistance." *States News Service* (June 20, 2010).

"What's for Dinner? Your Heart Is Asking for Vegetables: Antioxidants and Nutrients in Veggies Help Maintain Cardiovascular Health." *Health Advisor* 13, no. 4 (2010): S2.

ASPERGER SYNDROME

Autism spectrum disorders are a group of developmental disabilities that can cause significant social, communication, and behavioral challenges. According to 2007 figures released by the Centers for Disease Control and Prevention (CDC) following a comprehensive survey of autism in children, an estimated 1 in

110 children in the United States has autism. The surveys also found that boys were four times more likely to have autism than girls.

Like all autism spectrum disorders, Asperger syndrome (or Asperger's disorder) involves difficulties in three major areas: social interaction, communication, and behavior (Wing & Gould, 1979). While lower-functioning individuals with autism might show little desire for social interaction and spontaneous communication, those with Asperger syndrome are typically quite verbal and often eager to share information. It is the unusual quality of their language, their poor social skills, and their unusual habits or behaviors that distinguishes them. Because the symptoms are more subtle than those of classic autism, most children with Asperger syndrome are not diagnosed until elementary school, or even much later (Attwood, 1998).

A certain amount of debate exists among experts today about what, exactly, constitutes Asperger syndrome. The *Diagnostic and Statistical Manual of Mental Disorders* (*DSM-IV-TR*; American Psychiatric Association, 2000), which publishes the official criteria used by psychologists and psychiatrists in the United States, uses much of the same language to describe Asperger syndrome and autistic disorder (e.g., at least two symptoms of impairment in social interaction and one symptom of restricted, repetitive interests or behaviors). However, to receive the Asperger diagnosis, the individual may not have mental retardation and may not have had a significant delay in learning to talk. Given those criteria, many argue that Asperger syndrome is not, in fact, a separate disorder but a form of high-functioning autism.

Other experts argue, however, that Asperger syndrome has more distinct characteristics than those covered in the *DSM-IV-TR* criteria. Commonly mentioned ones include poor social skills, special interests, language peculiarities, sensory processing difficulties, gross and fine motor problems, and difficulties with self-help and organizational skills.

Social Skills While small children with Asperger syndrome may initially show little interest in playing with other children, they are generally described as being very attached to parents and family members. Older children and adults with Asperger syndrome generally *do* want to establish friendships and relationships, but they lack the ability to do so. Others may view them as quirky, shy, or, in some cases, even frightening. This is due to the fact that, while most people automatically develop an understanding of social rules and nonverbal communication, people with Asperger syndrome do not. They need to be explicitly taught.

Language Children with Asperger syndrome are often described as sounding like "little professors" because of their often extraordinary vocabularies and their tendency to lecture. While their speech may be superficially perfect, they often tend to be overly literal in their use and interpretation of language. Metaphors and idioms (e.g., "beating a dead horse") might be baffling. Others' inexact use of language, such as Mom asking, "Would you mind getting that?" when she really means "Get that!" can cause frustration and anger. The pragmatics (social aspects) of speech—such as the ability to carry on back-and-forth conversations—often do not come naturally to people with Asperger syndrome and must be explicitly taught. One distinctive language feature of many individuals with Asperger syndrome is their love of perseverative scripting—telling the entire story line of, say, a cartoon, video game, or movie, over and over again, complete with exact dialogue and, sometimes, speech inflections and accents.

Special Interests   Individuals with Asperger syndrome often have one or more all-encompassing special interests. These interests go far beyond those of a normal hobby and can interfere with social skills, academics, and work. The amount of information on a particular topic that an individual with Asperger syndrome may acquire can be quite staggering. Sometimes the area of interest may be typical for the person's age group—for example, baseball scores, video games, or cartoons—but the degree of interest sets the person with Asperger syndrome apart. Other interests can be quite unusual, such as vacuum cleaners or train schedules. When the person reads or views the same material over and over again, this is a form of perseveration.

Desire for Sameness   While many people love surprises, individuals with Asperger syndrome typically crave consistency. Sameness seems to provide comfort and security in a world with so many unwritten rules to decipher. Parents and teachers report that a change in routine—even a typically fun activity such as a party or school assembly—can often trigger a meltdown in a child with Asperger syndrome.

Sensory and Motor Difficulties   Many individuals with Asperger syndrome seem to be overly sensitive to light, sound, noise, smells, and/or touch. Clothing, especially tags and sock seams, may cause discomfort for them. Others seem to be less sensitive to sensory input than the average person and not even notice, say, a scraped knee that would set another child crying. Some seek out unusual sensory activities, such as spinning. These are all examples of difficulties with *sensory integration dysfunction* (also known as sensory processing dysfunction). Many people with Asperger syndrome also have difficulties with gross motor skills (e.g., running, jumping, riding a bicycle) and tend to be clumsy. Some also have difficulty with fine motor skills, such as handwriting.

Self-Help and Organizational Skills   Contrary to the *DSM-IV-TR* (American Psychiatric Association, 2000) criteria, clinicians today report that most individuals with Asperger syndrome have difficulties in self-help skills and adaptive behavior (Attwood, 2006). These difficulties extend logically from the other difficulties characteristic of individuals with Asperger syndrome. For example, tying shoes and getting dressed require fine motor skills; shopping at the supermarket requires an ability to adapt to change (as groceries are often rearranged or out of stock) and often some social interaction at the cash register. Going from class to class in middle school requires tolerating loud noise, being bumped into, and other students behaving in unpredictable ways. Many people with Asperger syndrome also have difficulties with executive functions (e.g., organizing and planning skills).

Not every person with Asperger syndrome manifests the same characteristics in number or degree. Therefore, it is important to keep in mind that Asperger syndrome is a spectrum disorder, ranging from relatively mild to quite severe. One person might be so impaired that he or she is unable to live independently while another might be able to hold down a job—even be quite talented and successful at it—but still have significant difficulties in interpersonal relationships.

Lisa Barrett Mann

See also Autism.

References

American Psychiatric Association. *Diagnostic and Statistical Manual of Mental Disorders,* 4th ed., text rev. Washington, DC: American Psychiatric Association, 2000.

Attwood, T. *Asperger's Syndrome: A Guide for Parents and Professionals.* London: Jessica Kingsley, 1998.

Attwood, T. "Is There a Difference between Asperger's Syndrome and High-Functioning Autism?" www.tonyattwood.com.au.

Myles, B. S., and R. L. Simpson. "Asperger Syndrome: An Overview of Characteristics." *Focus on Autism and Other Developmental Disabilities* 17, no. 3 (2002): 132–37.

Myles, B. S., G. P. Barnhill, T. Hagiwara, D. E. Griswold, and R. L. Simpson. "A Synthesis of Studies on the Intellectual, Academic, Social/Emotional and Sensory Characteristics of Children and Youth with Asperger Syndrome." *Education and Training in Mental Retardation and Developmental Disabilities* 36, no. 3 (2001): 304–11.

Powers, M. D. *Asperger Syndrome and Your Child: A Parent's Guide.* New York: Skylight Press, 2002.

Wing, L., and J. Gould. "Severe Impairments of Social Interaction and Associated Abnormalities in Children: Epidemiology and Classification." *Journal of Autism and Developmental Disorders* 9 (1979): 11–29.

ASTHMA

Asthma is a disease that affects breathing. It attacks and damages lungs and airways. Data from the Centers for Disease Control and Prevention (CDC) National Center for Health Statistics shows that in 2009 over 24 million Americans suffered from asthma (Akinbami, 2011). Asthma is described as like breathing through a straw; it can be a serious threat to persons of any age. Childhood asthma attracts attention because of its potential developmental consequences. Asthma is characterized by partially blocked airways. It can occur periodically or reactively, and attacks or events can range from mild to severe. The nose, sinuses, and throat can become constricted. Breathing becomes difficult and is accompanied by coughing and wheezing.

During an asthma event, the muscles around the breathing passages constrict. The mucous lining of the airways becomes inflamed and swollen. This further constricts air passages. These episodes can last for hours or days. They can be terrifying events for parents and children. Childhood asthma and its disproportionate impact on vulnerable populations is one of the foundational issues of environmental justice in the United States.

Causes of Asthma Asthma is a complex disease with many causes, some known, some contested, and some unknown. Each one presents its own issues. Environmental causes are controversial because they represent a broad, catchall category. Controversies about science, industry trade secrets, and unequal enforcement of environmental laws merge with a very high level of citizen concern. There is an emerging role for public health experts and advocates in urban environmental policies around childhood asthma. There is a greater incidence of asthma among children in U.S. inner cities.

Asthma often accounts for a large number of emergency room visits, especially in poor areas underserved by medical insurance. According to statistics from the U.S. Department of Health and Human Services, there were almost 2 million asthma-related emergency department visits and

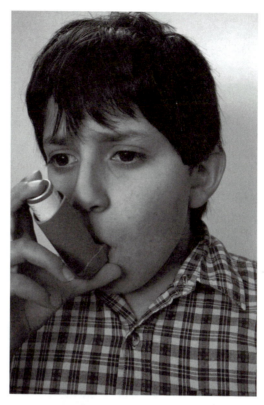

Young boy uses an asthma inhaler, a device used to provide relief from asthma symptoms. (Peter Elvidge/Dreamstime.com)

456,000 asthma hospitalizations in 2007 (CDC, 2011). Hospitals, health care administrators, and health insurance corporations are all very interested in the causes of asthma. Employers and educators know that a number of days in school or on the job are lost because of asthma. In 2008 persons with asthma missed 10 million school days and 14 million work days due to their asthma (Akinbami, 2011). They also have an interest in understanding the causes. Some stakeholders may fear liability for causing asthma. They have a strong interest in not being named as among those responsible.

Environmental Triggers What triggers an asthma attack? Indoor air contamination can be caused by dust mites, cockroach droppings, animal dander, and mold; all are among the environmental conditions that may cause asthma. Exposure to allergens alone may induce the onset of asthma. Exposure to secondhand tobacco smoke is also a contributor. Certain insecticides may also be triggers. Some researchers consider pesticides to be a preventable cause of asthma in children. The quality of indoor air in homes may be made worse by the increasing use of synthetic materials in the form of carpets, carpet glues, curtains, and building materials. There is concern that as these materials age, they release potentially dangerous chemicals.

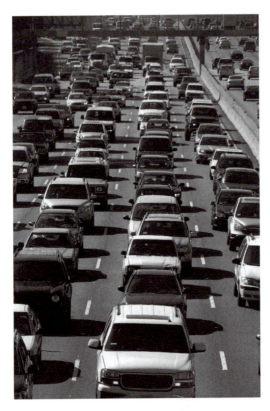

Automobile traffic congests a busy highway in Los Angeles, California. Across the nation, this type of frequent heavy traffic on roadways increases air pollution due to automobile emissions. (Roza/Dreamstime.com)

Manufacturers of these items strongly contest any conclusion that their products may be among the causes of childhood asthma. However, concern about release of toxins from synthetic materials has affected market trends in these products. Because many household products are believed to be possible causes of asthma, the marketplace or commerce in these products has become a point of discussion. Large big-box retailers such as Wal-Mart are accommodating these consumer concerns about causes of asthma that consumers can control, such as dust mites and animal dander.

There is strong evidence from longitudinal studies that ambient or outdoor air pollution acts as a trigger for asthma events among persons with this condition. Truck and automotive exhaust is a big part of the polluted air, especially in densely populated urban areas. Combined with industrial and municipal emissions and waste treatment practices (such as incineration), air quality becomes so degraded that the total polluted air load in some urban and nearby suburban areas is a threat to the health of children. It threatens them with the development of asthma due to long-time exposure and poses the risk of initiating an attack at any time.

It is clear that the increasing severity of asthma in the United States is concentrated in cities among children who live in poverty. Children are especially vulnerable to air pollution and other toxic exposures, partly because they have more skin surface relative to total body mass. According to Frederica Perera, director of the Columbia Center for Children's Environmental Health:

They consume more water, more food, and more air per unit body weight than adults by far. Today's urban children are highly exposed to allergens, such as cockroach and rodent particles, and pollutants, such as diesel exhaust, lead and pesticides. And these elements affect them even before they are born. Preliminary evidence shows that increased risk of asthma may start as early as in the womb before birth. (Perera & Herbstman, 2011)

The small particles of soot "are very easily breathed into your lungs, so they really exacerbate asthma," say Peggy Shepard, executive director of West Harlem Environmental Action, Inc., adding that she believes these diesel particles may also play a role in cancer. Shepard says that New York City is second in the nation when it comes to the amount of toxins released in the air, preceded only by Baltimore (Shepard, Vasquez, & Minkler, 2008).

David Evans, who runs the Columbia Center's "Healthy Home, Healthy Child" intervention campaign, maintains that cockroach particles pose a problem for urban areas nationwide. He says, "Simple housecleaning won't solve the problem, because the cockroach residue tends to be present in many city neighborhoods" (Evans, Fullilove, Green, & Levison, 2002). According to the Harlem Lung Center, childhood asthma rates increased 78 percent between 1980 and 1993 (Garg, Karpati, Leighton, Perrin, & Shah, 2003). And according to the Columbia Center, there are an estimated 8,400 new cases of childhood cancer each year nationwide.

Disparities in Care   Access to health care is an important aspect of the asthma controversy. Many low-income groups do not have health insurance and tend to use the emergency room instead of visiting a primary care physician. An asthma attack often presents that necessity. Language and cultural differences can make a tense medical situation worse. Even with regular medical intervention, differences in asthma treatment by race, gender, and class make this issue an ongoing one, and disparities in the burden and treatment of African Americans and Puerto Ricans with asthma are well documented.

Among African Americans and Puerto Ricans, rates of asthma, hospitalization, and death are higher compared with rates among whites. This is especially true among children. Different medicines are prescribed and used for different groups. Research shows that the use of long-term medications to control asthma is lower among African Americans and Puerto Ricans. Cost may be a factor, especially if there is no insurance coverage. Access to medical care is affected in many ways. Issues in minority communities are shortages of primary care physicians and trust about the role and usefulness of medications.

Costs of Asthma   Asthma is a cause of death among U.S. children. There are 247 deaths each year due to childhood asthma. It is the leading cause of hospital admission for urban children. Asthma is also the leading cause of days of school missed. It is estimated that about 30 percent of acute episodes of childhood asthma are environmentally related.

Air pollution is considered a major cause of asthma, and asthma and public health are major regulatory justifications for clean air laws. The U.S. Environmental Protection Agency (EPA) has estimated the cost savings that resulted from the Clean Air Act. For the years 1970 to 1990, the EPA calculated that the annual monetary benefits of reductions in chronic bronchitis and other respiratory conditions was $3.5 billion.

This figure represents health care costs that would have been incurred if there were no clean air regulations. There are other costs too, of course. Also, if there were no costs and if people with asthma could get free and accessible medical attention, the cost of human resources necessary to handle the scope of the problem could be large. Additional childhood asthma benefits are projected by the EPA to accrue over the years 1990 to 2010, assuming full implementation of the Clean Air Act Amendments of 1990 (Landrigan, Schechter, Lipton, Fahs, & Schwartz, 2002).

Emissions from traffic, industry, and heating and cooling systems are now part of the U.S. urban landscape. Environmentalists note that the law does not cover all the pollutants and is not enforced equally. Advocates of environmental justice consider childhood asthma as proof of at least one disproportionate environmental impact. Asthma generally has resulted in a substantial increase in the sales and profits of pharmaceutical companies. This controversy is structural in that it pits public health concerns against industrial emissions and is therefore of deep significance.

There will be many ongoing issues. The environmental controversies around childhood asthma will focus on air pollution and use other controversial methods such as ecosystem risk assessment or cumulative risk assessment. Childhood asthma is a big part of the new inclusion of cities by the EPA. In the early 1990s, EPA administrator Carol Browner called for reducing the level of particulate matter allowed in urban air districts, effectively banning many diesel and leaded gas vehicles. She started an urban air toxics policy task force to help engage cities and the EPA, along with several other successful policy initiatives. Asthma presents an ongoing public health challenge in the United States. Although more needs to be understood about preventing asthma from developing, the means for controlling and preventing symptoms are well established and include removing risks such as tobacco smoke, mold, and other environmental triggers.

Robert William Collin

See also Allergies; Environmental Health; Environmental Protection Agency (EPA); Health Insurance.

References

Akinbami, Lara J. "Asthma Prevalence, Health Care Use and Mortality: United States, 2005–2009." *National Health Statistics Reports* 32 (January 12, 2011). U.S. Department of Health and Human Services.

Akinbami, Lara J. *The State of Childhood Asthma in the United States, 1980–2005*. Hyattsville, MD: U.S. Department of Health and Human Services, 2006.

Bernstein, I. Leonard. *Asthma in the Workplace*. New York: Marcel Dekker, 1999.

Cherni, Judith A. *Economic Growth versus the Environment: The Politics of Wealth, Health, and Air Pollution*. London: Palgrave Macmillan, 2002.

Christie, Margaret J., and Davina French. *Assessment of Quality of Life in Childhood Asthma*. London: Taylor and Francis, 1994.

Evans, David, Mindy Thompson Fullilove, Lesley Green, and Moshe Levison. "Awareness of Environmental Risks and Protective Actions among Minority Women in Northern Manhattan." *Environmental Health Perspectives* 110, supplement 2 (April 2002): 271–75.

Garg, R., A. Karpati, J. Leighton, M. Perrin, and M. Shah. *Asthma Facts,* 2nd ed. New York: New York City Department of Health and Mental Hygiene, May 2003.

Institute of Medicine. *Clearing the Air: Asthma and Indoor Air Exposures.* Washington, DC: National Academies Press, 2000.

Landrigan, Philip J., Clyde B. Schechter, Jeffrey M. Lipton, Marianne C. Fahs, and Joel Schwartz. "Environmental Pollutants and Disease in American Children: Estimates of Morbidity, Mortality, and Costs for Lead Poisoning, Asthma, Cancer and Developmental Disabilities." *Environmental Health Perspectives* 110, no. 7 (July 2002): 721–28.

Naspitz, Charles K. *Pediatric Asthma: An International Perspective.* London: Taylor and Francis, 2001.

Perera, Federeica, and Julie Herbstman. "Prenatal Environmental Exposures, Epigenetics, and Disease." *Reproductive Toxicology* (2011), doi: 10.1016/j.reprotox.2010.12.055.

Shepard, P., V. Vasquez, and M. Minkler. "Using CBPR to Promote Environmental Justice Policy: A Case Study from Harlem, New York." *Community-Based Participatory Research for Health: From Process to Outcomes,* 2nd ed. Edited by M. Minklere and N. Wallerstein. San Francisco: Jossey-Bass, 2008.

ATKINS, ROBERT C.

Robert C. Atkins (1930–2003), founder of the famous Atkins diet has been denounced and celebrated since the 1972 release of his low-carbohydrate eating plan, which told dieters to switch carbohydrates for steak, eggs, and bacon. Atkins brought the U.S. nutrition battle between carbohydrates and fats to a head in the 1970s and pushed scientists to examine the low-fat versus low-carbohydrate question. Forty years later, researchers are still arguing. Now, study results such as those reported in the 2007 *Journal of the American Medical Association* suggest it may be time to give Atkins and his diet a second look (Gardner et al., 2007).

Born on October 17, 1930, in Columbus, Ohio, Atkins was the founder and executive medical director of the Atkins Center for Complementary Medicine in New York City. The center was founded in 1976 with the stated philosophy

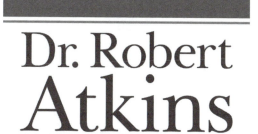
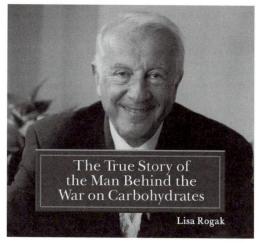

Cover of Robert Atkins's biography, published in 2005. Atkins was the founder of the low-carbohydrate diet craze that bears his name. (PRNewsFoto/Chamberlain Bros)

that "the best medicine integrates the safest and most effective therapies from all the healing arts, both traditional and alternative." Atkins was the author of several best-selling diet books, including *Dr. Atkins' Diet Revolution* (1972), *Dr. Atkins' New Diet Revolution* (1992), and *Dr. Atkins' New Diet Revolution: Revised and Updated* (1999). His last book was *Atkins for Life* (2003). He and his wife, Veronica, coauthored *Dr. Atkins' Quick and Easy New Diet Cookbook* (1997), and he wrote a guide to using vitamins, minerals, and other supplements titled *Dr. Atkins' Vita-Nutrient Solution: Nature's Answer to Drugs* (1998). He died from a fall in 2003 at the age of 73.

Many U.S. dieters are still following the Atkins diet today. It is a ketogenic diet—a high-protein, high-fat, and low-carbohydrate plan that causes rapid initial weight loss without limiting calories. However, the Atkins Center refers to its program as the Atkins Nutritional Approach, labeling it a controlled carbohydrate program for weight management and good health. The center objects to those who classify the diet as high-protein or ketogenic. Center spokespeople maintain that when the Atkins program is followed correctly, the amount of protein consumed is no higher than that in the typical U.S. diet.

A diet is ketogenic when the lack of carbohydrates for fuel triggers the body's production of large amounts of ketone bodies, a condition known as ketosis. Symptoms of ketosis include nausea, dehydration, constipation or diarrhea, and bad breath. Atkins Center representatives answer critics by saying a true ketogenic diet is 90 percent fat and 10 percent protein, while the first phase of the Atkins program is 60 percent fat, 30 percent protein, and 10 percent carbohydrates. They say the aforementioned symptoms are rare when individuals follow the program correctly.

In *Dr. Atkins' New Diet Revolution,* Atkins encouraged the onset of ketosis, calling it "one of life's charmed gifts" and a "dieter's best friend." Atkins maintained that, as long as an individual consumes sufficient calories from protein and fat, there is no health risk involved in ketosis. Both the original Atkins diet and the updated version start off with a two-week induction program designed, according to Atkins, to rebalance an individual's metabolism by causing ketosis. During the first 14 days, the plan allows dieters to eat liberal amounts of fat and protein; however, it restricts carbohydrates to 20 grams per day. That equals about three cups of salad vegetables such as lettuce, cucumbers, and celery.

Dietary intake recommendations from the U.S. Department of Agriculture (USDA) and the National Institutes of Health call for a daily intake of up to 300 grams of carbohydrates for an average, healthy adult male. Atkins argued that the USDA 300-gram recommendation has done nothing to help the growing number of Americans who are becoming fatter and fatter as well as the rising incidence of Type 2 diabetes. Atkins called these the "twin epidemics of diabesity."

However, this emphasis on an almost carbohydrate-free diet still worries critics like the National Cancer Institute, which urges Americans to eat five servings of fruits and vegetables each day to reduce the risk of certain kinds of cancers. The premaintenance phase of the Atkins program gradually adds one to three servings per week of carbohydrate-rich fruits and vegetables. The maintenance phase typically allows for 60 to 90 grams daily of carbohydrate foods.

Atkins began his study of medicine at the University of Michigan, where he earned a bachelor of arts degree in 1951. He received a medical degree from Cornell University in 1955. Atkins practiced as an internist and cardiologist for some 20 years before he published his first book and best-seller, *Dr. Atkins' Diet Revolution*. His diet was followed by another very popular high-protein, low-carbohydrate eating plan—*The Complete Scarsdale Medical Diet*, written in 1978 by physician and cardiologist Herman Tarnower.

Over the years, a number of leading medical and health organizations—including the American Medical Association, the American Dietetic Association, and the American Heart Association—denounced the Atkins diet. In 1973 Atkins was called to testify before the Senate Select Committee on Nutrition and Human Needs to answer charges that his diet would compromise the lives of unborn children. Appearing with his attorney, Atkins declared that he stood by everything in his book, including his recommendation that overweight women could follow the diet when pregnant. During testimony at the hearing, according to an April 13, 1973, *New York Times* article, a New York obstetrician cited extensive research evidence that the kind of diet Atkins recommended would compromise the well-being and possibly the life of an unborn child. Dr. Karlis Adamsons said, "If I were a fetus, I would forbid my mother to go on such a diet." Several other physicians, appearing in front of the Senate committee, said the full impact of such a low-carbohydrate diet may not become apparent until many years later and that obstetricians might not detect damage to a fetus until it was too late.

Over 30 years later, researchers analyzed data from 20 years of food diaries created by over 80,000 participants in the Nurses' Health Study and reported in 2006 that low-carbohydrate diets do not increase the risk of heart disease (Halton et al., 2006). The *Journal of the American Medical Association* also concluded that, compared to three other popular diets—the Zone, the Ornish, and the LEARN low-carbohydrate diet—the Atkins eating plan came out on top. That study randomly put 311 overweight or obese women on one of the four diets to discover which was the most effective over a year. The women on the Atkins diet had the greatest reductions in body mass index, triglycerides, and blood pressure (Gardner et al., 2007).

Critic of Atkins's diet plan include Dean Ornish, author of *Eat More, Weigh Less*, who said in a 2000 *Newsweek* interview, "The problem with low-carbohydrate diets is, even if you lose weight, you're mortgaging your health in the process" (Underwood, 2000). In answer to critics such as Ornish, Atkins Center representatives cite research at Harvard that found that excessive carbohydrate intake has been linked with an increased incidence of heart disease. The Atkins website, www.atkins.com, lists other studies as well as anecdotal evidence to further support the program.

The Atkins Diet The four-step diet begins with a two-week induction program, when dieters may eat liberal amounts of fat and protein while holding carbohydrate intake to just 20 grams per day. During this phase, meals are planned around Atkins's acceptable foods, such as beef, pork, bacon, fish, chicken, eggs, and cheese. Under the Atkins plan, cream is allowed but not skim milk, and sour cream can be eaten but not yogurt

Atkins encourages dieters on his plan to take vitamin supplements to correct any nutritional deficiencies they may encounter. In his book, he stressed that the early period of the diet is not a lifetime regimen unless the dieter has a particularly stubborn metabolic resistance. Following the induction period, a premaintenance period, known as the ongoing weight loss phase, is a time when weight loss is deliberately slowed in an effort to introduce more variety in foods. At this point dieters can choose from more vegetables, seeds and nuts, and low-glycemic fruits such as strawberries and blueberries. According to the Atkins plan, as long as weight loss continues, individuals can gradually increase their carbohydrate intake. The first week, they can eat 25 grams of carbohydrates per day; the second week, they move to 30 grams, and so forth until weight loss stalls. Finally, at the maintenance stage, dieters are allowed 60 to 90 grams of carbohydrates per day, which might include legumes and whole grains as well as other fruits.

By limiting carbohydrate intake, the Atkins diet eliminates many of the foods and food groups called for in the USDA Food Guide MyPlate. Those include fruits, cereals, breads, grains, starches, dairy products, and starchy vegetables. However, in direct contrast to the Atkins plan, the USDA encourages people to eat sparingly of foods high in fat, such as butter, oil, meat, poultry, fish, eggs, cheese, and cream, and instead suggests that a healthy diet should include five servings of fruits and vegetables each day.

In his book, Atkins stated that people who follow his plan and then return to eating their prediet amount of carbohydrates will find the pounds returning. The Atkins lifetime maintenance phase begins when dieters reach their goal weight. Then, depending upon age, gender, exercise level, and genetics, a person can decide how much carbohydrate to consume, usually from 90 to 120 grams per day. For most people, this means occasionally eating modest portions of foods such as potatoes, other starchy vegetables, whole-wheat pasta, and whole-grain bread without regaining weight. The Atkins diet is not recommended for lacto-ovo vegetarians, since it would be difficult to find enough nonanimal sources of protein to eat. And vegans cannot follow this diet since a vegan diet is very high in carbohydrates, according to Atkins. Instead, the Atkins Center recommends that vegetarians with a serious weight problem give up vegetarianism, or at least include fish in their diet.

Marjolijn Bijlefeld and Sharon Zoumbaris

See also Amino Acids; Carbohydrates; Dieting; MyPlate; Ornish, Dean.

References

Atkins, Robert C. *Atkins for Life*. New York: St. Martin's Press, 2003.
Atkins, Robert C. *Dr. Atkins' Health Revolution: How Complementary Medicine Can Extend Your Life*. New York: Houghton Mifflin Company, 1988.

Atkins, Robert C. *Dr. Atkins' New Diet Revolution.* New York: Avon Books, 1992.

Brody, Jane E. "Senate Nutrition Panel to Focus on Perils of Being Overweight." *New York Times* (April 13, 1973): 18.

"Fad Diets: Don't Look for Magic Bullets." *Consumers' Research Magazine,* July 2000, 24–26.

Gardner, Christopher D., Alexandre Kiazand, Sofiya Alhassan, Soowon Kim, Randall S. Stafford, Raymond R. Balise, Henela C. Kraemer, and Abby C. King. "Comparison of the Atkins, Zone, Ornish, and LEARN Diets for Change in Weight and Related Risk Factors among Overweight Premenopausal Women." *Journal of the American Medical Association* 297, no. 9 (2007): 969–77, doi: 10.1001/jama.297.9.969.

Halton, Thomas L., Walter C. Willett, Simin Liu, JoAnn E. Manson, Christine M. Albert, Kathryn Rexrode, and Frank B. Hu. "Low-Carbohydrate-Diet Score and the Risk of Coronary Heart Disease in Women." *New England Journal of Medicine* 355 (November 2006): 1991–2002.

"License Suspended, Dr. Robert Atkins." *Time,* August 23, 1993, 21.

Taubes, Gary. "The Soft Science of Dietary Fat." *Science* 291, no. 5513 (March 30, 2001): 2536–45.

"The Trendy Diet That Sizzles: A Counterintuitive Program Reaches Critical Mass." *Newsweek,* September 6, 1999, 60.

Underwood, Anne. "The Battle of Pork Rind Hill: When the Nation's Best-Selling Diet Gurus Squared Off in a Raucous Food Fight, One Thing Was Clear: There's No Easy Way to Shed That Ugly Flab. So Get Out the Jogging Shoes." *Newsweek,* March 6, 2000, 50–52.

Willett, Walter C. *Eat, Drink, and Be Healthy: The Harvard Medical School Guide to Healthy Eating.* New York: Simon & Schuster, 2001.

ATTENTION DEFICIT HYPERACTIVITY DISORDER (ADHD)

Attention-deficit hyperactivity disorder, sometimes called attention deficit disorder, is a condition characterized by a short attention span, excessive activity, and/or impulsive behavior. The symptoms begin at a young age and continue for a long time, sometimes lasting into adulthood. Some adults, however, do not realize that they have the disorder until they begin to face significant problems with such issues as disorganization and lack of focus in their careers or everyday life.

Depression is one of the most common coexisting conditions. By some estimates, up to 70 percent of those with ADHD will be treated for depression at some point in their lives.

About 3 percent to 5 percent of children have ADHD. Although the first signs of the disorder may show up in early childhood, it is difficult to make a diagnosis at that age, because even healthy preschoolers have short attention spans and limited control over their behavior. Often the condition is first diagnosed when children reach school age and ADHD symptoms begin causing problems in the classroom.

All children occasionally have trouble sitting still, blurt out things they don't mean to, or find it hard to pay attention. For children with ADHD, though, such behaviors occur more often than normal for their age. The behaviors are part of a long-lasting pattern, not just a temporary response to a short-term situation.

And they occur in a variety of settings, not just in one place such as the classroom or playground.

ADHD can affect children's ability to learn in the classroom, get along with others, and behave appropriately at home and at school. As a result, such children often wind up labeled as behavior problems. By their late teens, young people may grow out of some symptoms, such as hyperactivity. But other symptoms, such as being easily distracted, may be longer lasting. Thirty percent to 70 percent of those who had ADHD as children continue to experience some problems as adults.

Even when symptoms of ADHD subside as children grow older, earlier problems at home, school, and play can have far-reaching repercussions. That is why it is important to seek advice from a qualified medical or mental health professional if ADHD is suspected. If the disorder is diagnosed, several management options are available, including ADHD medication, behavioral therapy, and classroom interventions. When depression is also present, such approaches may be combined with cognitive therapy and/or antidepressants.

Criteria for Diagnosis   The symptoms of ADHD are defined by the *Diagnostic and Statistical Manual of Mental Disorders* (American Psychiatric Association, 2000) a diagnostic guidebook that is used by mental health professionals from many disciplines. By definition, ADHD starts early in life, with symptoms serious enough to cause problems appearing by age seven. The symptoms lead to significant impairment in school, work, or social functioning, and the problems occur in multiple settings. Symptoms of ADHD fall into two main categories: inattention and hyperactivity/impulsivity. To be diagnosed with the disorder, people must have six or more symptoms from at least one of these categories. The symptoms last for a minimum of six months and are inconsistent with what would be expected for individuals of that age.

Inattention   People who are inattentive have trouble keeping their mind focused on any one thing. Such individuals often (1) make careless mistakes or fail to pay close attention to detail; (2) have trouble staying focused on what they are doing; (3) do not seem to listen when spoken to; (4) do not follow instructions or finish tasks; (5) have problems getting organized; (6) dislike or avoid tasks that require sustained mental effort, such as studying; (7) lose necessary items, such as schoolbooks; (8) are easily distracted; and (9) act forgetful.

Hyperactivity/Impulsivity   People who are hyperactive always seem to be on the go, and those who are impulsive fail to think before they act. Such individuals often (1) fidget or have trouble sitting still, (2) leave their seat in the classroom or other places where they are supposed to stay seated, (3) run about or climb around in situations where it is inappropriate, (4) have problems engaging in quiet play or leisure activities, (5) seem to be in constant motion, (6) talk too much, (7) blurt out answers before the questions are finished, (8) find it hard to wait their turn, and (9) interrupt other people's conversations or butt into their activities.

Relationship to Depression   Left untreated, ADHD and depression often feed off each other. Children with ADHD may become demoralized and develop low self-esteem if they experience repeated failures at school or hear frequent criticism at home. As the negative experiences pile up, they may begin to feel helpless and hopeless. These feelings, in turn, can contribute to depression. Conversely, depression can make it harder to cope with the challenges of ADHD. It is a vicious cycle that can have serious consequences if allowed to continue unchecked. Fortunately, treatment can help break the cycle and create the conditions for turning failure into success.

Treatment of ADHD   When people have both ADHD and depression simultaneously, both conditions need to be addressed. The main treatment options for ADHD are medication, behavioral therapy, and classroom interventions.

Medication: Stimulant medications help decrease hyperactivity and impulsiveness as well as increase attention. Stimulants mainly affect dopamine. There is also a nonstimulant ADHD medication called atomoxetine, which affects the brain chemical norepinephrine.

Behavioral therapy: Behavioral therapy helps people with ADHD change their behavior to solve specific problems. Key elements include setting goals, rewarding desired behaviors, and monitoring progress. When children have ADHD, parents and teachers may learn to use these techniques for modifying behavior.

Classroom interventions: Classroom strategies that promote positive behavioral change include keeping a consistent routine, writing down assignments, and organizing books and supplies. If needed, extra tutoring or other special educational services can help keep students from falling too far behind.

Linda Wasmer Andrews

See also Depression.

References

American Academy of Family Physicians. *ADHD: What Parents Should Know* (November 2006), http://familydoctor.org/online/famdocen/home/children/parents/behavior/118.html.

American Psychiatric Association. *Diagnostic and Statistical Manual of Mental Disorders,* 4th ed., text rev. Washington, DC: American Psychiatric Association, 2000.

Attention Deficit Disorder Association, www.add.org.

Brown, Thomas E. *Attention Deficit Disorder: The Unfocused Mind in Children and Adults.* New Haven, CT: Yale University Press, 2005.

Children and Adults with Attention Deficit/Hyperactivity Disorder, www.chadd.org, www.help4adhd.org.

National Institute of Mental Health. *Attention Deficit Hyperactivity Disorder* (April 3, 2008), www.nimh.nih.gov/health/publications/adhd/complete-publication.shtml.

National Institute of Mental Health. "Can Adults Have ADHD?" (January 23, 2009), www.nimh.nih.gov.

National Institute of Neurological Disorders and Stroke. *NINDS Attention Deficit-Hyperactivity Disorder Information Page* (June 6, 2008), www.ninds.nih.gov/disorders/adhd/adhd.htm.

National Resource Center on ADHD. *AD/HD and Coexisting Conditions: Depression* (February 2008), www.help4adhd.org/en/treatment/coexisting/WWK5C.

National Resource Center on ADHD. *Psychosocial Treatment for Children and Adolescents with ADHD* (February 2004), www.help4adhd.org/treatment/behavioral/WWK7.

AUTISM

Autistic disorder, or autism, is currently understood as a developmental disability that begins before the age of three. Autism's three main areas of impact are in the domains of social interaction; communication; and restricted, repetitive, and stereotyped interests and behaviors. The psychiatric handbook of mental disorders, the *Diagnostic and Statistical Manual of Mental Disorders* (American Psychiatric Association, 2000), classifies autism as a pervasive developmental disorder (PDD)—a group of disabilities with similar core characteristics and a wide range of manifestation and prognosis. The other four diagnostic PDD labels include Asperger syndrome, childhood disintegrative disorder (also known as Heller's syndrome), Rett's disorder (also known as Rett syndrome), and pervasive developmental disorder-not otherwise specified (PDD-NOS, also known as atypical autism).

Camp for Children with Autism

Camp Gonnawannagoagain is a name that speaks for itself. That is fitting since a majority of this camp's participants may not be able to speak much at all. Camp Gonnawannagoagain is the summer program for children with autism started in 1993 by a group of parents of autistic children. Run under the auspices of the not-for-profit Families of Autistic Children of Tidewater in Virginia Beach, Virginia, this slice of summer lets kids try and be kids while offering parents and caretakers a safe place for their autistic child to meet new people and experience new activities.

Autism is a neurological disorder that robs individuals in many instances of their ability to communicate and interact with others. Diagnosed cases of autism are on the rise, and with those increasing numbers come a growing army of parents, siblings, and caretakers determined to stay connected and keep their autistic loved one engaged.

Camp Gonnawannagoagain is an example of that determination. Summer activities include field trips to places to play laser tag and go bowling and swimming, managed by adding an abundance of human contact through the use of volunteers and counselors. Not surprisingly, it isn't just the campers who love the camp. Every summer, all available spots fill up and so do the slots for volunteers and counselors. Volunteers are instrumental because each camper is assigned a non-disabled volunteer along with an adult counselor. Due to space limitations, campers can only attend up to three of the six one-week sessions offered. Which prompts many campers to complain that they "wannagoagain."

—*Sharon Zoumbaris*

Autism has been known by several other names over the past decades: early infantile autism, childhood autism, Kanner's autism, and classical autism. Individuals with autism present on a continuum of expression with cognition across all IQ levels and possession of individual strengths and needs. Some with autism have no language, have significant cognitive impairment, and are in need of constant care. Others have limited language and mild cognitive impairments but are in need of significant support. Still others have average to above-average intelligence and their difficulties are less noticeable. Common strengths in autism include visual/spatial abilities, systemizing skills, proclivity for routine-oriented behaviors, rote learning, and physical development. Some with autism have splinter skills, or unique talents and abilities that seem unusual when compared to adaptive or other functioning levels. For example, an eight-year-old child with autism may not be toilet trained but be able to do puzzles at amazing speed. Or an adult with autism may be nonverbal but be able to play a musical instrument with expertise.

Generally, those with autism have challenges with verbal and nonverbal communication, relating to others, and learning by traditional methods; are resistant to change; and insist on familiarity. Other concerns include possible co-occurring medical conditions, sensory processing difficulties, and behavioral deficits and/or excesses. Approximately one-third of those with autism experience seizures at some point. Some individuals with autism exhibit odd repetitive behaviors such as hand flapping, finger twisting, light filtering, body posturing, or complex movements of the body. It has been inferred that these behaviors are due to a need to respond to sensory input or as a means to deal with stress, anxiety, or confusion. Others with autism may have self-injurious or aggressive behaviors. These behaviors are often the result of inappropriate teaching, lack of positive supports, and the difficulties facing a person who may have limited communication and/or means to have needs met.

Today, many use the term *autism* to refer to an autism spectrum disorder (ASD) or the clustering of three of the most common PDDs (autism, Asperger syndrome, and PDD-NOS). The distinctions between these labels can be subtle, but generally those with PDD-NOS meet at least one of the criteria of autism but lack other criteria to qualify for the autism diagnosis. For example, a child with PDD-NOS might have average IQ and good social skills but significant and pervasive communication issues. Those with Asperger syndrome have average to above-average cognition and speech development that is typical but have social and behavioral impairments. For example, an adult with Asperger syndrome might have a high IQ, hold a job in a computer company, and be married but have intense social needs and anxieties as well as some repetitive and stereotyped behaviors.

Autism tends to be the most challenging of the group; many of those with the disorder have cognitive impairment (IQ less than 70); less or no verbal language ability; and more medical, sensory, and behavioral needs. For example, a teenager with autism might have cognitive impairment and limited adaptive skills, have no language ability, use limited sign language to communicate, have epilepsy, and display self-injurious behaviors. The previous examples are merely attempts at detailing the wide range of presentations for similar disabilities. Although each individual with autism has impairments in the three main areas (social, communication, and behaviors), each is unique in how the impairments and strengths are expressed, in personality and in potential. Today, many professionals use the terms PDD and ASD interchangeably.

Another ongoing debate in the field is whether Asperger syndrome is a distinct disability or just a form of high-functioning autism (HFA). HFA has been used to describe those with autism who are less impaired compared to those with severe cognitive impairment, individuals with autism who have an IQ above 70, or those with average or even superior IQ. Since Asperger syndrome was added to the *Diagnostic and Statistical Manual of Mental Disorders* in 1994 (American Psychiatric Association, 1994), there has been debate about whether Asperger syndrome and high-functioning autism are the same or different diagnoses.

Although autism has been one of the most studied disabilities of childhood, it remains one of the most perplexing. What causes autism is still beyond the understanding of scientists, although they are much closer today than when autism was first described in the literature by Leo Kanner in 1943. Autism has been conceptualized in a number of ways over the past 60 years. From the mid-1940s into the 1960s, autism was thought to be a psychogenic condition of childhood caused by parents' inability to bond with their children, and the negative term "refrigerator parent" (often the mother was implicated) was used to label the parents of children with autism.

Although Kanner and others first posited that autism was a condition that was present at birth or developed soon after, professionals missed some telltale signs (such as if parents could not bond with their child with autism, why did they have other children who developed without having autism?), and chose rather to blame the parent. From the 1960s onward, evidence was presented that began to overturn this unfortunate beginning. This evidence came in the form of family and twin studies, brain research, and other designs that described autism as a biological disorder that had genetic roots.

Even though most today agree that autism is a spectrum of disorders that range from mild to severe presentations, there is still debate on how autism develops. Some believe that autism is predetermined genetically and that the impact of the disability will depend on the number of genes affected in any one individual. Others believe that autism is caused by environmental factors that combine with affected genes to cause the disability. Still others believe that autism is caused when various environmental toxins get into a child's body, and the immune system is unable to process these materials. What most agree on is that the behavior, learning, and characteristics of individuals with autism are different from typically developing individuals because the biology of the brain is different due to genetic and environmental influences. Although biological in nature, there is currently no medical test for autism; it is diagnosed only after observations of the child and interviews with caregivers.

Autism was once thought an extremely rare condition of childhood. Initial prevalence statistics estimated that 4 to 5 out of 10,000 children had autism.

Currently, autism is one of the most diagnosed disabilities of childhood with a prevalence rate of approximately 1 in every 110 births and almost 1 in 70 boys. How and why the prevalence rate is changing are controversial questions; some blame the environment, and others conclude that the broadening of the autism spectrum accounts for the increase. Today the total autism population in the United States has been estimated at approximately 1.5 million children, youth, and adults (Autism Society of America, 2006). Both historically and currently, autism is much more common in males than females (4 to 1 for autism and as high as 9 to 1 for Asperger syndrome).

In the mid-1900s, psychotherapy and/or removal of the child with autism from the home were seen as possible treatments. Since that time, applied behavior analysis, special education, cognitive behavior modification, visual/environmental supports, structured teaching, positive behavior support, speech-language therapy, occupational therapy, physical therapy, counseling, and social skills training have all become avenues to teach individuals with autism. Historically, many individuals with autism were placed in institutions. Since the inclusion and de-institutionalization movements and passage of national laws, most individuals with autism now live at home and go to public schools. However, some children are homeschooled or attend special schools, and many families augment public school education by providing their children with private services at home.

The future for individuals with autism remains variable depending on education, supports, availability of services, early intervention, degree of strengths and impairments, and other factors. Although considered a lifelong disability, many with autism have made significant progress and contributions. For example, Temple Grandin, professor of animal sciences at Colorado State University, is one of the most well-known adults with autism in the United States. Grandin has become an expert in livestock handling and is known internationally for her expertise in this area as well as being a speaker and advocate for those with autism.

Since the controversy over the increased diagnosing of autism and related disorders in the 1990s to today, autism has become better known to the public. Television shows, magazine articles, newspaper stories, motion pictures,

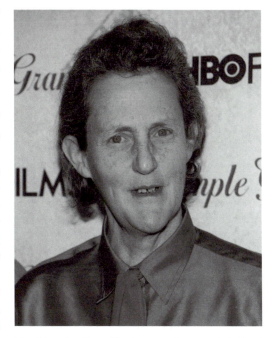

Dr. Temple Grandin is a professor of Animal Sciences at Colorado State University, a person with autism and an advocate for others with autism. (AP/Wide World Photos)

documentaries, and so forth have all helped to spread awareness about autism and its impact on individuals, families, educators, other professionals, and communities. For example, many people have seen or heard of the award-winning 1988 motion picture *Rain Man,* a portrayal of an adult with autism and his brother as they journeyed across the country.

A large and recent controversy regarding autism pertains to the question of potential cures for this disability. Some believe that those with autism can and should be cured. This remains highly controversial, and the ethical question of whether autism should be cured has been asked. Others—both those with autism and their advocates—have spoken out against curing autism. They believe that autism is a culture and that curing autism would be eradicating these persons and their way of life. They do not argue against helping and teaching persons with autism; however, they argue that curing autism would take away the uniqueness and future contributions of those with autism.

In the early 21st century, the autism research community was focusing on a number of areas, including, genetics, brain research, treatment and education, possible environmental contributors, and how autism develops. It is very possible that in the next 50 years the specific genes responsible for autism will be located and that therapies will be created to address these chromosomal differences both in utero and postnatally. Furthermore, continued advances in the field of brain studies may bring about treatments to change neurology. Environmental factors may be identified as contributors to autism, with appropriate responses following. Other new or existing methodologies will be identified as best practice for teaching those with autism. If an eventual cure for autism is discovered, the ethical question of whether autism should be cured will continue to be debated. Included within this discussion will be the moral imperative to treat those with this disability with dignity and respect.

Paul G. LaCava

See also Asperger Syndrome.

References

American Psychiatric Association. *Diagnostic and Statistical Manual of Mental Disorders,* 4th ed. Washington, DC: American Psychiatric Association, 1994.

American Psychiatric Association. *Diagnostic and Statistical Manual of Mental Disorders,* 4th ed., text rev. Washington, DC: American Psychiatric Association, 2000.

Autism Society of America. *What Is Autism?* [Brochure]. Bethesda, MD: Autism Society of America, 2006.

Centers for Disease Control and Prevention. "Facts About ASDs" (July 26, 2010), www.cdc.gov/ncbddd/autism/facts.html.

Frith, U., ed. *Autism: Explaining the Enigma.* Oxford: Blackwell, 1989.

Gillberg, C., and M. Coleman. *The Biology of the Autistic Syndromes,* 3rd ed. London: Keith Mac Press, 2000.

Grandin, T. *Thinking in Pictures and Other Reports from My Life with Autism.* New York: Vintage Books, 1995.

Herbert, M. R. "Autism: A Brain Disorder, Or a Disorder That Affects the Brain." *Clinical Neuropsychiatry* 2 (2005): 354–79.

Johnson, M. (producer), and B. Levinson (director). *Rain Man* [Motion picture]. United Artists, 1988.

Kanner, L. "Autistic Disturbances of Affective Content." *The Nervous Child* 2 (1943): 217–50.

National Research Council. *Educating Children with Autism.* Committee on Educational Interventions for Children with Autism. Division of Behavioral and Social Sciences and Education. Washington, DC: National Academy Press, 2001.

Powers, M. D. *Children with Autism,* 2nd ed. Rockville, MD: Woodbine House, 2000.

Quill, K. A. *Do Watch Listen Say: Social Communication Intervention for Children with Autism.* Baltimore: Brookes, 2000.

AYURVEDA

Ayurveda, life wisdom, is an ancient yet living discipline. Its theories and methods combine the ordinary with the extraordinary. Some regard it as more than a medical tradition; it is a comprehensive lifestyle, a way of life with choice and deliberation that reflects values and actions toward achieving optimal health in body, mind, and spirit.

Adherents of Ayurveda believe that its origins extend back at least 6,000 years. There is some inferential evidence to support this contention. Others say that a 3,000-year-old legacy is clearly verifiable. It would not be an understatement to regard Ayurveda as a world-class system of health and well-being. Health promotion and wellness are prime values.

Ayurveda, an ancient Sanskrit word (*Ayus*/living and *Veda*/revealed wisdom), derives from the traditions of the ancient Indian *rishis* (sages) and denotes the enlightened knowledge of all aspects of optimal, healthy, everyday living and longevity. Its adherents consider it a "fortress of wisdom."

A factor responsible for the slow recognition of Ayurvedic wisdom in the West may be the intentional ambiguity in form and content that has characterized its prehistory, history, and development. Its practical relevance for the Westerner may also be unclear. Eastern ideas have always been clothed in fluid boundaries, and their content may have appeared amorphous, intangible, impractical, and speculative, if not fanciful, to Western thinkers. A solid emphasis on self-inquiry and self-development, perhaps with a strong introspective, private, and very personal quality, has always been central.

Among Ayurveda's primary values are the concepts of *sattva* and of *dharma.* The Sanskrit word *sattva* refers to the ongoing attainment of ever-greater degrees of purity, harmony, balance, and goodness in one's life. For Hindus, the Sanskrit word *dharma,* an equally broad notion, refers to an individual's recognition of inherent lawfulness in the universe, assuming personal responsibility, and taking charge of one's own life in the world.

In the Buddhist tradition, which emerged out of Hinduism in the sixth century BCE, dharma has come to refer to the entire body of teachings, the corpus of enlightened life wisdom, ascribed to the Buddha. This denotes the cosmic law itself and also the words that the Buddha used to express it.

In fact, one of the great luminaries of Ayurveda, Nāgārjuna (ca. second century CE), was both an Ayurvedic physician and a Buddhist priest. The breadth of his wisdom not only enriched the Ayurvedic Materia Medica in a pragmatic way with the introduction of iatrochemistry (mineral-based medicine) but advanced the scope of Buddhism with contributions having profound philosophical and psychological significance. The inestimable significance and living historicity of Nāgārjuna's contributions attest to his continuing creative Ayurvedic presence, a golden thread stretching back two millennia.

Health and Disease Concepts   The concept of health and well-being (*swastha*) in Ayurveda grounds itself in the idea of fostering the balanced and normal functioning of the *doshas*—that is, restoring the *prakruti* to equilibrium when states of constitutional imbalance (*vikruti*) occur. The optimal functioning of each *dosha* in the body creates a homeostatic condition that is conducive to overall health and well-being. Ayurveda views health as a comprehensive state of physical, mental, and spiritual balance that includes the optimal quality, quantity, and functioning of the *doshas, dhatus* (tissues), *srotas* (channels), *malas* (waste products), *Agni* (digestive fire), and *Ojas* (immune system).

Disease is viewed as a state of imbalance (*vyadhi*) of component dimensions on all physical, mental, and spiritual levels that, when integrated, make up the entire person. Within an individual, disease takes hold when the *Agni* becomes impaired. Multiple factors both within and outside the person contribute to impaired *Agni*. *Agni* is the fire of conversion, digestion, and change within every aspect of an individual.

Subsequently, imbalances in the *doshas* produce further impairments in the functioning of the *Agni*, the channels, the tissues and organs, waste products, and the immune system. Terms for disease are *roga* and *amaya*. The commonly used term *roga* denotes that which causes pain and is derived from the Sanskrit root *ruj*, meaning to pain.

The word *duhkha* denotes suffering and usually accompanies descriptions of ill health and disease. It represents a fundamental Buddhist and highly significant Ayurvedic assumption. Man and woman's existence in the created world appears to be inextricably bound to fluctuating cycles both of pleasure and of unpleasure. The negative pole of these encompasses a broad experiential range from unpleasure, discomfort, unpleasantness, discontent, and unhappiness to pain, suffering, sorrow, and misery. Hence, the concepts of disease and *duhkha* reflect a disharmony in the integrity of the person as a biopsychospiritual being.

The antonym of *duhkha* is *sukha*, which translates as happiness, favorableness, or pleasantness. It is said that Charaka, the renowned Ayurvedic luminary, described disease as the condition in which "ease" is lost. The sense of this is understandable since the root *kha* suggests a space (similar to the notion of ether or *Akasha*) within the body, and *su* suggests a positive or favorable state, a condition of ease. The term *sukha* implies that bodily spaces such as the channels are in a positive or favorable condition.

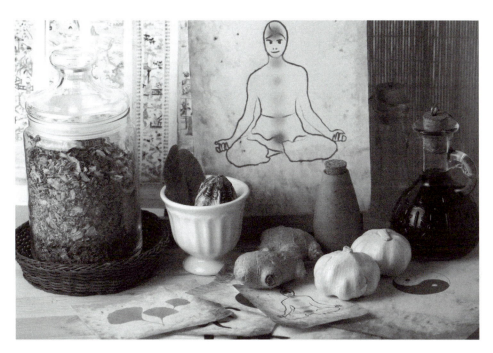

Herbs commonly used in the practice of Ayurveda. (Shutterstock)

The concept of health in Ayurveda also implies the condition of wholeness. This conceptualization has several connotations such as included in the term *samhita,* which means integrated compendium, and in the term *advaita,* meaning nonduality. Since the medical practice of Ayurveda, as its name implies, derives from the ancient tradition of the *Vedas,* a significant metaphysical dimension of the health concept is fundamental and complements its biological denotation.

The heart of the Ayurvedic concept of health contains the idea that the quality of one's consciousness should reflect wholeness, clarity, coherence, and integration. Consciousness here denotes the most intimate experience of awareness. It goes beyond a merely neurological description of alertness, orientation, and the cognitive capacity to concentrate.

The definition of disease in the Ayurvedic view suggests that any condition of impaired consciousness connotes a state of imbalance and some degree of disease, unhappiness, dysphoria, malaise, yearning, and a desire for the satisfaction of unfulfilled needs. This perspective demonstrates the intrinsic spiritual foundation of Ayurvedic thought. Although Ayurveda in theory and in practice places emphasis on the physical dimensions of man, a core spiritual underpinning, consciousness based, remains its central ballast.

Three Universal Causes of All Disease   Ayurveda describes three causes that contribute to all disease: *Prajna-aparadha, Kala-Parinama,* and *Asatmyendriy-artha Samyoga.*

Prajna-Aparadha   *Prajna-aparadha* is a concept that is variously translated as the mistake of the intellect, volitional transgression, or an error in wisdom; it is the loss of the memory of oneness. This default cognitive blindness is perpetuated, in part, by coercive habit/habituation over time—for example, repeating the same stereotyped thinking and behaviors in a reflexive, automatic manner without pause, introspection, and contemplative reflection.

Man's manifestation in the material world of flesh and blood constitutes his potential for rediscovering intrinsic unity within diversity by means of efforts toward repair, restoration, and the development of ever-greater expansions of consciousness. This is the meaning of *Moksha* (liberation) and *samadhi* (enlightenment). *Prajna-aparadha* is the universal human condition marked by a pervasive neglect or forgetting of the aforementioned interconnectedness of the essential unity of spirit and matter. With the original state of all being considered to be one of pure consciousness, birth into the world makes us oblivious of our origins. Most are distracted by the belief that only the conventionally discernible, material aspects of experience exist and, therefore, must constitute reality in its entirety. The assumption that man is, in fact, an integral composite of matter and spirit in an enormous, almost ineffable, universe of matter and spirit is the underpinning for positing the underlying cause of this cognitive distortion.

In the Ayurvedic view, material realities are not understood as being false or even as being bad. *Prajna-aparadha* maintains an everyday amnesia whose consequences result in forgetting the integrated field of existence of consciousness at the heart of matter. Ordinary cognition influenced by *Manas* (mind) experiences life as *Viparita-Bhavana*—that is, with the erroneous conviction that the visible world of appearances alone is the only reality. This given condition is explained by the influence of *Manas* on *Buddhi* (the discriminating intellect).

Intrinsic to the nature of *Manas* is a dulling of *Buddhi's* clarity. The epistemological term in Sanskrit for this misinterpretation is called *avidya* and is roughly translated as ignorance. The delusional understanding of reality that results from this become formalized in the Sanskrit term *Maya,* meaning the world as ordinarily experienced is a grand illusion.

The fundamental significance of *Prajna-aparadha* lies in the fact that the presence of *Manas* tends to produce an incorrect mind-set. This is the source of the perversions of desire that repetitively seek pleasure in an almost reflexive fashion. The upshot of this is the ordinary tendency to make wrong and unwholesome choices. In this view, wrong choices are ultimately caused by the puissant influence of *Prajna-aparadha* on the operation of *Manas.* The functioning of *Manas* is virtually synonymous with that of desire (*mara, raga, trishna,* and *iccha*) in almost every sense.

The natural, reflexive tendency of *Manas* is to divert attention to extremes. These focal extremes are points near the ends of the spectrum of indulgence and renunciation. *Manas* is always tempted to seek opposites. In fact, the middle path is suicide for *Manas. Manas* desiring life avoids the middle.

What must be clearly understood, if not stressed, is that *Manas,* per se, is not intrinsically bad or evil. *Manas* can be considered man's calling card, ticket of admission, and key to unlocking entry into the manifest world as ordinarily experienced. In this sense, *Manas* is neutral; it functions as an instrument that provides ample access to a world that can be experienced in perceptual, sensuous, and sensual ways. It provides information and opportunities that an individual is free to process in an unlimited number of ways.

If choices and behaviors that are more wholesome (*satmya*) continually discipline and healthfully shape *Manas,* then the functioning of *Buddhi,* the reality intellect, will be empowered, especially in the physical body (*sthula sharira*). This, in turn, will foster more wholesome, safe, and reality-based psychological choices (*pathya*) that are conducive to health. In this way, listening to the body and addressing its needs yield health; the mind or *Manas,* however, may continue to perpetuate ignorance, hedonistic choice, and thus disease.

Kala-Parinama *Kala-Parinama* refers to the transformations produced by the passage of time. It connotes the evolution and involution of states of order and disorder. This change over time refers to the activity of the *doshas.* When the normal level of a *dosha* is increased, this elevation is potentially unhealthful for the functioning of that *dosha.* When a *dosha* is decreased, this suggests less than optimal physiological functioning. Only in the condition of excess, elevated *doshas* and increased doshic functioning does a tendency toward significant imbalance and disease occur. This encompasses changes that may occur in three ways: (1) over the course of the life cycle, (2) during the course of the day, and (3) during the course of the seasonal shifts of the year.

Asatmyendriyartha Samyoga The distinctly Ayurvedic concept of *Asatmyendriyartha Samyoga* can be translated as the unwholesome contact of the sense organs with their sense objects (*vishaya*). The objects of the senses ordinarily denotes perceptions both of parts (qualities) and also of complete (whole) sensory objects. This conception has typically been understood to connote sensory perception referring to the inanimate world. An important, if not even more primary, psychological extension includes the mind's intellectual conceptions of and emotional links to the animate world of uniquely significant human objects.

These object relations, as they have been called in psychodynamic psychology, are sexual in the widest sense since human desire by definition instinctively seeks an object for pleasurable satisfaction. In this sense, sexual denotes attraction whose goal is attachment with reproducing this linking experience and even more novel experiences as an inextricable motivating force. The mind (*Manas*), therefore, is sexual by nature; hence, an important value resides in purifying sexuality and in refining the mind. Relations (*samyoga*) to other humans, moreover, constitute overriding psychodynamic meaningfulness.

They influence all aspects of the self's relationship to itself and to everything else. Love, hate, envy, greed, and jealousy, for example, are forged in this way. The functioning of the sense organs has great significance since it is the central nexus (yoga, *yukti*) between the individual and the outside world. The five sense organs—ears, skin, eyes, tongue, and nose—are called the *jnanendriyas,* the organs that ingest the objects of sensory perception, the sense objects.

When the contact of a sense organ and its object is proper or wholesome (*satmya*), the subtle half of the corresponding primary great Element grasped at that contact point is absorbed. These quanta of energy, the *sukshma Tanmatras,* then go on to feed the more immaterial sheaths (*koshas*), just as food and water feed the physical sheath of the body with the primary Elements.

The sense organs, therefore, are the physical vehicles through which the mind (*Manas*) and the discriminating intellect (*Buddhi*), in fact, effect the absorption of the *Tanmatras,* the subtle Essences, from experience of the outside world into the internal energetic dimensions of the individual. This energetic feeding not only replenishes the individual's own store of *Tanmatras.* The subsequently enhanced *Tanmatras* then go on to produce further vitalization of the body's own primary Elements, which, in turn, continue to nourish and replenish the bodily *doshas, dhatus* (tissues), and so forth.

Frank John Ninivaggi

See also Immune System/Lymphatic System; National Center for Complementary and Alternative Medicine (NCCAM); Yoga.

References

Anandamurti, S. S. *Discourses on Tantra,* Vol. 1. Bombay, India: Ananda Marga.

Anandamurti, S. S. *Discourses on Tantra,* Vol. 2. Bombay, India: Ananda Marga, 1994.

Bryant, E., and L. L. Patton. *Indo-Aryan Controversy: Evidence and Inference in Indian History.* London: Routledge, 2005.

Jee, H. H. Bhagvat Sinh. *Aryan Medical Science.* New Delhi: D. K. Publishers, 1993. Original work published 1895.

Johnson, W. *The Bhagavadgita.* Oxford: Oxford University Press, 1994.

Lele, A., S. Ranade, and A. Qutab. *Pancha-Karma and Ayurvedic Massage.* Pune, India: International Academy of Ayurveda, 1997.

Mishra, Lakshmi Chandra, ed. *Scientific Basis for Ayurvedic Therapies.* Boca Raton, FL: CRC Press, 2004.

Ninivaggi, F. J. "Attention/Deficit-Hyperactivity Disorder in Children and Adolescents: Rethinking Diagnosis and Treatment Implications for Complicated Cases." *Connecticut Medicine* 63, no. 9 (1991): 515–21.

Ranade, S., S. Ranade, A. Qutab, and R. Deshpande. *Health and Disease in Ayurveda and Yoga.* Pune, India: Anmol Prakashan, 1997.

B

BACK PAIN

Back pain plagues millions of Americans in one way or another, and, given the spine's complex structure, it's no wonder. Back pain can be caused by an injury, such as a sprain, strain, or spasm in a muscle or ligament. Too much strain or compression on the spine can lead to a ruptured or bulging disk, another common type of back pain. Arthritis, osteoporosis, and other degenerative conditions can also lead to lower back pain. Injuries to the back can occur in the upper, middle, or lower back, although back pain is most often experienced in the lower back. In fact, lower back pain affects some four out of five adults at least once during their lifetime. Back injury is the second most common neurological condition in the United States after headaches. Americans now spend some $50 billion each year on back treatments (National Institute of Neurological Disorders and Stroke, 2003). Fortunately, lower back injuries do improve in most cases, and only a few may take longer to heal or lead to more serious problems.

The human back is an intricate design of bones, muscles, and other tissues that stretches from the lower trunk to the upper neck. The center or spinal column plays many roles, including supporting the upper body's weight, covering the spinal cord, and acting as a conduit for the nervous system by carrying signals that control body movements and telegraph sensations. The spine includes more than 30 bones or vertebrae, and each has a round hole that creates the channel surrounding the spinal cord. The spinal cord begins at the base of the brain and reaches down to the bottom of the rib cage. The spaces between the vertebrae are separated by round, spongy pads of cartilage called disks. These provide a cushion for the bones as the body moves. Connecting pieces known as ligaments and tendons are attached the muscles of the spinal column and act to hold individual vertebra in place. The spine is divided into four regions: the cervical or neck vertebrae called the C1 to C7; the upper back vertebrae labeled the T1 to T12; the five lumbar vertebrae, also known as the lower back and labeled L1 to L5; and the sacrum, the bones at the base of the spine. Most back pain originates in lumbar region. Back pain may be caused by many different things, including injury when lifting something too heavy. Often when lifting is done by someone who does not have regular physical exercise, their muscles have lost tone and offer less protection to the spine as it twists and turns. Unfortunately, although the spine has great flexibility and range of movement, that movement creates many opportunities for injury. Many people experience damage to one or more of their disks.

Back pain becomes more common with normal aging because spinal disks dry out, shrink, and weaken over time. Chronic conditions such as fibromyalgia and arthritis are often accompanied by back pain and stiffness. Osteoporosis, a condition when bones have become thin and weak, can lead to compressed vertebrae as the person's posture becomes stooped over or hunched. However, osteoporosis is not painful to the back unless a bone fractures. A condition called sciatica, a severe pain that runs the length of the sciatic nerve, from the hip to the heel and down the leg, is estimated to affect some 10 percent of people with back pain. Back pain may be caused by a more serious medical problem such as cancer.

The duration of back pain depends on its cause. For example, back pain triggered by overexertion will improve gradually over several days or weeks. Back pain caused by a ruptured disk may require surgery if the pain fails to respond to other forms of treatment. While sudden back pain can seem very serious at first, most injuries will respond to over-the-counter medicines or prescription analgesics and a day of bed rest. However, doctors recommend against prolonged bed rest, which they believe can lead to loss of muscle and may make the situation worse. The use of hot or cold compresses has been shown in many cases to be effective in easing pain and inflammation. Cold packs or compresses should be applied as soon as possible following a back injury several times a day for two to three days. This should be followed by heat applied for brief intervals to help relax muscles and increase blood flow. Warm baths may also help relax the injured muscles. Of course, if there is no improvement in pain or inflammation after 72 hours of self-care, the injured person should contact his or her primary care physician.

Exercise is believed to be the best way to improve recovery and also to prevent initial back injuries. Abdominal muscle strength is very im-

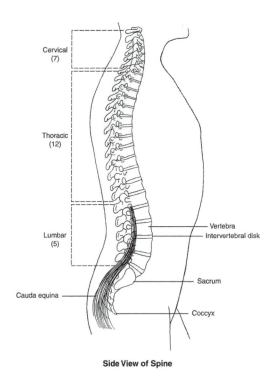

Side View of Spine

National Institute of Arthritis and Musculoskeletal and Skin Diseases graphic of side view of spine. (National Institutes of Health)

portant, and a routine of abdominal strengthening exercises is the best way to avoid problems before they start. Physical therapy, a medically approved form of exercise, involves strengthening as well as lifting under the direction of a trained therapist to avoid further injury and to heal some back injuries. Specific exercises designed to increase flexibility and strength, along with hydrotherapy or massage, may be included in the physical therapy program.

In cases of serious back injury, there are several options for surgery that can be performed in the doctor's office; others may require hospitalization. Invasive back surgery is a serious operation and is not always successful; it is recommended only in cases when other methods of treatment have failed. Types of back surgery include a discectomy, during which the surgeon removes a small piece of the spinal canal roof to relieve pressure on the nerve caused by a bone spur, bulging disk, or other injury. A foraminotomy is an operation designed to enlarge the hole of the spinal canal and relieve nerve pressure. Intradiscal electrothermal therapy utilizes thermal heat to reduce pain caused by a cracked or bulging disk. A special needle is inserted into the disk. The needle is heated, and the heat is used to seal the disk wall. This can, in some cases, reduce irritation of the spinal nerve.

Nucleoplasty is a treatment using radio frequency energy and a needle, which is guided through X-ray images. Once inserted into the disk, the needle creates a channel or space to allow disk material to be removed. Radio frequency lesioning is another type of surgery that uses electrical impulses to reduce or destroy nerve pain. The effects of this procedure can last up to one year. Spinal fusion is among the most serious of the surgical treatments. This involves removing disks between two or more vertebrae. The surgeon then fuses the vertebrae together with bone grafts or different types of devices. This method often means the patient loses flexibility in the spine. There is also a long recovery from this type of surgery as the grafts grow together. Spinal laminectomy or spinal decompression, another serious procedure, requires the removal of the lamina on both sides of the spine. The procedure allows the surgeon to increase the dimension of the spinal canal, which can relieve pressure and ease back pain.

When faced with back pain, more Americans are turning to alternative methods, including acupuncture, biofeedback, yoga, and hypnosis. Statistics show that 4 in 10 adults and 1 in 9 children have tried some form of complementary and alternative medicine (Buch & Browning-Blas, 2010). Acupuncture uses the body's energy to heal the injury or pain. The energy is released following the insertion of needles along precise points throughout the body.

Biofeedback is another alternative method of treatment that can be combined with traditional back treatments. Using relaxation techniques, patients are taught to work to change their response to pain and gain control over muscle tension and heart rate. Results from a study funded by the National Center for Complementary and Alternative Medicine found that individuals who practiced yoga were able to improve their pain, disability, and depression associated with long-term or chronic back pain (Williams et al., 2009). Massage is also thought to be preventive medicine for back pain by keeping soft tissue relaxed and improving blood flow, which can then help reduce muscle stress and strain. Researchers in a pilot study on the use of hypnosis in treating back pain reported a substantial reduction in pain intensity and pain interference. They concluded there was a need for more research to assess the long-term possibilities of back pain improvement from hypnosis treatment (Tan, 2010).

Scientists continue to search for different ways to effectively treat back pain. The National Institute of Neurological Disorders and Stroke (NINDS), part of the National Institutes of Health (NIH) and the U.S. Department of Health and Human Services, is a national resource for federal funding for research on nervous system disorders. The NIH supports pain research through the NINDS as well as through other institutes, including the National Center for Complementary and Alternative Medicine, the National Institute of Arthritis and Musculoskeletal and Skin Diseases, and the National Cancer Institute. Other federal organizations that offer research on low back pain include the Department of Veterans Affairs and the Centers for Disease Control and Prevention.

Research being funded includes a study by scientists using different drugs to treat chronic back pain lasting at least six months. Researchers are also comparing different treatment for the care of acute low back pain, including medical intervention versus acupuncture or massage therapy. The government-funded studies measure symptom relief, improvement of function, and changes in health-related quality of life among back patients.

Other researchers are studying the effects of low-dose radiation as a way to reduce scarring around the spinal cord and improve the outcome for back surgery patients. There is also research measuring the effects of spinal disk replacement surgery for patients with degenerative disk disease. Additionally, NIH-funded research at the Consortial Center for Chiropractic Research is working to encourage collaboration between conventional and chiropractic approaches to back pain and its treatment.

Since surgery is considered a serious, last resort in the treatment of back pain, many herbs and supplements are used for back pain management, but few have been scientifically studied. Before taking any supplements, an individual with back pain should consult with his or her primary care physician, since some supplements can interact with prescription medications and create problems or unintended consequences. Herbs that have been used but not scientifically studied for treatment of back pain include boswellia, capsaicin creams from cayenne pepper, devil's claw, kava, turmeric, valerian, and willow. Vitamin or mineral supplements used but lacking scientific study include calcium and magnesium.

Prevention remains an important ingredient in dealing with back pain. Lifestyle habits that can prevent back pain and injury include regular exercise; stretching before and after exercise; sleeping on one's side or on one's back with a pillow under the knees; stopping smoking; having good posture; using ergonomically designed furniture and tools; and choosing and wearing comfortable, supportive shoes that can cushion the weight load on the spine during standing and walking. It is also important to lift heavy objects safely. That means lifting from a squatting position, using the hips and legs to do the heavy work and not lifting with the back muscles. Safe lifting also requires getting close to the object to be lifted, placing feet shoulder-width apart, and tightening stomach muscles while lifting.

Another factor that can contribute to back pain is anxiety and emotional stress. Over time, emotional stress can contribute to back muscle spasms. The use of anxiety-reducing techniques such as yoga, meditation, and Reiki continue to grow in popularity among Americans and back pain sufferers around the world. According to recent research from London, there are growing numbers of individuals suffering from back pain injury across the United Kingdom (Harms, 2010). The United States and the United Kingdom are not the only countries seeing an increase in back pain. The World Health Organization (WHO) recognized lower back pain as a major cause of disability around the world and initiated an international effort to develop a comprehensive approach to low back pain treatment. A 1994 WHO symposium on back pain back brought together specialists from Japan, Brazil, Indonesia, Russia, and the United States. In 2003 the WHO issued a bulletin (Ehrlich, 2003) addressing its findings on the causes, treatment, and recommendations for dealing with back pain and continues to view back pain as a global issue.

Sharon Zoumbaris

See also Acupuncture; Exercise; Fibromyalgia; Primary Care Physicians; Yoga.

References

"Back Pain." *AltCareDex Medicine Modality* (May 2010), www.accessmylibrary.com/archive/435505-altcaredex-medicine-modality.html.

Buch, Linda J., and Kristen Browning-Blas. "Relief for Your Back Is at Hand: Alternative Remedies from Rolfing to Reiki Hold the Magic Touch Many Sufferers Seek." *Denver Post* (February 15, 2010): C-01, www.denverpost.com.

Ehrlich, George E. "Low Back Pain." *Bulletin of the World Health Organization* 81 (2003): 671–76.

Ernst, E., and A. White. "Acupuncture for Back Pain: A Meta-analysis of Randomized Controlled Trials."*Archives of Internal Medicine* 158, no. 20 (1998): 2235–41.

Harms, M. "Low Back Pain: What Determines Functional Outcome at Six Months? *BMC Musculoskeletal Disorders* 11 (2010): 236.

National Institute of Neurological Disorders and Stroke. "Low Back Pain Fact Sheet." NIH Publication No. 03-5161 (July 2003), www.ninds.nih.gov.

Tan, G. "Hypnosis Treatment for Chronic Low Back Pain." *International Journal of Clinical and Experimental Hypnosis* 58, no. 1 (2010): 53–68.

Williams, K., C. Abildso, L. Steinberg, et al. "Evaluation of the Effectiveness and Efficacy of Iyengar Yoga Therapy on Chronic Low Back Pain." *Spine* 34, no. 19 (2009): 2066–76.

BACTERIA

Bacteria are small, free-living, single-cell organisms without a true nucleus and bounded by a rigid cell wall composed of protein and carbohydrate components. These organisms reproduce asexually by binary fission (splitting). As a group they are among the most numerous and diverse organisms in the world. In fact, the average human body is made up of trillions of cells and houses nearly 10 times that number of bacterial cells. Individual bacteria, however, are only visible with the aid of the microscope. Bacteria are distinguished from other single-cell organisms such as yeasts, molds, and protozoa by the lack of an organized nucleus as well as by more subtle biochemical properties.

Researchers are looking at the interaction between the human immune system and the legion of bacteria on the skin in hopes of understanding what triggers many diseases and why allergic disorders such as eczema, hay fever, and asthma have dramatically increased over the past few decades. The $173 million Human Microbiome Project (HMP) is led by a dermatologist at the Center for Cancer Research at the National Cancer Institute and a geneticist at the National Institutes of Health. To increase their understanding, scientists are closely monitoring the microbial communities found on half a dozen body sites, including the gut, mouth, and skin. Up until now, only the hardiest and most numerous bacterial species were studied in the laboratory. However, recent discoveries and improvements in the study of DNA sequencing have improved the technology needed by the HMP.

The study of the unseen world of these organisms was first revealed through the use of the microscope, invented in the early 1600s. These early microscopes were simply single lenses of high curvature, such as small spherical glass beads of very short focal length. The best of these microscopes had a magnification of about 200 times.

The acknowledged pioneer in both microscope construction and careful observation was the Delft cloth merchant Anthony van Leeuwenhoek. Leeuwenhoek produced a series of landmark communications to the Royal Society of London that extended from 1673 until his death in 1723. Leeuwenhoek described what appeared to be little animals ("animalcules") in many seemingly pure substances, from melted snow and vinegar to extracts of spices from the Far East.

These are the first reports on the organisms we now take to be the subject of the field of microbiology. Not only did Leeuwenhoek note that these little animals had regular structures, which he arranged in a simple classification scheme, but he also reported that some were motile (able to move themselves) and that they seemed to increase in number, that is, to grow and multiply over time.

Although many objects that Leeuwenhoek described are now recognized as amoeba, paramecia, diatoms, and small multicellular organisms such as rotifers, some of the smallest objects appear to have been true bacteria. Leeuwenhoek's classification scheme is the distant precursor of the one in use today. He described four types of these tiny organisms based on shape and size: round cocci, rod-shaped bacteria (two sizes), and helical spirillia.

In 1773 Otto Friedrich Müller (1730–1784) published a treatise on "infusoria," the name for the collection of organisms that were found in various teas and other water extracts of plant and animal materials. Müller, using the improved microscopes of the 18th century, including the compound microscope with multiple lenses, recognized two main groups of infusoria—*Monas* and *Vibrio*—which contain bacterial forms.

Müller's scheme was used in the late 18th century and was extended in 1838 with the famous study by Carl Gustave von Ehrenberg (1795–1876), who published *Die Infusionthierchen als vollkemmene Organismen,* a large folio atlas with extensive hand-colored, engraved plates. Ehrenberg, like his predecessors, did not make a distinction between protozoa and bacteria. They were all classified as infusoria, and all were believed to have tiny stomachs and other parts analogous to those of larger animals. His classification scheme was detailed, complex, and extensive. Of relevant interest are his descriptions of the family Vibrionia, which was comprised of five genera: *Bacterium, Vibrio, Spirochaeta, Spirillum,* and *Spirodiscus.* Despite Ehrenberg's detailed descriptions, we cannot unequivocally identify many of his organisms with current microbial classifications.

Throughout the 19th century, the classification of microorganisms evolved and developed, but all attempts were limited by the fact that they were superficially descriptive, not physiologic, morphologic but without the aid of chemical stains, and mixtures rather than homogeneous samples of the organisms.

As soon as bacterial culture became routine, following the work of the 19th-century bacteriologists, it was noted that growth requirements and culture conditions were properties that were useful in characterizing the various bacterial types. These physiological studies paralleled the study of metabolism in both plants and animals and showed that bacteria were similar in many ways to higher forms of life.

Although bacteria share basic metabolic pathways with all other organisms, they are in general much more adaptable and exhibit a great diversity of special physiological and metabolic processes. As free-living, single-cell organisms, functional and biochemical specialization that is a hallmark of multicellular organisms is not usually available to them as a survival strategy.

The relationship of bacteria to disease, fermentation, and putrefaction was elucidated toward the end of the 19th century initially through the work of Louis Pasteur, Robert Koch, and their colleagues. So-called germ theories of disease provided an explanation for the specificity of various diseases while also explaining mechanisms of contagion, pathogenesis as a result of bacterial toxins, and, subsequently, immunity to infectious diseases.

Bacteria living in diverse environments have many special structures, chemicals, and metabolic pathways to exploit their particular ecological niches. Thus, the membrane lipids of bacteria living at low temperatures differ significantly from those of bacteria adapted to warm temperatures. The differing lipid compositions allow maintenance of membrane fluidity at different temperatures. The adaptive utilization of a wide variety of carbon compounds for energy, the presence or absence of the requirement for oxygen for energy production, and the production of secondary metabolites that are toxic to environmental competitors are all examples of this biological diversity. This diversity of bacterial metabolism has been exploited for many useful purposes, including such age-old processes as production of vinegar by *Acetobacter* and such recent discoveries as antibiotic production from *Streptomyces.*

Many bacteria have evolved special, mutually beneficial relationships with other organisms. The bacteria that inhabit the intestines of animals are supported by the food that the animal eats, but at the same time, the bacteria produce certain essential nutrients as by-products, which are absorbed by the animal host. One

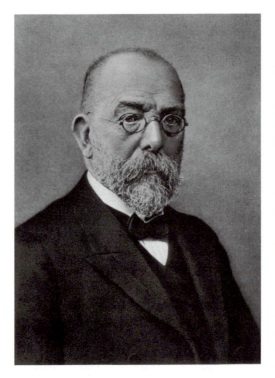

A physician and founder of bacteriology, Robert Koch was the first to prove that specific microorganisms caused specific diseases. (National Library of Medicine)

such example is the vitamin biotin. The intestinal bacteria *Escherichia coli* produces all the biotin needed by humans. In the case of certain animals that subsist on a diet of grass, such as cattle, special bacteria in their stomachs can digest cellulose to produce sugars, which are absorbed by the cattle as their main source of nutrition. These animals, called ruminants, are absolutely dependent on being colonized by these cellulose-digesting bacteria. A similar situation exists in some plants (legumes) that harbor bacteria in small root nodules. These bacteria are able to absorb atmospheric nitrogen and convert it (by a process called nitrogen fixation) into ammonia and related compounds, the most important of which are the amino acids. These amino acids are then provided to the plant for protein synthesis and growth. The process of nitrogen fixation is crucial to the existence of life on earth. An extreme case of this type of mutual benefit is represented by the subcellular organelles called mitochondria, which exist in most eucaryotic cells. There is strong evidence that mitochondria evolved from bacteria that long ago invaded the cytoplasm of some cells, became a useful source of oxidative energy production for the cell, and along the way lost the ability to live independently.

One type of growth process distinguishes bacteria from many higher organisms: the ability, when placed in unfavorable environments, to develop into a dormant state known as a spore form. Spores are living cells that are metabolically quiescent, surrounded by a durable wall, and relatively dehydrated in comparison with normal cells. Under normal growth conditions, spores germinate to produce normal vegetatively growing bacteria again. The spore forms of bacteria are highly resistant to drying, to temperature (they are not killed by boiling water temperature but require high-pressure steam above 120 degrees Celsius to be killed), and to ultraviolet light. Sporulation is a survival strategy that is common to bacteria that live in diverse environments and is less common in bacteria that inhabit more constant ecological niches, such as the mammalian intestine, for example.

The widespread presence of bacteria and their adaptability to many ecological niches provide them with the ability to move about in nature with speed and efficiency. Humans perceive such survival strategies as contagion and the basis for epidemic disease. Bacteria can often be spread by simple physical contact, which transfers a few organisms to a new location. Often, however, water or air currents serve to carry bacteria to new environments. Some bacteria have evolved to be carried by other organisms (called vectors) such as insects or other animals. One important example is the transmission of human plague bacteria by the bite of the rat flea.

Although bacteria do not have a membrane-bounded organelle, the nucleus in which the genetic apparatus of the cell resides, their genetic organization is similar to that of all other cellular life. Genes are encoded in DNA, and the genetic code of bacteria is identical to that of higher organisms (with a few interesting variations in the evolutionarily ancient *Archea*). Most bacteria reproduce by binary fission so they form clonal populations, all descended from a founder organism. However, some bacteria have evolved mechanisms for mating and genetic exchange as a way to increase genetic diversity and, presumably, evolutionary fitness. So-called bacterial sex has been a very useful tool for analysis of genetic mechanisms at the molecular level.

William C. Summers

See also Antibiotics; Immune System/Lymphatic System; Pasteur, Louis.

References

Dubos, René J., with an addendum by C. F. Robinow. *The Bacterial Cell in Its Relation to Problems of Virulence, Immunity and Chemotherapy.* Cambridge, MA: Harvard University Press, 1955.

Dyer, Betsey Dexter. *A Field Guide to the Bacteria.* Ithaca, NY: Cornell University Press, 2003.

Hughes, Virginia. "Our Body the Ecosystem: Even a Healthy Human Body Is Teeming with Bacteria. Studying the Subtle Interplay between Man and Microbe Could Help Doctors Understand Diseases That Affect Millions." *Popular Science* (March 2011): 54.

Ingraham, John L. *March of the Microbes: Sighting the Unseen.* Cambridge, MA: Belknap Press of Harvard University Press, 2010.

Maczulak, Anne Elizabeth. *Allies and Enemies: How the World Depends on Bacteria.* Upper Saddle River, NJ: FT Press, 2011.

Tomes, Nancy. *The Gospel of Germs: Men, Women, and the Microbe in American Life.* Cambridge, MA: Harvard University Press, 1999.

BARIATRIC SURGERY

Bariatric surgery, also called obesity surgery, is the last resort for severely obese people who have tried weight loss and exercise programs and have repeatedly failed. The different procedures include gastric-bypass surgery, the lap band procedure, vertical banded gastroplasty, and jejuoileal bypass. The theory behind all types of obesity surgery is simple: if the volume the stomach holds can be reduced, bypassed, or shortened, people will not be able to consume or, in some cases, absorb as many calories. Obesity surgery typically reduces the volume of food the stomach can hold from about four cups to about a half a cup. But these procedures are not a magic solution. There is a long-term failure rate of up to 50 percent, additional surgery is necessary in some cases, and many patients face daily complications such as intolerance to foods high in fats, lactose intolerance, vomiting, diarrhea, and intestinal discomfort.

Celebrities who have had bariatric surgery include Al Roker, Sharon Osbourne, Roseanne Barr, professional soccer player Diego Maradona, and singer Carnie Wilson. The singer had her surgery in 1999 but, like may others, has gained back a significant amount of her initial weight loss. According to Daniel Jones, doctor of the bariatric program at Beth Israel Deaconess Medical Center in Boston, at least 5 percent of surgery patients regain the weight they initially lost after surgery. Within the first two years, most patients who have the procedures can expect to lose up to 80 percent of their excess weight. Unfortunately, for many the factors that caused the initial overweight remain after the surgery. Counseling and other forms of psychological support are often needed.

Gastric-bypass surgery, developed in the 1960s, is a procedure in which surgeons sew the stomach shut to a fraction of its original size, then reattach that portion directly to the small intestine, limiting room for food and time for absorption. Patients must be carefully screened physically and psychologically for the operation, which is suggested only for people with 100 or more pounds to lose, and always as a last resort. The operation can be risky; stomach perforations, infection, allergic reaction to anesthesia, excessive bleeding or blood clots in the lungs, and heart attacks are among the serious, and sometimes fatal, complications. And because the surgery can affect absorption in the intestine, all gastric-bypass patients must take vitamins for the rest of their lives.

After the procedure, patients need to follow a lifelong diet, exercise, and behavior modification program, keeping in mind how important their food choices are now that they can literally fill up on a single piece of bread. Once patients return to eating solid food, poor choices leave them without necessary nutrients and can even make them physically ill. Foods to avoid include carbonated beverages, popcorn, nuts, fried foods, red meat, and sugar—meaning no pie, cookies, or cake. Still, some surgery patients experience a 10- to 20-pound weight gain once the new stomach stretches a bit, while others who do not adopt the necessary lifestyle and dietary changes find themselves returning to their preoperation weight.

The American Society for Metabolic and Bariatric Surgery (ASMBS) reports more than 15 million Americans are morbidly obese, and in 2009 an estimated 220,000 people had some form of bariatric surgery. Recent statistics released by the Bariatric Outcomes Longitudinal Database indicated that bariatric surgery, while invasive and risky, is becoming safer. Current figures show that 5 patients in 1,000 die from gastric-bypass surgery.

On the other hand, complications from obesity, such as diabetes, high blood pressure, and arthritis, cost consumers millions of dollars in related health care costs each year. Still, many health insurance companies do not cover the cost of the operation, which can range from $20,000 to $25,000. Figures from the National Institutes of Health say that almost 90 percent of dieters who use other methods regain the weight they lost within five years. But a 1995 study cited by the Gainesville, Florida–based chapter of the ASMBS reported that 14 years after the surgery, most bypass patients have managed to keep off more than 50 percent of their original weight loss, over 100 pounds in most cases.

The success rate for the surgery may be one reason the number of gastric-bypass operations performed in the past several years has jumped by as much as 25 percent. But this increased popularity can also be attributed to publicized surgeries such as the operation on Carnie Wilson, daughter of the Beach Boys' Brian Wilson and a member of the singing group Wilson Phillips. Wilson was morbidly obese and, after trying and failing at all sorts of diets, she dropped 150 pounds and almost 20 dress sizes following gastric-bypass surgery in August 1999. She even had the procedure broadcast live on the Internet as a way to educate people about the reality of morbid obesity. Although Wilson has gained and lost large amounts of weight since the operation, she continues to educate others about the realities of weight loss surgery.

The less invasive lap band procedure (short for laparoscopic adjustable gastric band), approved in June 2001 by the U.S. Food and Drug Administration, is intended for people with smaller weight loss requirements and involves the surgeon wrapping a band around the top part of the stomach to restrict how much food it can hold. The procedure is cheaper and faster than gastric-bypass surgery and requires a shorter hospital stay. Lap band surgery takes less than an hour and requires an overnight stay, compared to the more extensive bypass surgery that lasts two to three hours and requires a three-day hospital recuperation. The adjustable silicon band with a balloon at the end that is used in the lap band procedure can be adjusted or even removed if the patient experiences serious side effects—a reversal not possible with the gastric-bypass procedure.

Other obesity surgery procedures include vertical banded gastroplasty, where an artificial pouch is created using staples in a different section of the stomach. Plastic mesh is sutured into part of the pouch to prevent it from dilating. In this surgery, like the gastric-bypass operation, the food enters the small intestine farther along than it would enter normally, reducing the time available for absorption of nutrients and calories. Jejuoileal bypass involves shortening the small intestine. This procedure has a high occurrence of serious complications, such as chronic diarrhea and liver disease, and is thought to be the least effective of any of the procedures. It is rarely performed now and has been replaced by safer procedures.

Following obesity surgery, most patients are restricted to a liquid diet for up to three weeks. Patients then graduate to a diet of puréed food for about a month or two until they can tolerate solid food. High-fat food is especially hard to digest and causes diarrhea. Patients also must be careful not to eat too quickly or to ingest too much food or they can experience nausea, vomiting, and intestinal dumping, when undigested food is shunted too quickly into the small intestine, causing pain, diarrhea, and dizziness.

Meanwhile, researchers continue to study the complex system of brain and body chemicals that govern weight and appetite. Exciting new studies on the growth hormone ghrelin have some scientists suggesting that an effective weight loss drug is closer than ever before. The development and use of obesity drugs came under close scrutiny in 1997, when the FDA ordered the withdrawal of the drug combination fen-phen when it was discovered to have dangerous effects on the heart. Still, doctors say it may be a long time before obesity surgery becomes obsolete, and at this time it remains the best option for some patients who have tried everything else and failed.

Marjolijn Bijlefeld and Sharon Zoumbaris

See also Dieting; Ghrelin; Health Insurance; Obesity; Vitamins.

References

Abouzeid, Nehme E. "Insane Growth in Inquiries about Surgeries for Obesity." *Boston Business Journal* 21, no. 39 (November 2, 2001): 39–40.

Alexander, Cynthia L. *The Emotional First + Aid Kit: A Practical Guide to Life after Bariatric Surgery.* West Chester, PA: Matrix Medical Communications, 2009.

Crawford, Dan, and Jeff Bell. "This Lap Band Is No Opening Act at Polaris." *Business First-Columbus* 17, no. 48 (July 20, 2001): A3.

Davidson, Tish. "Obesity Surgery." In *Gale Encyclopedia of Medicine,* 1st ed., edited by Jacqueline L. Longe and Deidre S. Blanchfield, 2079–80. Detroit: Gale Research, 1999.

Davis, Garth. *Experts Guide to Weight Loss Surgery: Is It Right for Me? What Happens after Surgery? How Do I Keep the Weight Off?* New York: Hudson Street Press/Penguin, 2009.

Park, Alice. "Weight-Loss Surgery: Safe, But Does It Work?" *Time,* June, 25, 2009, www.time.com/time/health/article/0,8599,1907094,00.html.

Parker-Pope, Tara. "The Skinny on Fat." *O, The Oprah Magazine,* May 2010, 166–69.

BASAL METABOLISM

The secret to weight loss or to maintaining a healthy weight is calories in versus calories expended. Another key part of this equation is what is known as basal metabolism. For healthy adults, caloric needs equal calories for basal metabolism function plus calories burned in food processing plus calories used in physical activity. Basal metabolism is the number of calories burned by your body in carrying out basic functions while at rest such as breathing, circulating blood, adjusting hormone levels, growing, and repairing cells.

If the number of calories taken in goes above the number of calories needed, then an individual will gain weight. An individual's basal metabolism and the number of calories he or she uses each day depends on several factors, including body size, amount of muscle and fat, and sex (men usually have less body fat and more muscle and for that reason burn more calories while at rest). Another factor affecting basal metabolic rate is age. As people age, their amount of muscle decreases and fat increases and the body slows down its calorie consumption. The basal metabolic rate accounts for up to 75 percent of the calories burned each day (Mayo Clinic, 2009).

Metabolism is a constant process and is controlled by a series of chemical reactions. It can be influenced by temperature and has been shown to increase slightly in cold climates. More calories are burned if it is cold enough to cause shivering, which involves involuntary contraction and relaxation of muscles. A person's basal metabolism is somewhat inherited and can also be affected by certain diseases or metabolic disorders. Some medical conditions slow metabolism, such as Cushing's syndrome, polycystic ovary syndrome, Type 1 and Type 2 diabetes, and hyperthyroidism.

These metabolic disorders cause abnormal chemical reactions in the body's cells and usually involve enzymes or hormones and how they function. When the metabolism is blocked or ineffective, it leads to a toxic buildup of substances or a deficiency of those same substances, such as in the case of insulin with diabetes. While individuals do not have total control over the speed of their metabolism, they can burn more calories through physical activity such as aerobic exercise and strength training.

Sharon Zoumbaris

See also Aerobic Exercise; Diabetes; Dieting; Polycystic Ovary Syndrome (PCOS); Weight Training.

References

Karas, Jim. "The Easiest Way to Take off Pounds: If You Speed up Your Metabolism, You'll Burn More Calories Every Day and Lose Weight Every Week." *Good Housekeeping,* January 2005, 173–75.

Kinucan, Paige, and Len Kravitz. "Controversies in Metabolism: How Do Resistance Training, Diet and Age Affect Resting Metabolic Rate?" *IDEA Fitness Journal* 3, no. 1 (January 2006): 20–23.

Mayo Clinic. "Metabolism and Weight loss: How You Burn Calories" (2009), www.mayoclinic.com.

Powell, Cheryl. "Weight Loss and Metabolism Are Linked." *Seattle Times* (March 6, 2005), http://seattletimes.nwsource.com/html/health/2002197301_healthmetabolism06.html.

Ray, D. Claiborne. "Chilling Out: Burning Calories." *New York Times* (January 11, 2011): D2.

Watson, Cathy, Don Jewett, and Jon Richfield. "Middle-Age Spread." *New Scientist* 199, no. 2665 (July 19, 2008): 57.

BASIC FOUR (FOODS)

Nutrition and our understanding of it have changed quite a bit over the decades. Nowhere is that more obvious than in the government's restructuring and rewriting of the food groups. The Basic Four food guide was produced in 1956 by the U.S. Department of Agriculture (USDA) as a tool to educate the public on nutritional matters. The difficult part of the government's task was working with food growers and producers to support the sale of those agricultural products. This led some critics to question whether dietary guidelines such as the Basic Four were designed for optimum health or to sell more food. To answer that question, it is necessary to go back to the early days of the USDA.

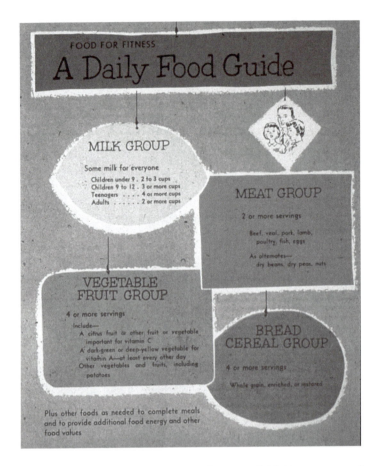

Food for Fitness: A Daily Food Guide, 1956. (U.S. Department of Agriculture)

The USDA published its first dietary recommendations as early as 1894. At that time, the study of vitamins and minerals was in its infancy and little was known about how to prevent nutritional diseases such as scurvy and beriberi. It was during these early days that W.O. Atwater, the original director of the Office of Experiment Stations in the USDA published the *Farmers' Bulletin*. In it, Atwater made the connecting between dietary intake and health. At this point, the government was still a long way from creating the Basic Four.

In 1916 the USDA released *Food for Young Children,* a guide that divided foods into five groups: milk and meat, cereals, vegetables and fruits, fats and fatty foods, and sugars and sugary foods. This work was updated several times into the 1920s, adding suggested amounts of food to purchase each week for the average U.S. household.

During the Great Depression, the USDA revised those plans into 12 major food groups and suggested which food groups to buy and use each week to meet basic health needs. President Franklin Roosevelt brought increased attention to the government's focus on nutrition in 1941 with his National Nutrition Conference for Defense. Out of his efforts came the first Recommended Dietary Allowances (RDAs) issued by the government. Included in the RDAs was a concept called the Basic Seven food guide, which was designed to help Americans cope with rationing during World War II.

It was not until 1956 that the Basic Four food guide was released with its four recommended groups of milk, meat, fruits and vegetables, and grains. The Basic Four would become the government's chief education tool for the next two decades. With its slogan of "Eat every day the four, four, two, two way," the Basic Four diet called for two cups or more daily from the milk group, two or more two-ounce servings each day from the meat group, four or more daily servings from the grains group, and four or more servings each day from the vegetable and fruit group (Storm, 1991). The government focus at this point was still on getting enough nutrients to Americans, an influence left over from the Depression and rationing of the war years.

It was in the 1970s that the government's message shifted from suggesting that Americans get enough to eat and began to consider that people were now getting too much to eat. In 1977, the *Dietary Goals for the United States* was released by the Senate Select Committee on Nutrition and Human Needs. The goals were meant to deal with the growing problem of chronic diseases caused by the United States' emerging obesity epidemic and its love affair with fat, cholesterol, sodium, and sugar.

This guide modified the Basic Four and added a new, fifth food group of fats, sweets, and alcoholic beverages. Just two years later, the Department of Health, Education and Welfare (now the Department of Health and Human Services) released a study that showed a strong link between nutrition and health. Those findings, published as *Healthy People: The Surgeon General's Report on Health Promotion and Disease Prevention,* made the case that excess fat, cholesterol, sodium, and sugar were factors in the country's growing disease rates. While this news was greeted with skepticism by the beef and dairy food industries, it led to the release of the first edition of the *Dietary Guidelines for Americans* in 1980. This time the government suggested numbers of servings from five of the six major food groups and called for reduced consumption of the sixth group—the fats, oils and sweets.

Since 1980 the *Dietary Guidelines for Americans* have been reissued every five years by the USDA as part of its consumer education program that also includes the food pyramid known as MyPyramid. The USDA and the Department of Health and Human Services released the 2010 *Dietary Guidelines for Americans* with an even stronger focus on portion sizes and the message of cutting back on overall intake of sodium and saturated and trans fats while increasing daily consumption of fruits, vegetables, and other high-fiber foods.

Another organization with its own take on the Basic Four food groups is the Physician's Committee for Responsible Medicine (PCRM), which unveiled its proposal in 1991. The PCRM plan, called the New Four Food Groups, emphasizes a plant-based, high-fiber diet. Its four groups are grains, legumes, vegetables, and fruits and leaves out any mention of meat and dairy products. At the time of its release, the PCRM called on Americans to abandon the USDA Basic Four and adopt its nutritional advice. Only time can tell what dietary guidelines will contain in the coming decades, as new technology and research reveal more about the makeup of a well-balanced diet. One thing, however, is for certain: the Basic Four has been replaced. Now, as Americans become more health and fitness conscious than at any other time in history, individuals can look to the government for nutrition information, keeping in mind the importance of weighing that information against the interests of the food producers.

Sharon Zoumbaris

See also Fats; MyPlate; Recommended Dietary Allowance (RDA); U.S. Department of Agriculture (USDA).

References

Brody, Jane. *Jane Brody's Nutrition Book: A Lifetime Guide to Good Eating for Better Health and Weight Control.* New York: W.W. Norton, 1981.

Cerrato, Paul L. "Goodbye Four Food Groups." *RN* 55, no. 12 (1992): 61.

Davis, Carole, and Etta Saltos. "Dietary Recommendations and How They Have Changed over Time." USDA Economic Research Service, www.ers.usda.gov/publications/aib750/aib750.pdf.

Gish, Jennifer. "Eat This: Forget the Food Pyramid, a Simple Message on Nutrition at Last." *Times Union* (Albany, New York; April 2, 2011), www.timesunion.com/default/article/Eat-this/1319537.php.

Sobel, Bruce Scott. "A New Balancing Act: Re-educating America about the Four Food Groups." *Total Health* (February 1993): 15.

Storm, Jackie. "A New Look at an Old Concept: Did Mother Know Best? The Four Basic Food Groups." *Women's Sports and Fitness* (January–February 1991): 18.

Strickland, David A. "New Food Groups: Data or Dogma? *Medical World News* (May 1991): 28.

U.S. Department of Agriculture. "Basic 4 Food Guide (1956–1979)," www.nal.usda.gov/fnic/history/asic4.htm.

BIOFEEDBACK

Biofeedback, developed in the 1960s, uses devices to amplify and provide feedback to an individual about the body's physiological processes. An individual undergoing biofeedback training is guided through a series of relaxation, breathing, or visualization techniques while receiving visual or auditory feedback from biofeedback devices to gain conscious awareness of and control over typically unconscious autonomic physiological states.

Biofeedback devices are used to monitor physiologic processes, including body temperature (using a thermistor or feedback thermometer), muscle tension (electromyography), blood pressure, heart rate or peripheral blood flow (photoplethysmograph), blood gases (capnometer), breathing patterns (pneumograph), and perspiration (electrodermograph or galvanic skin response). Neurofeedback provides information about brain waves through the use of electroencephalograph and neural activity using hemoencephalography.

Biodots (also known as stress dots) are made of heat-sensitive self-adhesive material that is attached to the skin. Biodots, which change color in response to changes in surface skin temperature, are used as a type of biofeedback to help control stress. Mood rings (which emerged in the 1970s) were a precursor of biodots.

Mind-body medicine is a holistic approach to healing based on interactions between the brain, mind, body, and behavior focusing on the ways spiritual, emotional, mental, and behavioral factors can influence physical health. Biofeedback is one of several mind-body techniques used to teach people how to decrease their level of stress or muscular tension, change breathing patterns, or modify their emotional state. Other mind-body therapies include relaxation training, cognitive-behavioral therapy, hypnosis, visual imagery, yoga, tai chi, qigong, and meditation.

Research has shown that learning to consciously control autonomic processes using mind-body techniques can sometimes decrease the severity of physical issues such as asthma, hypertension, and various stress-related disorders (Astin, Shapiro,

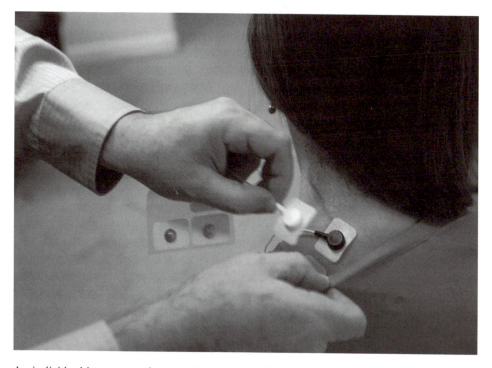

An individual is connected to monitors during a biofeedback therapy session at the Rehabilitation Institute of Chicago on January 31, 2008. (AP/Wide World Photos)

Eisenberg, & Forys, 2003). Biofeedback has been used to treat pain disorders such as headache, migraines, fibromyalgia, back pain, and chronic pain and to alleviate symptoms associated with cancer and chemotherapy (e.g., Sherman, 2004).

In addition to treating issues primarily regarded as physical, biofeedback has demonstrated efficacy in treating some cases of attention deficit hyperactivity disorder (Friel, 2007), substance abuse disorders (e.g., Scott, Kaiser, Othmer, & Sideroff, 2005), and some types of anxiety (Reed & Saslow, 1980). More research is needed to establish the effectiveness of biofeedback treatment for eating disorders (Pop-Jordanova, 2000) and test anxiety (Reed & Saslow, 1980).

Gretchen M. Reevy

See also Back Pain; Fibromyalgia; Meditation; Stress.

References

Astin, J.A., S.L. Shapiro, , D.M. Eisenberg, and K.L. Forys. "Mind-Body Medicine: State of the Science, Implications for Practice." *Journal of the American Board of Family Practice* 16 (2003): 131–47.

Friel, P.N. "EEG Biofeedback in the Treatment of Attention Deficit Hyperactivity Disorder." *Alternative Medicine Review* 12 (2007): 146–51.

Pop-Jordanova, N. "Psychological Characteristics and Biofeedback Mitigation in Preadolescents with Eating Disorders." *Pediatrics International* 42 (2000): 76–81.

Reed, M., and C. Saslow. "The Effects of Relaxation Instructions and EMG Biofeedback on Test Anxiety, General Anxiety, and Locus of Control." *Journal of Clinical Psychology* 36 (1980): 683–90.

Scott, W.C., D. Kaiser, S. Othmer, and S.I. Sideroff. "Effects of an EEG Biofeedback Protocol on a Mixed Substance Abusing Population." *American Journal of Drug and Alcohol Abuse* 31 (2005): 455–69.

Sherman, R.A. *White Paper: Clinical Efficacy of Psychophysiological Assessments and Biofeedback Interventions for Chronic Pain Disorders,* Association for Applied Psychophysiology and Biofeedback (2004), www.aapb.org/tl_files/AAPB/files/Whitepaper onPain.pdf.

BIPOLAR DISORDER

Bipolar disorder is sometimes known popularly as manic depression. It has been identified historically as one of many mood disorders. More recently the data suggest that it may be one of the forms of mental illness that is diagnostically more precisely defined as related to borderline personality syndrome with potential psychotic components. The symptoms of bipolar disorder are alternating patterns of mania and depression.

Mania is a form of hyperactivity, grandiosity, and schizoform euphoria that dissociates the patient from reality. It prompts such behavior as situation-inappropriate or uncharacteristic shopping sprees, megalomania, and obsessive collecting or hoarding. Frequently such patients have decreased sleep needs, racing thoughts, rapid speech, unlimited energy, and substantially increased sociability.

Bipolar Disorder Affects Many

Formerly known as manic depression, bipolar disorder includes a manic phase characterized by symptoms of euphoria, irritability, rapid thinking and speech, risky behavior, and sleeplessness. The other side of the illness is the depression, which may include irritability, excessive fatigue, slowed thinking, insomnia, sadness and lack of interest in life, and thoughts of suicide. The disorder affects millions of Americans. Award-winning actress Catherine Zeta-Jones publicly acknowledged in 2011 that she is undergoing treatment for bipolar II, a less severe type of the disorder.

The understanding of a difference between clinical depression and the combination of mania and depression or bipolar developed in the 1950s thanks to psychiatrist Karl Leonhard. Finally, in 1980 the term bipolar disease replaced manic-depressive disorder as a diagnostic term in the *Diagnostic and Statistical Manual of the American Psychiatric Association*. It was also in the 1980s that researchers realized there was a difference in adult and juvenile bipolar disorder.

A prominent authority in the field of bipolar disease is Kay Redfield Jamison, a psychologist who is professor of psychiatry at the Johns Hopkins University School of Medicine. Jamison has bipolar disorder herself and has written much on the subject, both for professionals and for the general public, including *An Unquiet Mind: A Memoir of Moods and Madness* (Knopf, 1995).

—*Sharon Zoumbaris*

Depression is a state of flattened affect or feeling in which the patient loses all resilience of mood, motivation, ability to carry on normal work, and to attend to schedules. Such patients normally lack social responsiveness and have no capacity for feeling mad, sad, glad, or scared. The depression is characterized by an inability to make decisions or concentrate, lack of self-confidence, feelings of emptiness, repressed libido, inadequate appetite, and loss of any sense of usefulness. Patients with depression tend to feel helpless and hopeless. This type of depression should not be confused with abject grief, in which the affect remains to some extent resilient, retaining some ability to be sad, mad, glad, or scared. Depressed patients may lose weight, draw religious ideation into their symptomology such as feeling they have done some unforgivable evil, and contemplate suicide.

The wave patterns of mania and depression may vary widely in length for a given person and between persons. Some patients may have long periods of mania followed by short periods of depression or vice versa. The variation pattern in each phase may be a matter of hours, days, months, or even years. Some persons suffering from this disorder experience only one of the two contrasting phases: mania or depression. This condition is referred to as a unipolar pattern, but the disease is the same and is technically still referred to as bipolar disorder.

Recent statistics released by the Centers for Disease Control and Prevention estimate that bipolar disorder affects approximately 5.7 million American adults, or about 2.6 percent of the adult population. The term *manic depression* was originally used to describe what is now known as bipolar disorder. Manic-depressive disorder was replaced in 1980 in the *Diagnostic and Statistical Manual of Mental Disorders* (*DSM*) of the American Psychiatric Association by bipolar disorder. The *DSM* provides a common language and standard criteria for the classification of mental disorders and is used in the United States and around the world.

The *Diagnostic and Statistical Manual of Mental Disorders,* fourth edition, text revision, discusses and defines bipolar disorder in detail (American Psychiatric Association, 2000, pp. 179–91). It delineates two categories of this disorder: bipolar I and II. The former includes single manic episode, most recent episode hypomanic, most recent episode manic, most recent episode mixed, most recent episode depressed, and most recent episode unspecified. Any of these types of suffering may be graded as mild, moderate, or severe. They may present with or without psychotic features. Bipolar II refers to conditions of partial or full remission. In keeping with the first type of bipolar II disorder, patients who have suffered mania only once are nonetheless diagnosed as having bipolar disorder.

Little is known about the cause of bipolar disorder, though there is overwhelming evidence that it follows familial patterns and so it is assumed to be genetically inherited and biochemically mediated. Fortunately, there are now medications for managing this form of dysfunction, though it is not curable. The Kline method of treatment employed lithium with moderately good results, but the side effects of dulling patient affect and depressing energy levels were counterproductive. More recently, patients treated with a consistent and lifelong regimen of divalproex sodium or similar medications usually maintain a normal and stable mood and affect. Some psychiatrists treat bipolar disorder with medications such as fluoxetine, which modulates serotonin uptake levels, but this usually increases the danger of inducing anxiety and mania reactions and incites more rapid cycling of the mood shift patterns.

In severe cases of bipolar disorder, the patient may experience hallucinations and delusions. In such instances, particularly when suicidal thoughts are at a critical stage, some practitioners recommend electroconvulsive therapy. Psychotherapy is of virtually no use in controlling bipolar mood shifts or managing the disorder but is crucial as an ancillary therapy for patients who are controlled by an appropriate medical regimen.

Psychotherapy is valuable in such cases for helping the patient rise out of and correct all the psychological bad habits created or adopted for coping with the bipolar disorder prior to its successful medical treatment. These usually have to do with fear, guilt, shame, and grief associated with the damaged self-esteem, broken relationships, financial mistakes, and social isolation and alienation that resulted from the suffering of the mania and/or depression.

Treatment of patients with bipolar disorder with medication and psychotherapy has proved relatively effective in making rehospitalization unnecessary and preventing relationship breakdown or employment dysfunction. Medication without psychotherapy proves generally somewhat less effective. Patients who are not treated with medication and/or psychotherapy suffer a high rate of recidivism.

J. Harold Ellens

See also Depression.

References

American Psychiatric Association. *Diagnostic and Statistical Manual of Mental Disorders,* 4th ed., text rev. Washington, DC: American Psychiatric Association, 2000.

"Bipolar Disorder." *The Columbia Encyclopedia,* 6th ed. New York: Columbia University Press, 2005.

"Burden of Mental Illness." Centers for Disease Control and Prevention, July 1, 2011, www.cdc.gov/mentalhealth/basics/burden.htm.

Goodwin, F. K., and K. R. Jamison. *Manic-Depressive Illness: Bipolar Disorders and Recurrent Depression,* 2nd ed. New York: Oxford University Press, 2007.

National Institute of Mental Health. "The Numbers Count: Mental Disorders in America: Bipolar Disorder," 2010, www.nimh.nih.gov/health/publications/the-numbers-count-mental-disorders-in-America/index.shtml#Bipolar.

Silverstein, Alvin, Virginia Silverstein, and Laura Silverstein Nunn. *The Depression and Bipolar Disorder Update.* Berkeley Heights, NJ: Enslow, 2009.

U.S. Census Bureau. *Population Estimates by Demographic Characteristics.* "Table 2: Annual Estimates of the Population by Selected Age Groups and Sex for the United States: April 1, 2000 to July 1, 2004" (NC-EST2004-02), www.census.gov/popest/national/asrh.

Whitaker, Robert. *Anatomy of an Epidemic: Magic Bullets, Psychiatric Drugs and the Astonishing Rise of Mental Illness in America.* New York: Crown, 2010.

BIRTH CONTROL

Birth control is the control of fertility, or the prevention of pregnancy, through one of several methods. Another common name for birth control is contraception, because that is precisely what the various birth control methods do; they prevent the viable sperm and egg from uniting to form a fertilized embryo. Though discussing birth control is no longer likely to lead to an arrest, as in the days of birth control pioneer Margaret Sanger, public debates remain. Some debates address which methods of birth control are the most effective at attaining one's reproductive goals, while others address whether insurance benefits should include the cost of birth control, the likely long- and short-term effects of their use, how to increase the use of birth control among sexually active young people, and questions over why there are still so many more methods that focus on women's fertility compared with those that focus on men's fertility.

Controlling fertility affects the well-being of women, men, children, families, and society by providing methods and strategies to prevent unplanned pregnancies. Planned fertility positively impacts the health of children, maternal longevity, and the empowerment of women. Access to birth control provides women and men with choices regarding family size, timing between pregnancies, and spacing

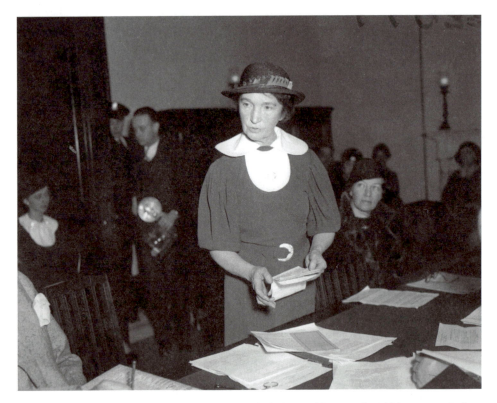

Margaret Sanger, who founded the American Birth Control League in 1921, appears before a Senate committee for federal birth control legislation in Washington, DC, on March 1, 1934. Sanger's legal appeals eventually prompted federal courts to grant physicians the right to give advice about birth control methods. (AP/Wide World Photos)

of children. Additionally, controlling fertility reduces the prevalence of chronic illness and maternal death from pregnancy-related conditions.

Globally, approximately 210 million women become pregnant each year. Of these pregnancies, nearly 40 percent are unplanned. In the United States, 49 percent of pregnancies are estimated to be unplanned. Research shows that unintended pregnancies can have devastating impacts on not only women but also on children and families. An unintended pregnancy places a woman at risk for depression, physical abuse, and the normal risks associated with pregnancy, including maternal death. Pregnancies that are spaced closely together present risks to children, including low birth weight, increased likelihood of death in the first year, and decreased access to resources necessary for healthy development. Unintended pregnancies can have devastating impacts on the well-being of the family unit. An unplanned pregnancy often pushes families with limited economic resources into a cycle of poverty that further limits their opportunities for success.

The period of fertility in a person's life spans approximately 30 years, and preferences for birth control methods and strategies vary among individuals, across the life course, and are influenced by multiple social factors. These factors may include socioeconomic status, religious or moral beliefs, purpose for using birth control (permanent pregnancy prevention, delay of pregnancy, or spacing between births), availability of birth control products, access to medical care, willingness to use birth control consistently, concern over side effects, and variability in the failure rates of different types of birth control products. Although the primary purpose of birth control is to control fertility, increases in the prevalence of sexually transmitted infections (STIs) and the human immunodeficiency virus, which causes AIDS, have created pressures to develop new pregnancy prevention options that combine contraception and STI prevention. The availability of contraceptive options allows women and men the opportunity to maximize the benefits of birth control while minimizing the risks of contraceptive use according to their needs.

The availability of birth control has raised important questions about reproductive control and the relationships between men and women. Traditionalists argue that pregnancy and child rearing are the natural or biologically determined roles of women, given their capacity to become pregnant and give birth. Opponents of this view argue that reproduction and motherhood are one of many choices available to women. Providing options to women and men that allow them to control their fertility has shifted pregnancy and motherhood from a position of duty to one of choice. This shift is a consequence of changes to the workforce, increased opportunities for women, and changes in the economic structure of contemporary families. These changes, along with ongoing developments in fertility control research, provide women and men today with many innovative choices concerning birth control. These choices allow women and men to tailor birth control to their individual needs and life circumstances.

Today, birth control debates focus on the advantages and disadvantages of different birth control methods. The most common debates focus on the merits of temporary versus permanent methods of pregnancy prevention. Other debates examine the benefits of natural versus barrier methods of controlling reproduction. Still other debates examine the advantages and disadvantages of male and female contraception. With the growing pandemic of AIDS in sub-Saharan Africa and Asia and the increasing prevalence of sexually transmitted diseases that threaten world health, contemporary debates about birth control focus on the feasibility and practicality of combining STI prevention and contraception.

Brief History of Contraception Although women have sought to control their fertility since ancient times, safe and effective contraception was not developed until the 20th century. The large influx of immigrants in the 1900s and the emergence of feminist groups working for women's rights helped bring to the forefront large-scale birth control movements in the United States and abroad. Ancient forms of birth control included potions, magic charms, chants, and herbal recipes. Ancient recipes often featured leaves, hawthorn bark, ivy, willow, and poplar, believed to contain sterilizing agents. During the Middle Ages, potions containing lead, arsenic, or strychnine caused death to many women seeking to control their fertility. Additionally, crude barrier methods were used in which the genitals were covered with cedar gum or alum was applied to the uterus. Later, pessary mixtures of elephant dung, lime (mineral), and pomegranate seeds were inserted into a woman's vagina to prevent pregnancy. Other barrier methods believed to prevent pregnancy included sicklewort leaves, wool tampons soaked in wine, and crudely fashioned vaginal sponges.

Later birth control developments were based on more accurate information concerning conception. Condoms were developed in the early 1700s by the physician to King Charles II. By the early 1800s, a contraceptive sponge and a contraceptive syringe were available. By the mid-1800s, a number of more modern barrier methods to control conception were available to women. However, it was illegal to advertise these options and most were available only through physicians and only in cases that were clinically indicated. Thus, early modern conception was limited to health reasons.

Modern contraceptive devices such as the condom, diaphragm, cervical cap, and intrauterine device (IUD) were developed in the 20th century and represented a marked advance in medical technology. Effectiveness was largely dependent on user compliance. While these methods represented a significant improvement over more archaic methods, contraceptive safety remained an issue. Other modern methods included the insertion of various substances (some toxic) into the vagina, resulting in inflammation or irritation of the vaginal walls, while other devices often caused discomfort.

The birth control pill, developed in the 1950s by biologist Charles Pincus, represented a major advance in fertility control. Pincus is credited with the discovery of the effects of combining estrogen and progesterone in an oral contraceptive that would prevent pregnancy. The development and mass marketing of the birth control pill provided women with a way to control not only their fertility but their lives.

Traditional Contraceptive Methods   Traditional contraception includes both temporary and permanent methods of controlling fertility. Temporary contraception provides time-limited protection from becoming pregnant. Permanent contraception refers to surgical procedures that result in a lasting inability to become pregnant. The choice of contraception takes into consideration several biological and social factors, including age, lifestyle (frequency of sexual activity, monogamy or multiple partners), religious or moral beliefs, legal issues, family planning objectives, as well as medical history and concerns. These factors vary among individuals and across the life span.

Traditional contraceptive methods provide varying degrees of protection from becoming pregnant and protection from STIs. While some of these methods provide noncontraceptive benefits, they require consistent and appropriate use and are associated with varying degrees of risks. Traditional contraception includes both hormonal and nonhormonal methods of preventing pregnancy and sexually transmitted diseases. These methods provide protection as long as they are used correctly, but their effects are temporary and reversible once discontinued. Traditional contraceptive methods include sexual abstinence, coitus interruptus, the rhythm method, barrier methods, spermicides, male or female condoms, IUDs, and oral contraceptive pills.

Sexual abstinence refers to the voluntary practice of refraining from all forms of sexual activity that could result in pregnancy or the transmission of sexually transmitted diseases. Abstinence is commonly referred to as the only form of birth control that is 100 percent effective in preventing pregnancy and STIs; however, failed abstinence results in unprotected sex, which increases the risks of unintended pregnancy and transmission of STIs.

Coitus interruptus is the oldest method of contraception and requires the man to withdraw his penis from the vagina just prior to ejaculation. Often referred to as a natural method of birth control, coitus interruptus is highly unreliable because a small amount of seminal fluid, containing sperm, is secreted from the penis prior to ejaculation and can result in conception. This method offers no protection from sexually transmitted diseases.

The *rhythm method* of birth control developed in response to research on the timing of ovulation. Research findings indicate that women ovulate approximately 14 days before the onset of their menstrual cycle. The rhythm method assumes that a woman is the most fertile during ovulation. To determine an individual cycle of ovulation, this method requires a woman to count backward 14 days from the first day of her menstrual period. During this time period, a woman should abstain from sexual activity or use another form of birth control (such as condoms) to avoid pregnancy. The rhythm method is another natural form of birth control that is highly risky. Few women ovulate at the exact same time from month to month, making accurate calculations of ovulation difficult. Additionally, sperm can live inside a woman for up to seven days, further complicating the calculations of safe periods for sex. Finally, the rhythm method does not provide protection from sexually transmitted diseases.

Barrier methods of contraception prevent sperm from reaching the fallopian tubes and fertilizing an egg. Barrier methods include both male and female condoms, diaphragms, cervical caps, and vaginal sponges. With the exception of the male condom, these methods are exclusively used by women. Barrier contraception is most often used with a spermicide to increase effectiveness. Spermicides contain nonoxynol-9, a chemical that immobilizes sperm to prevent them from joining and fertilizing an egg. Barrier methods of contraception and spermicides provide moderate protection from pregnancy and sexually transmitted diseases, although failure rates (incidence of pregnancy resulting from use) vary from 20 to 30 percent.

Condoms, a popular and nonprescription form of barrier contraception available to both men and women, provides moderate protection from pregnancy and STIs. The male condom is a latex, polyurethane, or natural skin sheath that covers the erect penis and traps semen before it enters the vagina. The female condom is a soft, loosely fitting polyurethane tubelike sheath that lines the vagina during sex. Female condoms have a closed end with rings at each end. The ring at the closed end is inserted deep into the vagina over the cervix to secure the tube in place. Female condoms protect against pregnancy by trapping sperm in the sheath and preventing entry into the vagina. Used correctly, condoms are between 80 and 85 percent effective in preventing pregnancy and the transmission of STIs. Risks that decrease the effectiveness of condoms include incorrect usage, slippage during sexual activity, and breakage. Natural skin condoms used by some men do not protect against the transmission of HIV and other STIs.

The diaphragm is a shallow, dome-shaped, flexible rubber disk that fits inside the vagina to cover the cervix. The diaphragm prevents sperm from entering the uterus. Diaphragms are used with spermicide to immobilize or kill sperm and to prevent fertilization of the egg. Diaphragms may be left inside the vagina for up to 24 hours, but a spermicide should be used with each intercourse encounter. To be fully effective, the diaphragm should be left in place for six hours after intercourse before removal. Approximately 80 to 95 percent effective in preventing pregnancy and the transmission of gonorrhea and chlamydia, the diaphragm does not protect against the transmission of herpes or HIV.

Cervical caps are small, soft rubber, thimble-shaped caps that are fitted inside the woman's cervix. Cervical caps prevent pregnancy by blocking the entrance of the uterus. Approximately 80 to 95 percent effective when used alone, effectiveness is increased when used with spermicides. Unlike the diaphragm, the cervical cap may be left in place for up to 48 hours. Similar to the diaphragm, the cervical cap provides protection against gonorrhea and chlamydia but does not provide protection against herpes or HIV.

Vaginal sponges, removed from the market in 1995 due to concerns about possible contaminants, are round, doughnut-shaped polyurethane devices containing spermicides and a loop that hangs down in the vagina allowing for easy removal. Sponges prevent pregnancy by blocking the uterus and preventing fertilization of the egg. Vaginal sponges are approximately 70 to 80 percent effective in preventing pregnancy but provide no protection against STIs. Risks include toxic shock syndrome if left inside the vagina for more than 24 hours.

Barrier methods of birth control provide moderate protection from pregnancy and STIs but are not fail-safe. Effectiveness is dependent on consistency and proper use. Advantages include lower cost, availability without a prescription, and ease of use (with the exception of the diaphragm). Disadvantages include lowered effectiveness as compared to other forms of birth control and little or no protection against certain STIs.

Two other traditional contraceptive methods are the IUD and oral contraceptive pills. Both of these methods are characterized by increased effectiveness if used properly. The IUD is a T-shaped device inserted into a woman's vagina by a health professional. Inserted into the wall of the uterus, the IUD prevents pregnancy by changing the motility (movement) of the sperm and egg and by altering the lining of the uterus to prevent egg implantation. The effectiveness of IUDs in preventing pregnancy is approximately 98 percent; however, IUDs do not provide protection from STIs. Oral contraceptive pills are taken daily for 21 days each month. Oral contraceptives prevent pregnancy by preventing ovulation, the monthly release of an egg. This form of contraception does not interfere with the monthly menstrual cycle. Many birth control pills combine progesterone and estrogen, but newer oral contraceptives contain progesterone only. Taken regularly, oral contraceptives are approximately 98 percent effective in preventing pregnancy but do not provide protection from STIs.

New Contraceptive Technologies   Despite the availability of a broad range of contraceptive methods, the effectiveness of traditional contraceptive methods is largely dependent on user consistency and proper use. Even with consistent and proper use, each method is associated with varying degrees of risk. Risks include the likelihood of pregnancy, side effects, and possible STI transmission. New developments in contraceptive technology focus on improvement of side effects and the development of contraceptives that do not require users to adhere to a daily regimen. These new technologies are designed to make use simpler and more suitable to users' lives. Additionally, many of the new technologies seek to combine fertility control with protection from STIs.

The *vaginal contraceptive ring* is inserted into a woman's vagina for a period of three weeks and removed for one week. During the three-week period, the ring releases small doses of progestin and estrogen, providing month-long contraception. The release of progestin and estrogen prevents the ovaries from releasing an egg and increases cervical mucus that helps to prevent sperm from entering the uterus. Fully effective after seven days, supplementary contraceptive methods should be used during the first week after insertion. Benefits include a high effectiveness rate, ease of use, shorter and lighter menstrual periods, and protection from ovarian cysts and from ovarian and uterine cancer. Disadvantages include spotting between menstrual periods for the first several months and no protection against STIs.

Hormonal implants provide highly effective, long-term, but reversible, protection from pregnancy. Particularly suitable for users who find it difficult to consistently take daily contraceptives, hormonal implants deliver progesterone by using a rod system inserted underneath the skin. Closely related to implants are hormonal injections that are administered monthly. Both hormonal implants and injections are highly effective in preventing pregnancy but may cause breakthrough bleeding. Neither provides protection from STIs at this stage of development.

Contraceptive patches deliver a combination of progestin and estrogen through an adhesive patch located on the upper arm, buttocks, lower abdomen, or upper torso. Applied weekly for three weeks, followed by one week without, the contraceptive patch is highly effective in preventing pregnancy but does not protect against the transmission of STIs. The use of the patch is associated with withdrawal bleeding during the week that it is not worn. Compliance is reported to be higher than with oral contraceptive pills.

Levonorgestrel intrauterine systems provide long-term birth control without sterilization by delivering small amounts of the progestin levonorgestrel directly to the lining of the uterus to prevent pregnancy. Delivered through a small T-shaped intrauterine plastic device implanted by a health professional, the levonorgestrel system provides protection from pregnancy for up to five years. It does not currently offer protection from STIs.

New contraceptive technologies are designed to provide longer-term protection from pregnancy and to remove compliance obstacles that decrease effectiveness and increase the likelihood of unintended pregnancies. The availability of contraceptive options provides users with choices that assess not only fertility purposes but also variations in sexual activity. However, until new contraceptive technologies that combine pregnancy and STI prevention are readily available, proper use of male and female condoms provides the most effective strategy for prevention of sexually transmitted diseases and HIV.

Abortion Abortion, defined as the intentional termination of a pregnancy, was legally established in 1973 with the Supreme Court decision in *Roe v. Wade* (410 U.S. 113). The decision spawned disparate and strongly held opinions among the U.S. public and the emergence of activist groups taking a variety of positions on abortion. The availability of elective abortion has called into question traditional beliefs about the relations between men and women, raised vexing issues about the control of women's bodies, and intensified contentious debates about women's roles and brought about changes in the division of labor, both in the family and in the broader occupational arena. Elective abortion has called into question long-standing beliefs about the moral nature of sexuality. Further, elective abortion has challenged the notion of sexual relations as privileged activities that are symbolic of commitments, responsibilities, and obligations between men and women. Elective abortion also brings to the fore the more personal issue of the meaning of pregnancy.

Historically, the debate over abortion has been one of competing definitions of motherhood. Pro-life activists argue that family, and particularly motherhood, is the cornerstone of society. Pro-choice activists argue that reproductive choice is central to women controlling their lives. More contemporary debates focus on the ethical and moral nature of personhood and the rights of the fetus. In the last 30 years, these debates have become politicized, resulting in the passage of increasingly restrictive laws governing abortion, abortion doctors, and abortion clinics. Currently, South Dakota is the only state that has passed laws making abortions illegal except in cases in which the woman's life is endangered. Other states are considering passage of similarly restrictive legislation.

The consequences of unintended pregnancy are well documented and contribute to the need for the continued development of contraceptive options that will meet the needs and goals of diverse populations whose reproductive needs change throughout their life course. By definition abortion is not a type of contraception but is an option when contraceptive efforts did not prevent pregnancy.

Permanent Contraception Permanent contraception refers to sterilization techniques that permanently prevent pregnancy. Frequently referred to as sterilization, permanent contraception prevents men from impregnating women and prevents women from becoming pregnant.

Tubal ligation refers to surgery to fuse a woman's fallopian tubes, preventing the movement of eggs from the ovaries to the uterus. The procedure is considered permanent and involves the cauterization of the fallopian tubes. However, some women who later choose to become pregnant have successfully had the procedure reversed. The reversal of tubal ligation procedures are successful in 50 to 80 percent of cases.

Hysterectomy refers to the complete removal of a woman's uterus or the uterus and cervix, depending on the type of procedure performed, and results in permanent sterility. Hysterectomies may be performed through an incision in the abdominal wall, vaginally, or by using laparoscopic incisions on the abdomen.

Vasectomy refers to a surgical procedure for men in which the vas deferens are sealed and cut apart to prevent sperm from moving out of the testes. The procedure results in permanent sterility, although the procedure may be reversed under certain conditions.

Permanent contraception is generally recommended only in cases in which there is no desire for children, family size is complete, or in cases where medical concerns necessitate permanent prevention of pregnancy.

Emergency Contraception   Emergency contraception, commonly referred to as postcoital contraception or the morning after pill, encompasses a number of therapies designed to prevent pregnancy following unprotected sexual intercourse. Emergency contraception is also indicated when a condom slips or breaks, a diaphragm dislodges, two or more oral contraceptives are missed or the monthly regimen of birth control pills are begun two or more days late, a hormonal injection is two weeks overdue, or a woman has been raped. Emergency contraception prevents pregnancy by preventing the release of an egg from the ovary, by preventing fertilization, or by preventing attachment of an egg to the uterine wall. Most effective when used within 72 hours of unprotected sex, emergency contraception does not affect a fertilized egg already attached to the uterine wall. Emergency contraception does not induce an abortion or disrupt an existing pregnancy; it prevents a pregnancy from occurring following unprotected sexual intercourse.

Conclusion   Ideally, birth control should be a shared responsibility between a woman and her partner. In the United States, approximately 1.6 million pregnancies each year are unplanned. Unplanned pregnancies position women, men, and families in a precarious situation that has social, economic, personal, and health consequences. An unintended pregnancy leaves a woman and her partner facing pregnancy termination, adoption, or raising an unplanned child—often under less-than-ideal conditions. Contraceptive technologies and research developments in the transmission of sexually transmitted diseases represent increased opportunities for not only controlling fertility but also improving safe sex practices.

Jonelle Husain

See also Acquired Immunodeficiency Syndrome (AIDS); Sexually Transmitted Diseases (STDs)

References

Connell, Elizabeth B. *The Contraception Sourcebook.* New York: McGraw-Hill, 2002.

Ginsberg, Faye, D. *Contested Lives: The Abortion Debate in an American Community.* Berkeley: University of California Press, 1989.

Luker, Kristen. *Abortion and the Politics of Motherhood.* Berkeley: University of California Press, 1984.

Maxwell, Carol J.C. *Pro-Life Activists in America: Meaning, Motivation, and Direct Action.* Cambridge, England: Cambridge University Press, 2002.

Weschler, Toni. *Taking Charge of Your Fertility.* New York: Harper Collins, 2006.

BLOOD PRESSURE

Blood pressure is defined as the force of the blood pushing against the walls of the arteries as the heart muscle contracts. Stephen Hales, an English country parson, first discovered this phenomenon around 1733. Hales connected a glass tube to the artery of a horse and noted the height the blood rose and fell in the tube when the heart beat and relaxed.

Although noninvasive measures of blood pressure were developed in the late 19th century, it was not until 1905 that Russian surgeon, N.C. Korotkoff, developed the modern method of measuring blood pressure. This required the use of both a sphygmomanometer (blood pressure measuring device) and stethoscope placed on the inside of the elbow to hear the pulse. In this method, a wide inflatable rubber cuff is wrapped around a person's upper arm. Attached to the cuff is a mercury column to measure pressure. Air is added to the cuff until the pulse is no longer detected. As air is released from the cuff, the pressure indicated on the mercury column, when the heartbeat is first heard (*systolic*), is noted. The pressure when the heart beat disappeared (*diastolic*) is also noted. Today blood pressure is measured in a similar manner, often with automatic devices.

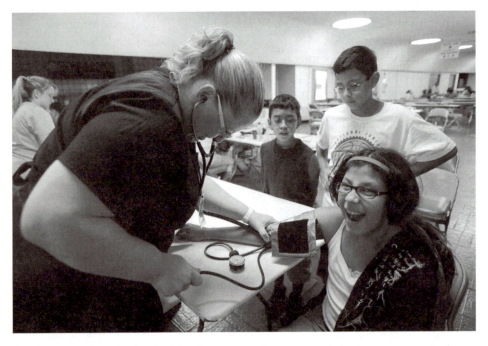

A volunteer nurse checks the blood pressure of a young girl during a free medical care clinic sponsored by the nonprofit group Remote Area Medical in California, August 2009. (AP/Wide World Photos)

Table 1. Classification of Blood Pressure Levels in mmHg

Classification of Blood Pressure	Systolic (top number)		Diastolic (bottom number)
Normal	< 120	and	< 80
Prehypertension	120–139	or	80–89
Hypertension			
Stage 1	140–159	or	90–99
Stage 2	160 or higher	or	> 100

Blood Pressure Classifications   Blood pressure is recorded with the systolic pressure on the top and diastolic pressure on the bottom of a line, such as 120/80 mmHg. The unit in which blood pressure is measured is millimeters of mercury (mmHg).

The following table shows classifications of blood pressure in adults.

High Blood Pressure   High blood pressure is sometimes called the silent killer because it generally has no warning signs or symptoms so most people do not know they have it. About one in three adults in the United States has hypertension. For over 85 percent of people, the cause of their high blood pressure is not known; this called *primary* or *essential* hypertension.

Secondary hypertension is caused by a known health condition such as kidney disease, sleep apnea, steroid therapy, thyroid or parathyroid disease, and some other medical conditions. Common over-the-counter medications such as antihistamines used to treat cold symptoms or asthma medications can increase blood pressure. Women who take hormones to reduce symptoms of menopause and young women who take birth control pills may also experience a rise in blood pressure. While taking any medication that may increase blood pressure, it is recommended that frequent blood pressure measurements be taken.

Risk Factors   Both environmental and hereditary factors increase the risk of developing high blood pressure. Some risk factors can be controlled, such as lifestyles changes, while others, such as gender and age, cannot.

Age   The risk of developing hypertension increases in those over 45 years of age. Almost half of all Americans over the age of 60 have hypertension. Of this age group, two out of three will have systolic pressures above 120. This is termed *isolated systolic hypertension*. Due to an increased rate of obesity among youth, an increased trend in hypertension has been observed.

Alcohol   In some individuals, heavy or even moderate alcohol consumption can cause hypertension.

Ethnicity or race   A higher rate of hypertension is found among individuals with African or Native American ancestry compared to those with European or East Asian ancestry in the United States African Americans develop hypertension earlier in life, and their average blood pressures are much higher compared to European Americans. In addition, they have higher rates of premature death from hypertension-related complications such as kidney failure, coronary heart disease, and strokes.

Those with Hispanic ancestry have a higher incidence of diabetes and obesity compared to non-Hispanic Americans. These higher incidences of hypertension among African and Hispanic Americans may be due to poor diet, stress, or hereditary factors.

Family history and heredity Individuals who have close family members (parents or siblings) with high blood pressure are more likely to be at risk for the condition. This increased risk is likely to be genetic, although environmental factors such as constant stress, poor diet, and smoking are contributing factors for those with a genetic predisposition for hypertension. High cholesterol levels, and especially high levels of LDL ("bad") cholesterol and low levels of HDL ("good") cholesterol have a hereditary component. The retention of salt (sodium chloride) in some people that contributes to hypertension has a genetic basis.

Gender Both men and women age 45 to 54 are at equal risk for hypertension. After age 55, women are more likely to have high blood pressure compared to men.

High-fat diet A diet high in saturated fat such as red meats, butter, lard, and cheese can contribute to obesity and high cholesterol. High cholesterol, in turn, can cause the formation of plaque and arthrosclerosis, which causes a narrowing of the arteries and thus an increase in blood pressure.

High sodium intake A diet high in salt (sodium chloride) can predispose some individuals to hypertension

Lack of exercise and sedentary lifestyle A lack of exercise can lead to obesity, which is a risk factor for hypertension.

Obesity and overweight Being overweight or obese (having too much weight in the form of fat) is a risk factor for many health problems, including hypertension. A measure of overweight or obesity is the body mass index (BMI), a measure of body fat based on height and weight. An individual with a BMI of 25 to 29.9 is overweight, and a BMI of 30 or greater is obese. Both of these conditions increase the risk of hypertension and other diseases, including diabetes, heart disease, and some cancers.

Stress Individuals with constant environmental stress, heightened anxiety, anger, and suppressed expression of anger are often at risk for developing high blood pressure.

Tobacco Nicotine is a stimulant that increases blood pressure. Smoking and chewing tobacco can lead to hypertension and other health issues such as cancer.

Dangers of Hypertension Hypertension can contribute to many chronic and fatal illnesses.

Acute coronary syndrome This condition includes pain in the chest, angina, and heart attack (myocardial infarction). It is the result of the narrowing of the coronary arteries in the heart, usually from atherosclerosis (thickening of the arterial walls by waxy cholesterol plaques) and/or build up of blood clots.

Cardiovascular disease (heart disease) and coronary artery disease
Hypertension is a major risk factor for heart disease, the leading cause of death in the United States among both men and women. The most common type of heart disease is coronary artery disease, where the arteries are thickened through the process of atherosclerosis.

Heart failure Chronic hypertension can lead to an enlarged heart. This reduces the heart's ability to adequately pump blood, which can cause symptoms of fatigue, shortness of breath, or fluid buildup in the abdomen and legs.

Renal (kidney) failure Chronic hypertension can lead to renal failure or the slow deterioration of kidney function. In addition to diabetes, hypertension is the primary risk factor for this condition.

Stroke (cerebral vascular accident) This debilitating and often fatal condition happens when a blood vessel in the brain suddenly bursts (cerebral hemorrhage) or is blocked by a blood clot (cerebral thrombosis). Brain cells in the area of the broken blood vessel die due to a lack of oxygen. Paralysis, inability to speak, and death can occur. Strokes are the third leading cause of death in the United States.

Prevention and Treatment A change in lifestyle can help prevent or even treat hypertension.

Alcohol Drink moderately no more than one drink per day for women and no more than two drinks a day for men. A drink is 12 ounces of beer, 5 ounces of wine, or a jigger (1.5 ounces) of spirits. In some people a small amount of alcohol can reduce blood pressure, and numerous studies have shown a lower risk of heart disease by those who consume a moderate amount of alcohol.

Dietary approaches to stop hypertension (DASH) eating plan Adopt a diet rich in fruits, vegetables, and whole grains in addition to protein from legumes, low-fat dairy products, chicken, and fish. Reduce consumption of foods high in saturated fat.

Dietary sodium reduction Reduce sodium intake by avoiding processed foods and not using salt in cooking. Potassium chloride salt, readily found in the supermarket, can be used instead of regular salt.

Maintain a healthy weight As weight is lost among overweight individuals, blood pressure also tends to fall. The BMI should be under 25.

Minerals Adequate amounts of calcium, potassium, and magnesium can reduce blood pressure. Although controversial, supplements of these minerals are sometimes recommended.

Monitor blood pressure For people with hypertension or its risk factors, frequent monitoring of blood pressure is advised. This can be accomplished at a health care professional's office, pharmacy, or at home with the use of an automatic blood pressure machine.

Physical activity and exercise Regular physical activity (30 minutes per day most days of the week) not only lowers blood pressure but can also reduce the risk of other chronic health problems

Stress management Relaxation, exercise, meditation, listening to music, yoga, reading, or other activities can reduce stress and in turn blood pressure.

Tobacco   Stop smoking, chewing, and dipping and avoid secondhand smoke.

Drug Treatment   Numerous classifications of drugs are used to treat hypertension.

ACE inhibitors cause blood vessels to relax, and so blood pressure goes down.

Alpha blockers reduce nerve impulses that constrict blood vessels. This allows blood to flow more easily, causing the blood pressure to go down.

Alpha-beta blockers work the same way as alpha blockers but also slow the heartbeat, causing decrease in blood pressure.

Angiotensin antagonists shield blood vessels from angiotensin II, which causes narrowing of arteries. As a result, the blood vessels relax and widen and there is a decrease in blood pressure.

Beta blockers reduce nerve impulses to the heart and blood vessels. This makes the heart beat slower and with less force. Blood pressure drops and the heart does not work as hard.

Calcium channel blockers keep calcium from entering the muscle cells of the heart and blood vessels. This causes the blood vessels to relax, and so blood pressure goes down.

Diuretics (water pills) flush excess water and sodium from the body, which often lowers blood pressure.

Nervous system inhibitors relax blood vessels by controlling nerve impulses, which causes the blood vessels to become wider and the blood pressure to decrease.

Vasodilators relax the muscle in the vessel walls, causing the blood pressure to go down.

In summary, keeping blood pressure at normal levels should first start with lifestyle changes. If these are not effective, various classifications of medication can be prescribed. However, like most drugs, they have side effects.

Ruth C. Engs

See also Alcohol; Body Mass Index (BMI); Exercise; Hypertension; Obesity; Smoking.

References

American Heart Association. *Heart Disease and Stroke Statistics—2011 Update: A Report from the American Heart Association* (December 15, 2010), http://circ.ahajournals.org/cgi/content/full/123/4/e18?maxtoshow=&hits=10&RESULTFORMAT=&fulltext=2011+update&searchid=1&FIRSTINDEX=0&resourcetype=HWCIT.

Booth, Jeremy. "A Short History of Blood Pressure Measurements." *Proceedings of the Royal Society of Medicine* 70, no. 11 (November 1977), www.ncbi.nlm.nih.gov/pmc/articles/PMC1543468/.

Centers for Disease Control and Prevention. "High Blood Pressure" (July 7, 2011), www.cdc.gov/bloodpressure.

Engs, R.C. "Women, Alcohol and Health: A Drink a Day Keeps the Heart Attack Away." *Current Opinion in Psychiatry* 9, no. 3 (1996): 217–20, www.indiana.edu/~engs/articles/women.html.

Genest, J., E. Koiw, O. Kuchel, R. Boucher, W. Nowaczynski, and J.M. Rojo-Ortega, eds. *Hypertension: Physiopathology and Treatment.* New York: McGraw-Hill, 1977.

National Heart, Blood, and Lung Institute. "Calculate Your Body Mass Index," www.nhl bisupport.com/bmi.

National Heart, Blood, and Lung Institute. "Types of Blood Pressure Medications," www. nhlbi.nih.gov/hbp/treat/bpd_type.htm.

National Heart, Blood, and Lung Institute. "What Is High Blood Pressure?" (April 1, 2011), www.nhlbi.nih.gov/health/dci/Diseases/Hbp/HBP_WhatIs.html.

U.S. Department of Health and Human Services. Reference Card from the Seventh Report of the Joint National Committee of Prevention, Detection, Evaluation, and Treatment of High Blood Pressure (JNC7)" (May 2003), www.nhlbi.nih.gov/guidelines/hyperten sion/phycard.pdf.

BLUEBERRIES

James Joseph, a nutrition researcher at the Human Nutrition Research Center on Aging at Tufts University, begins his days by drinking a glass of pomegranate juice and eating a cup of wild blueberries. According to a 2008 article in *Psychology Today,* after studying blueberries for years, Joseph is convinced that they help the brain and the body fight the seemingly endless number of problems associated with aging. While blueberries contain traditional nutrients, such as carbohydrates, fiber, vitamins C and E, and manganese, they also have anthocyanidins (dark flavonoid phytochemicals), which fight oxidative stress and inflammation. "Cumulatively, the berries produce antioxidant effects, neutralizing cellular damage created by free radicals of oxygen and blocking pathways by which oxidative stress damages cells. Perhaps more important, they function as anti-inflammatory agents to preserve cardiovascular as well as brain integrity" (Marano, 2008, pp. 59–60).

In a 2004 interview with the *Seattle Post-Intelligencer,* Joseph said that the old neurons in the brain are like couples who have been married a long time—they no longer communicate. Blueberries change that dynamic. They enable neurons to once again converse. "Blueberries have compounds that boost neuron signals and help turn back on systems in the brain that can lead to using other proteins to help with memory or other cognitive skills" (Condor, 2004).

In his research on rats and mice, Joseph has found that rats that eat blueberries have fewer cases of Alzheimer's disease and lower instances of arthritis-related inflammation. He and his colleagues have also determined that blueberries may be useful for those undergoing radiation therapy. Blueberries reduce the effects on cognitive and motor skills and may "even eliminate radiation-induced nausea" ("Eating Blueberries to Battle Alzheimer's," 2004). Rats that were fed a diet containing 2 percent blueberry extracts before undergoing radiation did far better than those rats who received no blueberries before their radiation treatments. "Irradiation causes deficits in behavior and signaling in rats which were ameliorated by an antioxidant diet." Possibly, "the polyphenols in these fruits might be acting in different brain regions" (Shukitt-Hale et al., 2007)

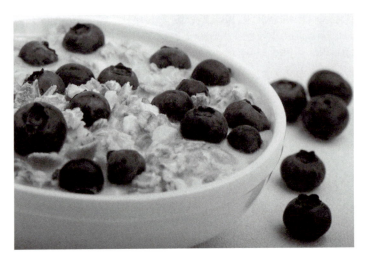

Blueberries are added to cereal for an extra dose of antioxidants. (Arnel Manalang/Dreamstime.com)

Joseph has even observed that blueberries tend to work best when eaten with certain high-fat foods such as walnuts, which contain polyphenols and omega-3 fatty acids. Working together, the blueberries and walnuts make nerve cell membranes more responsive. As a result, "the efficacy of all transactions" is improved. In addition, the combination of blueberries and walnuts "may help block inflammation at the cellular level, a process now implicated in cardiovascular disease, Alzheimer's disease, and other degenerative processes of aging" (Marano, 2008, pp. 59–60).

Cardiovascular Health   A Canadian study led by Wilhelmina Kalt, a researcher with Agriculture and Agri-Food Canada, reported in 2008 in the *British Journal of Nutrition* that pigs who were fed a 2 percent blueberry diet experienced reductions of total, LDL, and HDL cholesterol. The 2 percent blueberry diet is equivalent to two cups of blueberries in the human diet. Why is this significant? Pigs and humans have similar levels of LDL cholesterol. They are also prone to diet-related vascular disease and atherosclerotic plaques in the carotid artery and aorta. Furthermore, their heart rate and blood pressure resemble human heart rate and blood pressure ("Research: Diets with Blueberries Show Promise in Lowering Cholesterol," 2008). A 2008 article in *Grocer* states that, as a result of her research, Kalt advises people to eat at least four ounces of blueberries every day ("Blueberries Reduce Cholesterol in Pigs," 2008).

Cancer   In a 2006 study published in the *Journal of Agricultural and Food Chemistry*, Navindra Seeram, assistant director of the UCLA Center for Human Nutrition and assistant professor at the David Geffen School of Medicine at UCLA, reported that the extracts of common berries, such as blueberries, which are filled with antioxidants, inhibit the growth of in vitro mouth, prostate, breast, and colon cancer cells. Seeram and his colleagues also determined that higher amounts of berries inhibit larger numbers of cancer cells. "With increasing concentration of berry extract, increasing inhibition of cell proliferation in all of the cell lines were observed, with different degrees of potency between cell lines" (Seeram et al., 2006).

Another study, published in 2007 in *Clinical Cancer Research,* describes research conducted by scientists at Rutgers University and the U.S. Department of Agriculture (USDA) on the relationship between pterostilbene, a naturally occurring antioxidant in blueberries, and colon cancer. During the study, rats were given a compound to induce colon cancer. Half of the rats were then placed on a balanced diet; the other half were given the same diet, but it was supplemented with pterostilbene. At the end of eight weeks, when compared to the control group, the rats that had consumed supplemental pterostilbene had 57 percent fewer precancerous colonic lesions. Researchers concluded that the "study suggests that pterostilbene, a compound present in blueberries, is of great interest for the prevention of colon cancer" (Suh et al., 2007).

Agnes Rimando, a researcher with Natural Products Utilization Research in Mississippi, a division of the USDA Agriculture Research Service, has found similar results. In her studies, Rimando has noted that pterostilbene may impair the ability of enzymes to activate chemical carcinogens. So cells that might otherwise turn cancerous do not (Pons, 2006).

Antiaging and General Well-Being   It has been well established that there is a strong relationship between oxidative stress and chronic illness and aging. Moreover, the antioxidants in blueberries are known to fight that oxidative stress. A research study published in 2007 in the *Journal of the American College of Nutrition* found that it is not only important for people to eat blueberries and other antioxidant foods; it is also significant *when* they eat them. To reduce oxidative stress throughout the day, the researchers recommend eating blueberries or other antioxidant foods with each meal (Prior et al., 2007).

A 2006 study published in *Neurobiology of Aging* addressed the fact that as people age, the heat shock proteins in the brain, which, like antioxidants, support healthy brain functions, decline. Could eating blueberries reverse this decline? For 10 weeks, researchers fed a blueberry-enhanced diet to young and old rats and compared them to a control group of old rats, who were fed a diet without blueberries.

As expected, after 10 weeks the brains of the young rats were found to contain large amounts of heat shock proteins, and the brains of the old rats who did not eat blueberries had low amounts of heat shock proteins. However, the heat shock proteins of the old rats who ate blueberries were completely restored. Researchers concluded that blueberries may play a serious role in protecting against the neurodegenerative processes that often are associated with aging (Galli et al., 2006).

A 2005 article in *Nutrition Today* summarizes the many reasons for including blueberries in the diet. "The blueberry is becoming more widely recognized for its flavor, nutrition, and health benefits. Both production and consumption in the United States have more than doubled in the last 20 years. Not only are blueberries ranked among the highest in antioxidant activity when compared to other fruits and vegetables, they are also one of the richest sources of anthocyanins" (Lewis & Ruud, 2005). And there is very strong evidence that the consumption of anthocyanins reduces the risk the heart disease, cancer, and other problems associated with aging.

Marjolijn Bijlefeld and Sharon Zoumbaris

See also Antioxidants; Cancer; Cholesterol.

References

"Blueberries Reduce Cholesterol in Pigs." *Grocer* 231, no. 7869 (August 23, 2008): 54.

Bone, Kerry. "Blue Is the Healthy Color: The Health Benefits of Anthocyanins." *Dynamic Chiropractic* 26, no. 4 (February 12, 2008): S25–S26.

Condor, Bob. "Living Well: Blueberries Trigger Neurons That Keep the Brain Sharp." *Seattle Post-Intelligencer* (September 6, 2004), http://seattlepinwsource.com/health.

"Eating Blueberries to Battle Alzheimer's: 'Getting the Blues' May Also Help Lower Cholesterol and Reduce the Side Effects of Radiation Treatment." *Tufts University Health and Nutrition Letter* 22, no. 11 (December 2004): 3.

Galli, Rachel L., Donna F. Bielinski, Aleksandra Szprengiel, et al. "Blueberry Supplemented Diet Reverses Age-Related Decline in Hippocampal HSP70 Neuroprotection." *Neurobiology of Aging* 27, no. 2 (February 2006): 344–50.

Kalt, W., Kim Foote, and S.A.E. Fillmore. "Effect of Blueberry Feeding on Plasma Lipids in Pigs." *British Journal of Nutrition* 100, no. 1 (July 2008): 70–78.

Lewis, Nancy, and Jaime Ruud. "Blueberries in the American Diet." *Nutrition Today* 40, no. 2 (March/April 2005): 92–96.

Marano, Daniel A. "The Smartest Food: Phytochemical-Rich Berries Can Multiply Their Own Brain-Saving Effects When Eaten with Certain Fat-Rich Foods." *Psychology Today* 41, no. 3 (May–June 2008): 59–60.

Pons, Luis. "Pterostilbene's Healthy Potential: Berry Compound May Inhibit Breast Cancer and Heart Disease." *Agricultural Research* 54, no. 11–12 (November–December 2006): 6–7.

Prior, Ronald L., Liwei Gu, Xianli Wu, et al. "Plasma Antioxidant Capacity Changes Following a Meal as a Measure of the Ability of a Food to Alter In Vivo Antioxidant Status." *Journal of the American College of Nutrition* 26, no. 2 (April 2007): 170–81.

"Research: Diets with Blueberries Show Promise in Lowering Cholesterol." *Food & Beverage Close-Up* (June 26, 2008).

Seeram, N.P., L.S. Adams, Y. Zhang, et al. "Blackberry, Black Raspberry, Blueberry, Cranberry, Red Raspberry, and Strawberry Extracts Inhibit Growth and Stimulate Apoptosis of Human Cancer Cells in Vitro." *Journal of Agricultural and Food Chemistry* 54, no. 25 (December 13, 2006): 9329–39.

Shukitt-Hale, Barbara, Amanda N. Carey, Daniel Jenkins, et al. "Beneficial Effects of Fruit Extracts on Neuronal Function and Behavior in a Rodent Model of Accelerated Aging." *Neurobiology of Aging* 28, no. 8 (August 2007): 1187–94.

Shukitt-Hale, Barbara, Rachel L. Galli, Vanessa Meterko, et al. "Dietary Supplementation with Fruit Polyphenolics Ameliorates Age-Related Deficits in Behavior and Neuronal Markers of Inflammation and Oxidative Stress." *AGE* 27, no. 1 (March 2005): 49–57.

Suh, Naajoo, Shiby Paul, Xingpei Hao, et al. "Pterostilbene, An Active Constituent of Blueberries, Suppresses Aberrant Crypt Foci Formation in the Azoxymethane-Induced Colon Carcinogenesis Model in Rats." *Clinical Cancer Research* 13 (January 1, 2007): 350–55.

U.S. Highbush Blueberry Council, www.blueberry.org.

Wild Blueberries, www.wildblueberries.com.

BODY IMAGE

The modeling and magazine industries frequently come under fire for promoting what many describe as an unhealthy and unrealistic body image. On a monthly basis, magazines publish airbrushed images of very thin women and chiseled men and present them as the ideal of beauty. On fashion runways, thin models under pressure to maintain their looks and size, have resorted to dangerous diets and other unhealthy eating behaviors in order to maintain a body image of thin perfection. Several high-profile models, actresses, and entertainers have died in recent years as a result of their unhealthy, body-conscious activities.

Possessing a healthy body image is defined as accurately perceiving and accepting one's bodily features. This image is due in part to personal experiences as well as social standards and personality. Due to society's standards of thinness, a growing number of men and women now view their bodies in ways other than how the world sees them. For example, a person with an eating disorder perceives himself or herself as being fat when actually they are thin. This poor body image and distorted view of their shape and size brings with it a sense of shame and anxiety, which leads to other problems, including eating disorders and depression (National Women's Health Information Center, 2009).

In a popular children's fairy tale, the queen asks, "Mirror, mirror on the wall, who is the fairest of them all?" Many women who look in the mirror struggle with their body image and how to accept what they see in their reflection. In fact, every individual must reconcile his or her physical features with an ideal of beauty based on cultural norms and foundations. While some body characteristics can be controlled, other physical characteristics are beyond control and are a part of what makes each individual unique.

Achieving a healthy body image is important to overall wellness. Loving oneself and accepting one's own one-of-a-kind qualities are part of having a healthy body image, healthy self-esteem, and good mental health. This can be achieved through adopting positive lifestyle choices. Behaviors such as eating

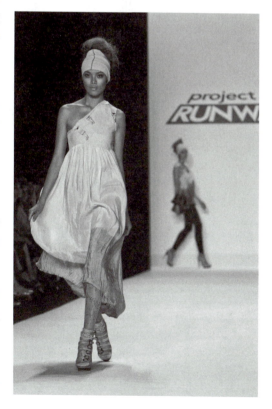

Project Runway model walks the catwalk during a fashion show in New York, on September 9, 2010. The fashion industry has been criticized for promoting an unhealthy body image. (Kurniawan1972/Dreamstime.com)

healthy foods, practicing good hygiene, avoiding cigarettes and excess alcohol can help individuals nurture a healthy body and body image. Exercise and proper amounts of sleep are a part of a daily regimen that can ensure strong bones, a healthy body weight, heart health, and low stress (National Women's Health Information Center, 2009). Being physically active is connected to a positive body image as well.

Technology and the influence of entertainment and social media reach citizens in a number of countries who are adopting more American ways of thinking about their appearance and, by extension, their bodies. A study released by the University of Haifa in Israel found that adolescent girls in that country developed an increasingly negative body image and various eating disorders in proportion to the time they spent looking at Facebook (Siegel-Itzkovich, 2011).

Thanks to media images and messages that showcase unrealistic body types, youngsters are also being influenced by the adults in their lives who may have their own negative body images or may be struggling with unhealthy eating habits or fad diets. For example, research shows that daughters are more likely to have opinions and thoughts on dieting if they have mothers who are constantly dieting. The study concluded that girls who perceived that their mothers thought thinness was important wanted to be thinner (Field et al., 2005).

This can be especially difficult for teens. The adolescent years can be challenging enough, but when teens adopt a poor body image, they can develop eating disorders, self-esteem issues, or depression. This can also lead to poor school performance and other unhealthy social and physical behaviors (National Women's Health Information Center, 2009).

Parents can help their children avoid a negative body image by acknowledging their child's talents and gifts, supervising the amount and content of media they consume, and helping them understand that weight gain and physical growth are normal parts of adolescence. Above all, because parents and older siblings are primary role models for younger children, those role models must adopt and display their own healthy behaviors (National Women's Health Information Center, 2009).

Organizations are hoping to improve body image among U.S. youngsters. By targeting children and teens with more positive messages, groups are working to combat the effects of the media on body image. One example is the Dressing Room Project (DRP), which uses social media and the Internet to educate girls and women about healthy body image and how their perceptions may be influenced by media-imposed standards of beauty. Launched in 2000 by Emerging Women Projects, a nonprofit organization for teen girls' empowerment, the DRP continues to offer girls and women a message of self-acceptance.

The good news is that body image is fluid, not fixed, and can change at any age. Body image can be enhanced by challenging body distortions and misleading assumptions about appearance. In other words, individuals can identify natural strengths that represent their best qualities, let compliments reinforce positive feelings about themselves, and focus on what they are good at to help build self-esteem.

The Dressing Room Project

The Dressing Room Project (DRP) uses social media and the Internet to educate girls and women about healthy body image and how their perceptions may be influenced by media-imposed standards of beauty. Launched in 2000 by Emerging Women Projects (EWP), a nonprofit organization for teen girls' empowerment, this initiative began as one woman's response to the mainstream media's portrayal of women.

Mimi Kates, founder and director of EWP and the Dressing Room Project, developed the project as a way to take positive action to shift girls' perceptions of their bodies. The project encourages girls to post cards with affirming statements on dressing room mirrors to remind other girls and women about the importance of feeling comfortable in their own, unique bodies. Kates maintains that unrealistic ideals depicted in magazines, movies, and television contribute to the prevalence of negative body image, eating disorders, and other unhealthy behaviors in girls and women, especially in the United States.

According to Kates, the DRP is a global effort thanks to its website. The positive information on the site is available to women all over the world and is shared at interactive workshops and other events for girls presented by over 200 registered DRP action teams. Additionally, the DRP does collaborative work with other like-minded organizations to promote positive body image and prevent eating disorders.

Mary Pipher, author of *Reviving Ophelia—Saving the Selves of Adolescent Girls,* commends the initiative and called the Dressing Room Project "an inspired idea that could change the ways girls think about themselves when they look in the mirror. This could be revolutionary." Information about the project and how to get involved is available from www.TheDressingRoomProject.org.

—*Sharon Zoumbaris*

While websites like the Dressing Room Project can support a positive body image, other websites offer unhealthy viewpoints. There are Internet sites that promote anorexia and bulimia and discuss the latest techniques to avoid calories and hide the behavior from concerned family members and friends. Pro-ana and Pro-mia are names that proponents of eating disorders have given themselves.

Reality TV shows constantly display the insecurities of everyday people and their pursuit of perfection, often through plastic surgery. Ideal candidates for cosmetic surgery procedures, according to the American Society of Plastic Surgeons, should possess a healthy, positive, and strong self-image. Their interest in surgery should focus on a characteristic they would like to have changed or enhanced, or a birth defect or cosmetic flaw that has negatively affected their self-esteem over the course of their lives.

However, people with unrealistic expectations about how a procedure can change their lives, such as those who desire to look like a particular celebrity, are not appropriate cosmetic surgery candidates. Patients in crisis and people with a mental illness should also not have cosmetic surgery. Neither should those individuals who are never pleased with their surgical results and keep returning for more, some of whom may suffer from a condition known as body dismorphic disorder (National Women's Health Information Center, 2009).

Body dismorphic disorder (BDD) is a serious condition where people are obsessed with minor or imaginary physical flaws of the skin, hair, or nose and repeatedly seek cosmetic surgery to correct them. These flaws can produce a lot of anxiety and be a point of constant focus. Unfortunately, cosmetic surgery can make BDD worse. Plus, individuals with BDD are often dissatisfied with the results of their procedures, then seek additional surgery for further correction or change their focus to another area of the body. BDD is treated with antidepressants plus cognitive-behavioral therapy that focuses on stopping the behavior and changing the patient's perception about his or her body (National Women's Health Information Center, 2009).

Eating disorders are associated with poor body image. According to the National Eating Disorders Association (NEDA), more than 10 million females and 1 million males are battling anorexia or bulimia in United States (NEDA, 2011). Anorexia nervosa is a life-threatening eating disorder involving starvation and dangerous weight loss. Bulimia nervosa is also life-threatening and involves binging on food, and in come cases purging or vomiting after eating.

In addition to eating disorders, overexercising is another behavior in which those with a poor body image engage. Body image issues are often masked as a desire to be healthy and physically fit. However, pushing the body to perform extremely strenuous activities for a long period may result in injury. The *American Journal of Sports Medicine* suggests pulled muscles, stress fractures, knee trauma, shin splints, strained hamstrings, and ripped tendons can all be consequences of overexercising. Moderation in exercise is the key. Too much of anything, even exercise, can be unhealthy. In addition, when a behavior interferes with normal life activities, it is a sign that a person needs to evaluate that behavior (National Women's Health Information Center, 2009).

Pregnancy is a natural condition that creates negative body images for some American women. There is increasing pressure for pregnant women to return quickly to their pre-pregnancy weight evident by the articles in popular magazines that prominently showcase celebrity moms who quickly get back into shape. Unlike celebrities, most women do not have access to personal trainers or chefs. The bodily changes that come during and after pregnancy are natural and are important for a healthy pregnancy and baby.

Activities such as prenatal yoga and massage can ease tension and help women appreciate their pregnant bodies. After birth, mom-and-baby classes offer new moms the opportunity to exercise with their babies in appropriate ways. Concentrating on the baby and taking steps to prepare for its arrival can help new mothers feel better about body changes. Above all, reading and learning about what to expect during and after pregnancy are healthy ways to feel empowered about the process of pregnancy and childbirth (National Women's Health Information Center, 2009).

When body image concerns during pregnancy are ignored, the consequences can be dire. Pregnant women can develop eating disorders, which can prevent future pregnancies. Eating disorders can also be responsible for premature labor, causing babies to be born underdeveloped or, worse, stillborn (National Women's Health Information Center, 2009).

Men are not immune to body image issues. Popular culture and society put pressure on American men to appear a certain way in order to be considered attractive and masculine. While women feel pressure to appear thin, men must bulk up. One indication of how men are paying greater attention to their appearance is the increase in men having cosmetic surgery. According to the American Society of Plastic Surgeons, men accounted for almost 10 percent of cosmetic procedures in 2010, a number that continues to increase (Forshee, 2011). This focus on body image has captured the attention of the fitness and cosmetic industries, which now actively target men, as well as psychologists and researchers (Silva, 2006).

Research indicates that men are expressing dissatisfaction with their bodies in greater numbers, and there is a corresponding increase in the number of men who suffer from eating disorders. Women work hard to hide the symptoms of their eating disorders, and medical experts suggest that men go even further to do so. One characteristic of men that has not changed is the need to be strong and silent. Under pressure to hold in their feelings, men are even less likely to share the things that may be hurting them (Silva, 2006).

When men have a poor body image, they may also suffer from low self-esteem and depression. In their drive to appear more athletic, they may experiment with steroids, which can cause heart disease and liver damage and impair the immune system. While building the appearance of muscles, steroids shrink testicles and can cause infertility and baldness. Telltale signs of steroid abuse include extreme mood swings and aggression. Studies have shown that steroid abusers have instances of hostility where they commit violent acts, including crimes against property, physical fighting, theft, or armed robbery (National Institute on Drug Abuse, 2011).

While there are some changes that individuals can safely make to enhance their appearance, nothing beats a healthy body image, self-acceptance, and learning to embrace the unique qualities that make individuals interesting and integral to their family and friends.

Abena Foreman-Trice

See also Adolescence; Anorexia Nervosa; Eating Disorders; Liposuction; Steroids.

References

Cleveland Clinic Foundation. "Fostering a Positive Self-Image" (1995–2009), http://my.clevelandclinic.org/healthy_living/mental_health/hic_fostering_a_positive_self-image.aspx.

Field, Alison E., et al. "Weight Concerns and Weight Control Behaviors of Adolescents and Their Mothers." *Archives of Pediatric & Adolescent Medicine*. 159 (December 2005): 1121–26.

Forshee, Stephanie. "More Men Getting Plastic Surgery." *Los Angeles Daily News* (May 19, 2011), www.dailynews.com/health/ci_18096994.

Kearney-Cooke, Ann. "Be Your Own Cheerleader: Psychologist Ann Kearney-Cooke Shares Three Ways to Get Your Inner Voice to Do Less Criticizing and More Complimenting." *Shape* (April 2011): 96.

National Eating Disorders Association. *Global Eating Disorders News* (2011), www.nationaleatingdisorders.org/in-the-news/in-the-spotlight.php.

National Institute on Drug Abuse. *Research Report Series—Anabolic Steroid Abuse* (2011), www.drugabuse.gov/ResearchReports/Steroids/anabolicsteroids4.html.

National Women's Health Information Center, U.S. Department of Health and Human Services Office on Women's Health. *Body Image: Loving Yourself Inside and Out* (2009), www.womenshealth.gov/bodyimage/.

Norton, Amy. "Many Young Women May Misjudge Their Weight." *Reuters Health* (November 23, 2010), www.reuters.com/article/2010/11/23/us-misjudge-weight-idUSTRE6AM6C020101123.

Siegel-Itzkovich, Judy. "Link Found between Facebook Use and Eating Disorders." *Jerusalem Post* (February 1, 2011), www.jpost.com/Health/Article.aspx?id=206145.

Silva, Marc A. "Body Image Dissatisfaction: A Growing Concern among Men." Milwaukee School of Engineering (April 2006), www.msoe.edu/life_at_msoe/current_student_resources/student_resources/counseling_services/newsletters_for_mental_health/body_image_dissatisfaction.shtml.

BODY MASS INDEX (BMI)

Researchers developed the body mass index (BMI) to help people gauge a healthy weight range for their age. However, for children and teens who are still growing, the BMI should be used more as a guideline than to determine risk level. Here's how to calculate it:

- Multiply your weight in pounds by 704.5.
- Multiply your height in inches by your height in inches.
- Divide answer 1 by answer 2.

The BMI has been used by the World Health Organization as the standard measurement for obesity since the early 1980s. In the United States, most private health insurance plans use a high BMI as a cutoff point for insurance rates and in some situations will implement surcharges where a subscriber with a high BMI pays an additional penalty for insurance coverage.

The basic problem with using the BMI as a primary measure of obesity, especially in the case of athletes, is that muscle weight contributes to BMI. Professional athletes may fall in the obese range even though they carry little fat. BMI

Table 1. Body Mass Index

If Your BMI Is:	Your Risk Level Is:
19–24	Minimal to low
25–26	Low to moderate
27–29	Moderate to high
30–34	High to very high
35–39	Very high to extremely high
40 or more	Extremely high

has also been used as a measure of underweight for those suffering with eating disorders such as anorexia nervosa and bulimia nervosa.

Marjolijn Bijlefeld and Sharon Zoumbaris

See also Anorexia Nervosa; Bulimia Nervosa; Obesity; World Health Organization (WHO).

BONE HEALTH

Bones are more than mere puzzle pieces that, when connected, form a skeleton to hold bodies together. They are also complex structures containing various types of cells and substances responsible for their own overall maintenance and health. According to the American Society for Bone and Mineral Research, bone is as light as wood yet possesses the same strength as cast iron. In addition to supporting the body, bones are a type of connective tissue that attaches muscles, protects vital organs, and stores bone marrow and minerals.

Three types of cells play important roles in the bone-building process. Osteoblasts and osteocytes are support cells that grow and help maintain bone. In particular, osteocytes have long tentacles that can reach out to other cells and counter the effects of bone stress. Osteoclasts are cells that aid in absorbing and removing excess bone, thereby remodeling growing bones.

Bone marrow, found deep inside some bones, produces red, white, and yellow blood cells. Red blood cells carry oxygen throughout the body. Yellow blood cells store fat, and white blood cells help fight infections. Bone marrow also contains platelets that aid in blood clotting.

Most of the body's minerals—especially calcium and phosphorous—can be found in bones. Calcium is required for proper function of the heart, muscles, and nerves. In bones, calcium is joined by phosphorus to create calcium phosphate. The remaining phosphorus is distributed throughout the body and in all cells, such as in the form of (adenosine triphosphate, which is the main energy chemical in the body. Phosphorus is also a main component of the genetic materials DNA and RNA, which are found in every cell and help keep bones hard.

Sometimes things can go wrong with bone development. These problems come in the form of bone conditions that people are born with and bone diseases that form due to disease or improper nutrition. One of the most familiar bone conditions, scoliosis, results in a spine curvature that can vary in degrees of severity.

There are three types of the condition: degenerative, neuromuscular, and functional. Functional scoliosis is a condition where an abnormal curve develops because of a problem elsewhere in the body. For example, one leg being shorter than the other or muscle spasms in the back can cause the condition. Neuromuscular scoliosis occurs when there is a problem with bone formation of the spine. The bones may either not form completely, or they stay fused together. This type of scoliosis is seen in individuals with conditions such as birth defects, muscular dystrophy, cerebral palsy, or Marfan's disease. When scoliosis is present at birth, it is known as congenital and often requires treatments more aggressive than other forms of scoliosis. Degenerative scoliosis is seen in older adults and is caused by arthritis.

Rickets is a disease that weakens bones in children. There are three types: nutritional rickets, hypophosphatemic rickets, and renal rickets. Nutritional rickets is caused by insufficient amounts of vitamin D and can be treated with nutritional supplements. Hypophosphatemic rickets, a genetic condition caused by insufficient levels of phosphate, is painful and makes bones soft and bendy. This type is treated with phosphate and calcitriol. Renal rickets is caused by the presence of a kidney disorder. Individuals with kidney disease often have trouble regulating the amounts of electrolytes lost through urine, including calcium and phosphate. People suffering with this type of rickets have symptoms that mimic the nutritional type. Renal rickets can be treated by improving the underlying kidney problem and giving nutritional supplements. The disease also affects dark-skinned children who have limited sun exposure, infants who only receive breast milk, and children on vegan diets.

Osteoporosis is a disease characterized by an increased risk in fractures affecting mobility and quality of life. It occurs mainly in women, but not always. According to the Centers for Disease Control and Prevention, the average woman has acquired most of her bone mass by the age of 20. A large decline in bone mass for women ensues

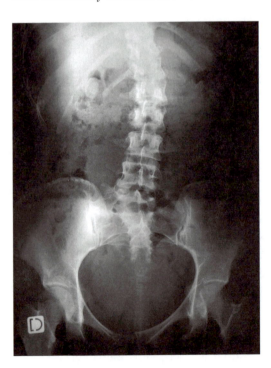

Young girl's spine shows scoliosis in an X-ray. (Ldambies/Dreamstime.com)

during menopause, which normally begins in a woman's 40s and can progress for up to a decade in some women. An associated decline in bone mass can lead to osteoporosis.

Adult men can be affected by osteoporosis as well. Typically when osteoporosis is present in men, it signals other conditions such as low testosterone or low calcium and vitamin D. While osteoporosis is treatable with medications, it is possible to avoid the condition through diet and exercise.

Fractures and broken bones occur when an individual falls, especially due to age-related issues, sports, or accidents. These types of injuries are often very painful and may result in an inability to use the affected body part. Treatment depends on the type and location of the fracture as well as the presence of other injuries.

There are two major types of fractures: closed and open. Closed fractures remain completely covered by the skin without any type of opening. Open fractures are not completely covered by skin, and there may be bone fragments that stick out or the bone may be exposed. An open fracture increases the victim's risk of infection. Types of fractures can become more detailed depending on their severity. A complete fracture is a break that results in the bone being in two or more pieces. When a bone is not broken in a way resulting in two or more separate pieces, it is called an incomplete fracture. A greenstick fracture, named because it simulates the breaking of a green stick from a tree, has a break on one side and a bend on the opposite side. This primarily happens in children because their bones are still growing. When a bone is broken in three or more pieces, it is called a comminuted fracture.

Some fractures are the result of bones being driven into each other. These are called impacted fractures and occur mainly in the wrist and hip. When this occurs in the spine area, it is called a compression fracture. If a piece of broken bone becomes misaligned, it is known as a displaced fracture. Sometimes fractures can happen without any known injury; these are known as pathological fractures. Pathological fractures often occur in bones weakened by disease. Stress fractures are very tiny breaks of the bone and many times are the result of overuse injuries. Ribs and skulls are also vulnerable to fractures due to direct blows. A hairline fracture is a minor fracture between two segments of a bone. The segments remain aligned and the fracture may not extend completely through the bone.

Considering all of the ways bones protect the human body, it is clear why people should take steps to keep their bones healthy. Bones change with age. To maintain healthy bones throughout a lifetime, there are specific ways each age group can protect their bones, including through proper diet and physical activity. In later years, medications are available to help maintain bone health. By young adulthood, individuals do not add any more calcium to their bones. At that point, the human body will maintain what is already stored. In fact, by the time teens finish growing, 90 percent of their adult bone mass is established. For this reason, it is never too soon to adopt behaviors that can optimize bone strength.

Building strong and healthy bones begins in childhood and in the "tween" and teen years. Tweens are youngsters between the ages of 9 to 12 years old who are older than young children but not yet teens, and this age span is when bones grow

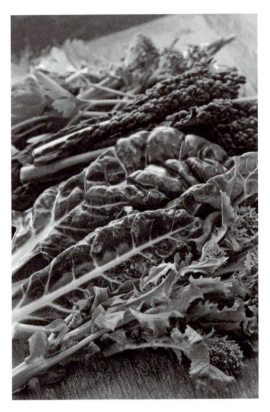

Green vegetables lay on a cutting board. Dark leafy green vegetables like broccoli, kale, and collard greens are a good source of calcium, which supports bone health. (Elena Elisseeva/Dreamstime.com)

the fastest. To avoid bone problems later in life, young people especially in this age range should get plenty of calcium. Since the body cannot produce calcium, it must be absorbed through food. Calcium is found in a variety of foods, including dairy products such as milk and cheese. Dark green, leafy vegetables such as spinach, broccoli, and bok choy also are optimal ways of getting the calcium needed for strong bones. Other options include foods that have calcium added to them, such as tofu, orange juice, soy beverages, and breakfast cereals.

The body constantly removes and replaces small amounts of calcium from its bones. If more calcium goes out than comes in, bones can weaken. When high amounts of the mineral are received, the body does not have to rob bones for calcium it needs to stay healthy. Vitamin D also plays an important role in healthy bone development. Vitamin D helps in the absorption of calcium, an important reason why milk is fortified with vitamin D.

Weight-bearing exercises and physical activity also help build bone mass. Special cells that help bones rebuild in response to stress can kick into high gear under the "good" stress of exercise and heavy activity. This also increases strength. When muscles push and tug against bones during physical activity, the two become stronger together. Some examples of weight-bearing physical activities include walking, jogging or running, stair climbing, jumping rope, basketball, dancing, hiking, and, most notably, weight lifting. It is recommended that adults receive at least 30 minutes of moderate physical activity, preferably every day. Children should engage in at least 60 minutes of moderate physical activity every day of the week to help keep their bones healthy and strong.

Abena Foreman-Trice

See also Calcium; Minerals (Food); Osteoporosis.

References

American Society for Bone and Mineral Research. "Bone Structure and Function" (January 16, 2004), http://depts.washington.edu/bonebio/ASBMRed/structure.html.

Eunice Kennedy Shriver National Institute of Child Health and Human Development, "Bone Health" (August 17, 2010), www.nichd.nih.gov/health/topics/bone_health.cfm.

International Osteoporosis Foundation. "Basic Bone Biology" (January 2011), www.iof bonehealth.org/health-professionals/about-osteoporosis/basic-bone-biology.html.

MedicineNet.com. "Fracture," www.medicinenet.com/fracture/page4.htm.

MedicineNet.com. "Rickets (Calcium, Phosphate, or Vitamin D Deficiency)," www.medi cinenet.com/rickets/article.htm.

MedicineNet.com. "Scoliosis," www.medicinenet.com/scoliosis/article.htm.

MedlinePlus, "Bone Marrow Diseases," www.nlm.nih.gov/medlineplus/bonemarrowdis eases.html.

Mosby's Medical Dictionary, 8th edition. Amsterdam: Elsevier, 2009.

WebMD, "Living with Osteoporosis," www.webmd.com/osteoporosis/living-with-osteo porosis-7/default.htm.

BREAST-FEEDING

Every so often, news stories circulate in the media about women who breast-feed in public. A breast-feeding woman is escorted off a plane, another is asked to leave a restaurant, a woman in a shopping mall is asked to nurse her infant in the public bathroom. These stories raise many questions. Why is breast-feeding widely unaccepted in U.S. culture? Why don't the women just give the infant a bottle? Why is it such a big deal? Not all of these questions can be addressed here, but the advantages and disadvantages of breast-feeding will be discussed. It is important to note that the debate about breast-feeding is multifaceted—part of it deals with health issues and the medical field, part of it deals with formula companies and marketing techniques, and other parts of it deal with aspects of social support. The issue of breast-feeding is quite complicated, but it is useful to begin with an overview of current recommendations regarding infant feeding.

Expressing Breast Milk and Terminology   Many women use a breast pump to express breast milk. Many women combine work and breast-feeding in this way, and it also allows the father to be more involved in the feeding of young infants. However, expressing milk is also challenging—it requires time to pump, careful cleaning of the components, and attention to storage details. Additionally, pumps can be quite expensive. Because pumping milk and then giving breast milk in a bottle is common, it is important to distinguish between bottle feeding and formula feeding. Bottle feeding can refer to either breast milk or formula, but formula feeding refers only to feeding an infant formula.

Breast-feeding in the United States   The American Academy of Pediatrics and the Centers for Disease Control and Prevention, among other organizations, recommend that infants are breast-fed. The current recommendation is to include only breast milk in a baby's diet for the first six months and to begin offering supplements such as baby cereal at six months. Breast milk should remain in the baby's diet for at least a year, and it is beneficial to continue to breast-feed as long as it is mutually desired by both the mother and the infant.

These recommendations are based on an abundance of literature about the health benefits of breast-feeding. Breast-fed babies tend to have fewer ear infections, fewer hospital admissions, and fewer cases of diarrhea than formula-fed infants. Human milk is designed specifically for humans, and therefore it contains the nutritional properties that babies need and that babies can digest. Breast-feeding may also offer some protection against sudden infant death syndrome, diabetes, and obesity.

In addition to the benefits for infants, breast-feeding can be beneficial for the mother. It seems to reduce the risk of ovarian cancer, breast cancer, and osteoporosis. While those are somewhat long-term advantages, there are also short-term health benefits for women. Breast-feeding helps the uterus contract after giving birth, and it generally seems to help women lose more of their pregnancy weight faster because of the calories expended to create the milk. Another important health aspect to breast-feeding is the psychological bond that is developed between the mother and the infant.

Breast-feeding is recommended for all of the above reasons, but few women in the United States are breast-feeding as suggested. According to the Centers for Disease Control and Prevention, approximately 74 percent of women in the United States will breast-feed during the early postpartum period. Approximately 42 percent are breast-feeding at six months, and 21 percent are breast-feeding at a year. When looking at rates of exclusive breast-feeding, the rates drop to only about 30 percent at three months and 12 percent at six months. Exclusive breast-feeding refers to not offering the baby any supplemental foods or liquids; however, one limitation of research in this area is that the term *exclusive* is often not well defined.

Breast-feeding rates also vary by mother's age, educational attainment, race, income level, and the mother's geographic location within the United States. Women are more likely to breast-feed if they are older when the child is born; women under age 20 are the least likely to breast-feed, whereas women over

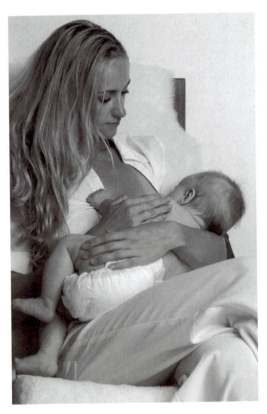

A mother nurses her baby. (Tatyana Gladskikh/ Dreamstime.com)

age 30 are the most likely. As far as educational attainment, women who have a high school degree are the least likely to breast-feed, and women who have graduated from college are the most likely to do so. Asian women are the most likely to breast-feed, and African American women are the least likely to do so. Women in lower income brackets are less likely to breast-feed than wealthier women. Women in rural areas are less likely to breast-feed than those in suburban areas. Additionally, women in the south central United States have the lowest rates of breast-feeding (Centers for Disease Control and Prevention, 2011.

Challenges of Breast-feeding There are many reasons why women stop breast-feeding before it is recommended to do so, and reasons for stopping vary with the infant's age. According to the Pregnancy Risk Assessment and Monitoring System, when women stop breast-feeding within the baby's first week, 34 percent of women did so because they experienced sore, cracked, or bleeding nipples, and 48 percent cited the baby having difficulty nursing as a reason for stopping. When women stopped nursing the baby between one and four weeks old, the most common reason given was because they were not producing enough milk. When women stopped nursing after the baby was four weeks old, the most common reason given was because the baby was not satisfied with breast milk. In addition to sore nipples and difficulties with the baby getting enough milk, many women stop breast-feeding because of work or school responsibilities.

Another difficulty women have with breast-feeding is the limitations it places on them as far as what they can eat and drink. Everything that is in a mother's system can be passed on to the infant through breast milk, so mothers must be careful about what they consume. Some say that breast-fed babies will eat a wider variety of food because they were exposed to more flavors through the mother's breast milk, but this situation can also cause a great deal of stress for a mother. Babies can have allergies to things in the mother's diet, such as dairy, and sometimes foods such as broccoli cause an infant to have painful gas. Some women go on elimination diets and keep food diaries while they are breast-feeding to try to find the source of the infant's discomfort. In addition to everyday foods such as green vegetables and dairy, women are restricted in the amount of caffeine they should consume and the amount of alcohol they can drink. Breast-feeding mothers can drink alcohol, but it is recommended that they drink one drink for every two hours the baby won't nurse. If a baby won't nurse again for four hours, it is generally considered safe for the mother to drink two alcoholic beverages. These limits placed on a mother's consumption can frustrate some women and can be seen as a disadvantage of breast-feeding.

Another important aspect to consider when looking at breast-feeding rates in the United States is the acceptability of breast-feeding in public. According to the Healthstyles 2000 national mail survey, 31 percent of respondents felt that one-year-old children should not be breast-fed, and 27 percent felt it was embarrassing for a mother to breast-feed in front of others. More negative attitudes toward breast-feeding were held by people with lower household incomes and less education and by those who were nonwhite and who were under 30 years old or over 65 years old (Li, Fridinger, & Grummer-Strwn, 2002). Many women do not feel comfortable nursing in public because of other people's reactions and will instead go to public restrooms or to their cars, carefully time trips out, or give the baby a bottle when they are in public. Women who nurse older children in public are even more likely to experience a feeling of inappropriateness based on other's looks, comments, or body posture, and women have said that their experiences nursing in public have lessened the enjoyment of breast-feeding.

Overall, breast-feeding is the recommended way to feed an infant because of its numerous health benefits. However, many variables, such as mother's age, race, and income level influence the decision to breast-feed. Many women stop breast-feeding because of sore or cracked nipples, milk supply concerns, and returning to work, and restrictive diets and nursing in public also complicate the breast-feeding experience.

Many people tend to think of breast-feeding as a very personal decision, and there are many influences on a mother's decision. Ultimately, each woman must decide what she feels is best for her and her family in their situation, but many things, both individual and societal, influence that decision.

Jeanne Holcomb

See also Allergies, Food; Centers for Disease Control and Prevention.

References

Ahluwalia, I., B. Morrow, and J. Hsia. "Why Do Women Stop Breastfeeding? Findings from the Pregnancy Risk Assessment and Monitoring System." *Pediatrics* 116, no. 6 (2005): 1408–12. http://pediatrics.aappublications.org/cgi/reprint/116/6/1408.

American Academy of Pediatrics. "Children's Health Topics: Breastfeeding," www.aap.org/healthtopics/breastfeeding.cfm.

Blum, L. *At the Breast: Ideologies of Breastfeeding and Motherhood in the Contemporary United States.* Boston: Beacon Press, 1999.

Centers for Disease Control and Prevention. "Breastfeeding Practices—Results from the National Immunization Survey" (August 1, 2011), www.cdc.gov/breastfeeding/data/NIS_data/index.htm.

Hausman, Bernice. *Mother's Milk: Breastfeeding Controversies in American Culture.* New York: Routledge, 2003.

Kellymom. "Pumping & Bottle Feeding," www.kellymom.com/bf/pumping/index.html.

La Leche League International. www.llli.org/.

Li, R., F. Fridinger, and L. Grummer-Strwn. "Public Perceptions on Breastfeeding Constraints." *Journal of Human Lactation* 18, no. 3 (2002): 227–35.

Sears, W., and M. Sears. *The Breastfeeding Book.* New York: Little, Brown, 2002.

Stearns, Cindy A. "Breastfeeding and the Good Maternal Body." *Gender and Society* 13, no. 3 (1999): 308–25.

Weiss, Robin Elise. *The Better Way to Breastfeed: The Latest, Most Effective Ways to Feed and Nurture Your Baby with Comfort and Ease.* Beverly, MA: Fair Winds Press, 2010.

Wiessinger, Diane. *The Womanly Art of Breastfeeding.* New York: Ballantine Books, 2010.

World Health Organization. "Breastfeeding," www.who.int/topics/breastfeeding/en/.

BULIMIA NERVOSA

Bulimia nervosa is an eating disorder characterized by a binge-and-purge eating pattern. Either by forcing oneself to vomit, taking laxatives or diuretics, or giving oneself enemas, the person with bulimia is purging to rid him- or herself of the food eaten. There is also a nonpurging form of bulimia characterized by some other method of keeping the weight off, such as compulsive exercising or fasting.

Binges and purges can range from once or twice a week to several times a day. What is visible to family and friends, however, may only be stringent dieting. Symptomatic of the disorder is the excessive amount of food being eaten. Someone with bulimia will eat more food and more frequently than most people. Often, while eating, the person seems to lack control or feels as if he or she can't stop eating. For example, normal food intake for women and teens is between 2,000 and 3,000 calories per day. But bulimic binges are often more than that in a span of less than two hours. Some people with the disorder have reported consuming up to 20,000 calories in binges lasting up to eight hours.

Binge-eating disorder, a newly recognized variation of bulimia, may affect many Americans who eat large amounts of food but do not purge afterward. Another recognized variation, disordered eating, differs from bulimia in that sufferers practice severe calorie restriction. This is a growing problem especially for female athletes in sports where they are judged by build and endurance, such as running, gymnastics, and figure skating. In this instance, the athlete becomes obsessed with his or her weight and may exercise excessively or even vomit to maintain an unrealistic low body weight as he or she seeks to improve performance. While this condition is seen largely in female athletes, the number of U.S. males with eating disorders may be as high as 25 percent of all Americans with an eating disorder, according to information released by the National Association for Males with Eating Disorders, Inc. (2011).

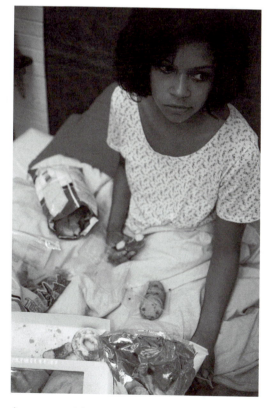

A woman with an eating disorder eats a variety of unhealthy food. Binge eating is one characteristic of bulimia. (PhotoDisc, Inc.)

Results from a national survey released in 2007 suggested that people with bulimia or binge-eating disorder had their condition for about eight years each. The average duration of anorexia was 1.7 years, which researchers say may reflect how difficult it is for people with chronic anorexia to participate in a study. The study, funded by the National Institute of Mental Health (2008) found that 15 percent of adult women and 5 percent of adult men reported having bulimia some time in their lives.

Rapidly purging food through abuse of laxatives, enemas, and diuretics or through induced vomiting upsets the body's balance of chemicals, including sodium and potassium. The result is often fatigue, irregular heartbeat, thinner bones, and seizures. Repeated vomiting can also damage the stomach and esophagus, erode tooth enamel, and result in skin rashes and broken blood vessels in the face.

Bulimia typically begins during adolescence and can continue for years undetected by others. The longer someone with an eating disorder waits to seek help, the more ingrained her or his eating habits become and the more difficult the recovery.

Marjolijn Bijlefeld and Sharon Zoumbaris

See also Anorexia Nervosa; Eating Disorders.

References

Abraham, Suzanne. *Eating Disorders.* New York: Oxford University Press, 2008.

"Anorexia and Bulimia: What You Should Know." *American Family Physician* 77, no. 2 (January 15, 2008).

Bennett, Jessica. "It's Not Just White Girls." *Newsweek,* September 15, 2008, 96.

Bulik, Cynthia M. *Crave: Why You Binge Eat and How to Stop.* New York: Walker, 2009.

"Eating Disorders." *The Columbia Encyclopedia,* 6th ed. Farmington Hills, MI: Gale Group, 2000.

James, Delores C.S., ed. "Female Athlete Triad." *Nutrition and Well-being A-Z,* 2 vols. New York: Macmillan Reference USA, 2004.

National Association for Males with Eating Disorders, Inc. "Statistics" (2011), www.namedinc.org/statistics.asp.

National Institute of Mental Health, "Eating Disorders" (2008), www.nimh.nih.gov/health/publications/eating-disorders.

Neumark-Sztainer, Dianne, Marla Eisenberg, Jayne Fulkerson, Mary Story, and Nicole Larson. "Family Meals and Disordered Eating in Adolescents." *Archives of Pediatrics and Adolescent Medicine* 162, no. 1 (2008): 17–22.

Orr, Tamra. *When the Mirror Lies: Anorexia, Bulimia and Other Eating Disorders.* New York: Franklin Watts, 2007.

C

CAFFEINE

As a chemical compound, caffeine is an alkaloid purine belonging to the group of organic compounds called methylxanthines. Pure caffeine is a white, crystalline, bitter-tasting compound. Caffeine is found in a number of plants, principally coffee and tea plants, as well as cola and cacao nuts. In plants, caffeine functions as a natural pesticide to deter insects.

The consumption of caffeine dates back thousands of years. Tea was consumed in China several thousand years BCE but quite possibly was used in India before that and introduced into China. Coffee consumption is believed to have started in the Kaffa region of Ethiopia around 800 CE and over time spread to Arabia, Turkey, and other parts of the Middle East. The port city of Mocha on the Red Sea in Yemen became a principal coffee-growing region and area of export in the Middle East. Rulers in coffee-growing areas imposed strict laws against the exportation of coffee plants to exercise their monopolies over the lucrative product. Coffee plants spread throughout the world from successful smuggling.

Tea and coffee were introduced into Europe in the 17th century, well after its use in other parts of the world. Chocolate drinks from cacao beans (cocoa is often used for the drink or powder product made from the cacao beans) were being concocted by native populations in Central and South America several hundred years BCE. The Spanish explorer Hernando Cortés (1485–1587) brought cocoa back to Spain around 1528.

Only a small amount of caffeine is found in the cacao plant and chocolate. The principal alkaloid in the cacao plant is theobromine, which is almost identical to caffeine but differs by having one less methyl group. Theobromine does not contain bromine but derives its name from the genus *Theobroma* of the cacao tree. Theobroma's Greek translation is "food of the gods." Another compound almost identical to caffeine in tea is theophylline. It also contains one fewer ethyl group.

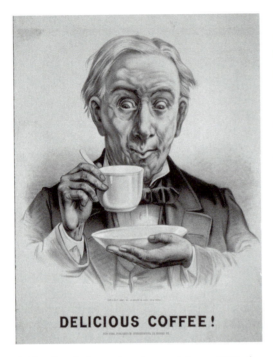

DELICIOUS COFFEE!

A Currier & Ives advertisement from 1881 depicts a man enjoying a cup of coffee. (Library of Congress)

The discovery of caffeine is attributed to Friedlieb Ferdinand Runge (1795–1867), a German physician and chemist. Runge was working in the laboratory of Johann Wolfgang Döbereiner (1780–1849), when Döbereiner's friend, Johann Wolfgang von Goethe (1749–1832), paid a visit. Runge performed an experiment for Goethe in which he dilated a cat's eye with an extract from a nightshade plant. Goethe awarded Runge with a sample of rare coffee beans and challenged him to determine the compound that gave coffee its stimulating effects. After several months, Runge isolated caffeine from coffee in 1819. Caffeine derives its name from the Kaffa region of Ethiopia and from the German *kaffeine,* which in turn is derived from the German word for coffee, *kaffee.* In 1827, a compound isolated from tea was named theine, but this was eventually shown to be caffeine.

Caffeine is a stimulant to the central nervous system and cardiac muscle and is a mild diuretic. Caffeine's physiological effects are thought to be the result of caffeine's interference with adenosine in the brain and body. Adenosine moderates nerve transmissions. As adenosine builds up while a person is awake, it produces a self-regulating mechanism to inhibit nerve transmission. As adenosine receptors in the brain acquire more adenosine, the reduction in nerve transmission induces sleep. Caffeine competes with adenosine and interferes with the neural modulation function of adenosine. This is why coffee has a tendency to keep people awake.

The effects of coffee and caffeinated drinks vary widely among individuals. Generally, moderate consumption leads to restlessness and tends to energize individuals. Caffeine increases blood pressure and has been indirectly associated with heart and pregnancy problems; it increases stomach acid, which can lead to ulcers. Regular users of caffeinated drinks can experience withdrawal side effects such as anxiety, nervousness, fatigue, and headaches. The effects of caffeine last several hours after consumption. It is carried by the blood to all parts of the body and is eliminated primarily through the urine after a half-life of 4 to 10 hours in most adults.

Health experts advise that moderated amounts of caffeine from 100 to 300 milligrams per day are acceptable. Adult Americans consume approximately 250 milligrams of caffeine per day. The LD50 (the lethal dose that kills 50% of a test population of individuals subjected to a substance) of caffeine for humans is estimated between 150 and 200 milligrams per kilogram of body weight. The amount of caffeine in some popular food items is given in Table 1.

Coffee beans are the primary source of caffeine. These beans are obtained from a variety of plants but can be broadly grouped into two classes: arabica and robusta. Arabica is obtained from the species *Coffea arabica* and robusta from the species *Coffea canephora*. Robusta, as the name implies, is more robust than arabica coffee but produces an inferior taste.

Arabica plants are grown globally, but robusta plants are grown only in the Eastern Hemisphere. Coffee beans contain 1 to 2 percent caffeine, with robusta varieties generally containing twice the content of arabica varieties. Other sources of caffeine contain various amounts: kola nut (1 to 3.5%), tea leaves (1.4 to 4.5%), and cacao (0.1 to 0.5%).

Some food processors add caffeine to their products (soft drinks), but others remove caffeine and advertise the product as decaffeinated. Coffee was first decaffeinated in 1906 in Germany through a process founded by the coffee merchant Ludwig Roselius (1874–1943). Roselius's team sought to decaffeinate coffee without destroying the aroma and flavor. Roselius fortuitously worked on beans that had been soaked with seawater during a storm and found a method to remove 97 percent of the caffeine in coffee beans without destroying the flavor. Roselius then marketed the product under different names in various European countries.

Table 1. Approximate Caffeine Content of Selected Food and Medicine Items

	Caffeine Content (in Milligrams)
Coffee (8 ounces)	30–140
Mountain Dew (12 ounces)	54
Coca-Cola (12 ounces)	45
Pepsi-Cola (12 ounces)	37
Tea (brewed) (8 ounces)	20–100
Red Bull (8.2 ounces)	80
Häagen-Dazs coffee ice cream (1 cup)	58
Hot chocolate (8 ounces)	5
Excedrin (2 tablets)	130
NoDoz (1 tablet)	200
Anacin (2 tablets)	64

In France, the name of the decaffeinated coffee was Sanka, which is derived from *sans* caffeine (*sans kaffee*). Sanka was introduced in the United States in 1923. The traditional method of decaffeinating coffee beans involved steaming the beans and then extracting the caffeine in an organic solvent such as freon, chloroform, methylene chloride, or ethyl acetate. Because of the environmental problems and costs associated with organic solvents, green decaffeination techniques have been developed in recent years. One popular method is to use supercritical carbon dioxide to extract caffeine.

Caffeine has widespread therapeutic use. It is widely used in headache (migraine) remedies such as aspirin and other analgesics. Caffeine is a mild vasoconstrictor, and its ability to constrict blood vessels serving the brain explains its use to relieve headache. Individuals who consume caffeine regularly through medications and food are susceptible to what is known as a rebound headache or caffeine rebound. This occurs when regular caffeine intake is suddenly reduced and the vessels dilate. Caffeine is a common substance in medications to treat apnea in premature infants. Apparently, the area of the brain controlling respiration in premature infants is not fully developed and caffeine helps to stimulate this portion of the brain. The combination of caffeine and ephedrine is used in dietary and athletic supplements, and their role as appetite suppressant and energy boosters has been extensively studied. Some individuals claim that a modest dose (200 milligrams) of caffeine can enhance athletic performance, but its exact effect is unclear. Caffeine is used for the treatment of attention deficit hyperactivity disorder, but health experts do not recommend its use for this condition.

Richard L. Myers

See also Attention Deficit Hyperactivity Disorder; Ephedra/Ephedrine.

References

Aftalion, Fred. *A History of the International Chemistry Industry,* 2nd ed. Philadelphia: Chemical Heritage Foundation, 2001.

Baird, Colin, and Michael Cann. *Environmental Chemistry,* 3rd ed. New York: W.H. Freeman, 2004.

"Chemical & Engineering News." *Top Pharmaceuticals* 83, no. 25 (June 20, 2005): 44–139. Special issue devoted to reports on 46 of the most important drugs for human society.

Kent, James A. *Riegel's Handbook of Industrial Chemistry,* 10th ed. New York: Kluwer Academic/Plenum, 2003.

May, Paul. *The Molecule of the Month.* www.chm.bris.ac,uk/motm/motm.htm.

Mayo Clinic. www.mayoclinic.com/health/site-map/smindex.

The Merck Index, 12th ed. Whitehouse Station, NJ: Merck, 1996.

Myers, Richard L. *The Basics of Chemistry.* Westport, CT: Greenwood Press, 2003.

Snyder, Carl H. *The Extraordinary Chemistry of Ordinary Things,* 3rd ed. New York: John Wiley, 1998.

Tobin, Allan J., and Jennie Dusheck. *Asking about Life.* Fort Worth, TX: Saunders College, 1998.

Walsh, Christopher. *Antibiotics: Actions, Origins, Resistance.* Herndon, VA: ASM Press, 2003.

CALCIUM

Calcium is everywhere these days—added to orange juice, cereal, dairy products, and a host of other prepared foods. This important mineral is needed for the development of bones and teeth. Plus, muscles, nerves, and all parts of the human body need calcium for optimum health. Due to this key role in dental health and the prevention of bone diseases such as osteoporosis, calcium is now a popular supplement. Even though it has been increasingly added to foods and made into supplements, calcium can easily be found naturally in many foods, including dairy products, green leafy vegetables, and soy products, including tofu.

Calcium requirements are highest for adolescents, whose bones are growing rapidly, and for pregnant and lactating women. The National Institutes of Health Office of Dietary Supplements in its 2010 fact sheet listed calcium requirements based on age with a few other noted factors. It recommended that preteens and adolescents should consume 1,300 milligrams per day of calcium. Adults from age 19 to age 50 should get 1,000 milligrams per day, and adults over 51 years old should increase their intake to 1,200 milligrams each day. Finally, pregnant teens need the same amount as their regular teen counterparts with 1,300 milligrams per day, and adult women who are pregnant and breast-feeding need 1,000 milligrams daily. The government recommendations also suggest exercise as an

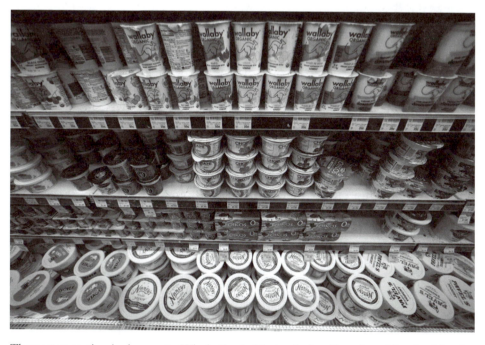

The yogurt section is shown at a Whole Foods Market in San Francisco, Monday, May 24, 2010. An explosion of yogurt options has given Americans bold new choices, from goat's milk to Greek-style to soy and even coconut milk yogurts. (AP/Wide World Photos)

important partner for achieving maximal peak bone mass, and stress that fat-reduced dairy products such as skim milk are just as nutritious for older children. In fact, starting around age 9, kids need twice the daily amount of calcium as younger children.

How can U.S. teens, renowned for their often poor nutrition, get enough calcium? One way is by consuming four to five glasses of low-fat milk per day. Other milk products are also good sources of calcium. Besides dairy products, green leafy vegetables, such as kale, collards, beets, and turnip tops are excellent natural sources of calcium. So are tofu, dried peas and beans, the soft bones of canned fish, and calcium-fortified orange juice.

Without enough from a daily diet of calcium rich foods or beverages, the human body turns to bones to find the calcium it needs. For people who do not eat enough calcium for a variety of reasons including lactose intolerance, calcium supplements are available, especially for anyone at particularly high risk for osteoporosis. Read the label of a calcium supplement carefully to find the amount of elemental calcium. There are different kinds of calcium supplements—including calcium citrate (which is generally the most easily absorbed), calcium carbonate, and calcium phosphate—that include other elements such as vitamin D, which help with absorption. Because of its ability to neutralize stomach acid, calcium carbonate is found in some over-the-counter antacid products.

Factors that affect calcium absorption include age, since young children and infants have a higher rate of absorption than adults. Vitamin D intake can improve calcium absorption when skin is exposed to a certain amount of sunlight. Research shows that other, competing nutrients in foods can actually slow the body's ability to absorb calcium. For example, foods with high levels of oxalic acid such as spinach, collard greens, sweet potatoes, or rhubarb can slow absorption because the oxalic acid in the foods binds to calcium.

A lack of calcium can also occur when calcium is regularly eliminated from the body in large quantities through waste and sweat. Those who regularly eat or drink high levels of sodium, protein, or caffeine can expect increased calcium loss. The opposite is true of a diet of fruits and vegetables; these foods, when metabolized, help reduce calcium loss by shifting the acid/base balance of the body and producing bicarbonate, which studies have shown reduces calcium excretion. While more calcium is generally better, too much is not good. Overdoses of calcium can interfere with the absorption of other nutrients, such as zinc and iron.

Bone loss, otherwise known as osteoporosis, is a long-term effect of low calcium intake, although symptoms may not be visible for years. Along with taking calcium supplements, bone mass and overall bone health can be improved by regular weight-bearing exercise, such as dancing and running, which can rebuild bone mass and strength. Unhealthy activities, such as smoking, alcohol use, and a poor diet contribute to losing bone mass.

According to the National Institute of Child Health and Human Development, supplementing the daily diets of girls ages 12 to 16 with an extra 350 milligrams of calcium produced a 14 percent increase in bone density. Researchers say this is a striking difference, because for every 5 percent increase in bone density, the risk of later bone fracture declines by 40 percent. Calcium requirements rise again during the second and third trimester of pregnancy—the period during which the fetal skeleton is developing quickly. The general recommendation for pregnant women is that calcium intake should be increased by 400 milligrams per day.

Other examples of calcium's effect on health include the possibility that it lowers blood pressure and reduces the likelihood of forming kidney stones. Researchers say calcium from food does not increase the risk of calcium oxalate stones, which are the most common type of kidney stones. People who form calcium oxalate stones are advised to include 800 milligrams of calcium-rich foods in their diet every day. However, if they take calcium supplements, they should be taken at the same time oxalate-rich foods are eaten. Studies have shown that calcium supplements may increase the risk of calcium oxalate stone formation when taken alone.

Scientists are also studying whether the recommended amount of daily calcium might lower the chance of developing colon cancer in adults. While it is too early to tell, there is research underway. As for heart health, an adequate supply of daily calcium has been shown to help muscles, especially the heart muscle, do the work of contracting and relaxing. Plus, calcium appears to help the nervous system regulate the level of pressure in arteries.

Sharon Zoumbaris

See also Dental Health; Dietary Supplements; Lactose Intolerance; Minerals (Food); Osteoporosis; Sodium.

References

"Fitness Fuel." *Good Health* (July 7, 2010).

Mangels, Reed. "The Latest News on Protein and Bone Health." *Vegetarian Journal* 29, no. 3 (July–September 2010): 13.

Mulhall, Douglas, with Katja Hansen. *The Calcium Bomb: The Nanobacteria Link to Heart Disease and Cancer.* Cranston, RI: Writers' Collective, 2005.

National Institutes of Health. "Optimal Calcium Intake." *NIH Consensus Statement* 12, no. 4 (June 6–8, 1994):1–31, http://consensus.nih.gov/1994/1994OptimalCalcium097PDF.pdf.

National Institutes of Health. "Osteoporosis." NIH Osteoporosis and Related Bone Diseases National Resource Center, Institutes of Health (August 9, 2010), www.niams.nih.gov/Health_Info/bone/Osteoporosis/default.asp.

Pratt, Steven, and Kathy Matthews. *Superfoods Healthstyle: Proven Strategies for Lifelong Health.* New York: William Morrow, 2006.

Schwartz, Joseph A. *An Apple a Day: The Myths, Misconceptions, and Truths about the Foods We Eat.* New York: Other Press, 2009.

Tweed, Vera. "Improving Bone Density." *Better Nutrition* 72, no. 3 (March 2010): 12.

U.S. Department of Agriculture, Center for Nutrition Policy and Promotion. "MyPlate" (2011), www.choosemyplate.gov/.

U.S. Department of Agriculture, Agricultural Research Service. *National Nutrient Database for Standard Reference, Release 22* (2009), www.ars.usda.gov/ba/bhnrc/ndl.

CALORIES

A calorie is a measurement of heat needed to raise one kilogram of water one degree Celsius. Since food stokes the furnace of our bodies, foods have assigned calorie values. The number of calories in a food can be found on the nutrition facts label on any packaged food. Realize, however, that these are calories per serving. If the nutrition label claims the package has two servings—by eating it all, you've eaten double the calories that the label says.

Fat and alcohol are high in calories. Foods high in both sugars and fat contain many calories but often are low in vitamins, minerals, and fiber. Numerous calorie counters are readily available—online and often in cookbooks. A reduction in caloric intake will result in weight loss. An increase in the amount of calories consumed will cause weight gain. One pound equals 3,500 calories. So to lose a pound in, say, a week, an individual would have to consume 3,500 calories less, burn 3,500 calories in exercise, or some combination of the two during the course of the week (or 500 calories per day).

It is possible to estimate about how many calories per day must be eaten to maintain body weight. Use the formula below to calculate that number. For those seeking to lose weight, cut the calories or increase the overall level of activity.

Moderately active men should multiply their weight in pounds by 15. For example, if a man weighs 170 pounds, he needs about 2,500 calories per day. Moderately active women should multiply their weight by 12. A 130-pound woman needs about 1,560 calories per day.

However, those who are not regularly active will need to use a different formula because the number of calories needed per day decreases with the level of activity. In other words, if an individual burns fewer calories a day, he or she will need fewer of them to maintain current weight. Relatively inactive men should multiply their weight by 13 pounds, and women in that category should multiply their weigh by 10. So a 170-pound man who is relatively inactive needs 2,210 calories, and a 130-pound inactive woman needs 1,300 calories to maintain body weight.

Calories from Fat Numerous health and government authorities, including the U.S. Surgeon General, the National Academy of Sciences, the American Heart Association, and the American Dietetic Association, recommend reducing dietary fat to 30 percent or less of total calories. However, that doesn't mean giving up all high-fat food products. For example, peanut butter with sugar added has 200 calories in a two-tablespoon serving. Of those 200 calories, 140 calories are from fat—70 percent. Add that peanut butter to two slices of whole wheat bread, which have 120 calories and 20 calories from fat, and the equation is different: now the fat is down to about 48 percent. It's still higher than the recommendation, but by adding a glass of skim milk and an apple, the fat drops down to a healthy level.

Keep in mind that the information on nutrition labels is based on a 2,000-calorie-per-day diet. So if daily average caloric intake is lower, the overall percentage of fat is higher than what's listed on the label. For example, back to the peanut butter with its 16 grams of total fat and 3 grams of saturated fat. The total fat is 25 percent of the daily value and the saturated fat is 15 percent of the daily value—based on a 2,000-calorie diet, which calls for less than 65 grams of total fat and less than 20 grams of saturated fat per day. Now for an inactive person they would need only 1,300 calories per day to maintain their body weight.

According to figures released by the Centers for Disease Control and Prevention (CDC), Americans have steadily increased their rate of calorie consumption, and the rate of increase is three times greater in women than men. Diet analysis published in 2004 showed women went from 1,542 calories per day to 1,877 between 1971 and 2000. Men increased 7 percent from 2,450 calories per day to 2,618 calories over the same period. The study was based on data from the National Health and Nutrition Examination Survey collected by the CDC's National Center for Health Statistics.

Eating more frequently is encouraged by numerous environmental changes: a greater variety of foods, some with higher caloric content; the growth of the fast-food industry; the increased numbers and marketing of snack foods; and a growing tendency to socialize with food and drink.

At the same time, there are fewer opportunities in daily life to burn calories: children watch more television daily; many schools have done away with or cut back on physical education; many neighborhoods lack sidewalks for safe walking; the workplace has become increasingly automated; household chores are assisted by labor-saving machinery; and walking and cycling have been replaced by automobile travel for all but the shortest distances.

Consider this: the American Institute for Cancer Research says Americans' snack-food intake has tripled in the last 20 years. An average American now consumes 16 to 20 pounds of snack food, or 40,000 snack calories, per year.

Calories Burned during Exercise Exercise burns calories. For example, walking briskly can burn off about 100 calories per mile. Bicycling for half an hour at nearly 10 miles per hour will burn about 195 calories. The specific number depends on the person's weight and the intensity of the activity. A variety of interactive exercise counters, available on the Internet, allows anyone to plug in their weight and age, and change variables such as the length of time and intensity of the activity. For someone working to lose weight, the combination of exercise and a healthy diet works more effectively than either method by itself. Eat less and lose weight. Exercise more and lose weight, tone muscles, and build aerobic endurance. Do both and they will complement each other.

The more an individual weighs, the more calories he or she will burn. The reason is the heart has to pump harder to get the blood to the different parts of the body. So a 130-pound person doing medium-intensity aerobic dancing for 30 minutes will burn about 174 calories. A 150-pound person will burn about 201 calories in the same amount of time.

Table 1. Calories per Hour Expended in Common Physical Activities

Moderate Physical Activity	Approximate Calories Burned per Hour by a 154-Pound Person
Hiking	370
Light gardening/yard work	330
Dancing	330
Golf (walking and carrying clubs)	330
Bicycling (< 10 miles per hour)	290
Walking (3.5 miles per hour)	280
Weight lifting (general light workout)	220
Stretching	180
Vigorous Physical Activity	
Running/jogging (5 miles per hour)	590
Bicycling (> 10 miles per hour)	590
Swimming (slow freestyle laps)	510
Aerobics	480
Walking (4.5 miles per hour)	460
Heavy yard work (chopping wood)	440
Weight lifting (vigorous effort)	440
Basketball (vigorous)	440

Source: Adapted from the 2005 DGAC (Dietary Guidelines Advisory Committee) Report. Courtesy USDA Guidelines for Americans 2005, www.cnpp.usda.gov/dietaryguidelines.htm.

Note: Some examples of physical activities commonly engaged in and the average amount of calories a 154-pound individual will expend by engaging in each activity for one hour. The expenditure value encompasses both resting metabolic rate calories and activity expenditure. Some of the activities can constitute either moderate- or vigorous-intensity physical activity depending on the rate at which they are carried out (for walking and bicycling).

Calories burned per hour will be higher for persons who weigh more than 154 pounds (70 kilograms) and lower for persons who weigh less.

The Austin (Texas) Diagnostics Clinic put together this list of calorie-burning levels of different activities in the spring 1998 issue of its fitness publication, *Classics Club Quarterly.* Many such listings and online calculators exist to help provide a more precise gauge on calories burned.

Let's say you eat 2,000 calories' worth of food. But your physical activity only uses 1,500 of these. The extra calories are stored in your body—as fat. When you exercise, your body uses fuel, which comes from one of two forms: stored carbohydrates called glycogen or stored body fat. Stored body fat is found in fat cells and is also stored in small droplets in the muscles.

Most activities use both carbohydrates and fat for fuel. Lower-intensity workouts, such as walking, use fat as the primary fuel. As the workout intensifies, the fuel reserves come increasingly from carbohydrates. But that doesn't mean that walking burns more fat than running. When the carbohydrate or glycogen source runs low, the body releases fats for fuels. Also, a higher-intensity workout, such as running, continues to burn fat even after the physical activity itself is over. As the body works to restore glycogen, it continues to use fat to do so. And because higher-intensity workouts burn more calories overall, even though the mix of carbohydrates and fats may be different, it is possible to burn more fat in the workout.

Marjolijn Bijlefeld and Sharon Zoumbaris

See also Carbohydrates; Exercise; Fats.

References

Beil, Laura. "Fat Chance: Scientists Are Working on a Way to Rev Up the Body's Gut-Busting Machinery." *Science News* 178, no. 1 (July 3, 2010): 18–22.

Gallagher, Julie. "Americans Lack Dietary Knowledge." *Supermarket News* 58, no. 28 (July 12, 2010).

Keane, Maureen. *What to Eat If You Have Cancer: Healing Foods That Boost Your Immune System.* New York: McGraw-Hill, 2007.

Nestle, Marion. *What to Eat.* New York: North Point Press, 2006.

Pagano, Joan. *Strength Training for Women: Tone Up, Burn Calories, Stay Strong.* London: New York: Dorling Kindersley, 2005.

Park, Alice. "Fat Bug, Thin Bug." *Time,* December 7, 2009, W6.

Schwarcz, Joseph A. *An Apple a Day: The Myths, Misconceptions, and Truths about the Foods We Eat.* New York: Other Press, 2009.

Springen, Karen. "The Truth about Eating." *Newsweek,* November 3, 2008, 72.

Taubes, Gary. *Good Calories, Bad Calories: Challenging the Conventional Wisdom on Diet, Weight.* New York: Knopf, 2007.

Weisenberger, Jill. "The Skinny on Foods and Metabolism." *Environmental Nutrition,* 33, no. 7 (July 2010): 1–2.

CANCER

Cancer is a complex family of diseases characterized by cells that divide and grow without normal control. The study and treatment of cancer is known as oncology. The various types of cancers are named for the cells in the body where they begin. Carcinomas originate in epithelial cells that line or cover the surfaces of organs such as the lung, breast, and colon. Sarcomas start in connective or supportive tissues of the body such as bone, cartilage, fat, connective tissue, and muscle. Lymphomas are cancers that come from the lymph nodes and tissues of the body's immune system. Leukemias are cancers of the blood cells.

Interactions between the environment and a person's individual genetic predisposition can play an important role in the development of cancer. Carcinogens and environmental or extrinsic factors that have been implicated in causing cancer include viruses, chemicals, and radiation. These agents can directly or indirectly cause mutations or genetic damage within a cell that result in uncontrollable cell division and, eventually, a tumor.

Another set of factors, what we will call endogenous factors (of the body), also contribute to cancer. These endogenous influences are comprised of certain hormones and inflammatory molecules. Thus, there are three parts to the cancer-causing equation: each person's unique set of genes, his or her exposure to extrinsic or environmental factors, and his or her own health history relating to hormones and inflammation.

Environmental Risk Factors The International Agency for Research on Cancer keeps track of known carcinogens or agents that cause cancer, along with comprehensive evaluations on the health risk posed by these agents. The National Cancer Institute also maintains a website informing the public of environmental risk factors: www.cdc.gov/nceh/. At the turn of the millennium, Richard Doll and his colleague Richard Peto, while working at the Radcliffe Infirmary in Oxford, England, estimated the proportions of cancer deaths caused by avoidable environmental factors. They estimated that tobacco smoke, which is a source of chemical carcinogens, causes 25 to 40 percent of cancer deaths.

Our diet is considered to cause between 10 percent and 70 percent of cancer deaths. Infections from viruses are thought to cause 10 percent to 15 percent of all cancer. Chemical carcinogens in the workplace are thought to be responsible for 2 percent to 8 percent of cancer deaths. Radiation, the most common type being ultraviolet radiation from sun exposure, is reputed to be responsible for 2 percent to 4 percent of cancer deaths. Pollutants in air, water, and food are estimated to cause less than 1 to 5 percent of cancer deaths; and certain medicines cause 0.3 percent to 1.5 percent of deaths (Doll, 1998a; Doll & Peto, 1981; Nelson, 2004).

Lessons from Chimney Sweeps Many chemical carcinogens were first identified in the workplace. Beginning in the 1700s, doctors realized that workers within particular industries developed tumors at much higher rates than the rest of the population. The physicians rightly associated the tumors with industrial exposure to particular chemicals.

The earliest investigation of an occupational neoplasm examined the connection between soot and scrotal cancer (Pott, 1775; CA Journal, 1974). Sir Percivall Pott, who was a highly respected surgeon at Saint Bartholomew's Hospital in London in the 1700s, first described an occupational cancer in chimney sweeps, cancer of the scrotum. He noted "the disease, in these people, seems to derive its origin from a lodgment of soot in the rugae or folds of the scrotum." The chimney sweeper's cancer or "soot-wart" as it was called, produced a superficial, painful, ragged sore with hard and rising edges. Originally, this was thought to be a type of venereal or sexually transmitted disease and was treated with mercurials without success.

Pott also reported a case of cancer on the hand of a gardener who spread soot on the garden to protect the plants from slugs as part of his duties. He even observed cancer development in a man who merely stayed with a chimney sweep who stored bags of soot and tools in his home. These observations ultimately led to additional studies that identified a number of occupational carcinogenic exposures and led to public health measures to reduce cancer risk.

What Is in a Cigarette? Tobacco use is unfortunately the largest voluntary carcinogen exposure experiment in history, and is still ongoing (Wogan et al., 2004).

The most common exposure to known chemical carcinogens comes from tobacco products. Smoking and chewing tobacco, as well as inhalation of secondary smoke, all cause cancer. Tobacco smoke contains more than 60 known carcinogens, including polycyclic aromatic hydrocarbons or PAHs, nitrosamines, aromatic amines, acetaldehyde, and phenols, among others. Unburned tobacco, such as chewing tobacco and snuff, contains nitrosamines and small amounts of PAHs. The study of these chemicals and their tumorigenic potential was performed by chemical analysis of cigarette smoke. The different chemicals were applied to mouse skin to determine if they cause cancer, similar to the experiment performed by Yamagiwa and Ichikawa in 1915 (Hecht, 2003).

The Yin and Yang of Hormones Scientists have come to recognize that some of the natural molecules in the body indirectly promote tumorigenesis. While many of the carcinogens discussed previously can directly mutate DNA, some endogenous molecules have the potential to promote cancer formation by indirectly increasing the chances of mutation. These endogenous factors, hormones and inflammatory molecules, normally regulate healthy physiology. However, they may circulate in the blood at unhealthy, high levels in certain cases. Some hormones may be elevated in obese individuals, and inflammatory regulators may be elevated in patients with chronic inflammation. Prolonged, elevated levels of these naturally occurring chemicals can promote the development of neoplasia.

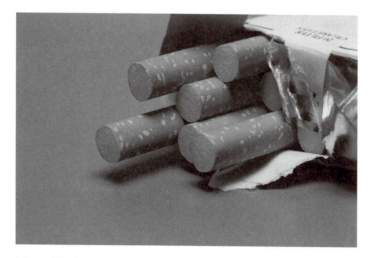

The addictive properties of nicotine make it difficult for many smokers to quit. The nicotine in cigarettes has been linked to lung cancer. (PhotoDisc, Inc.)

Estrogen Physicians and scientists have long recognized that sustained levels of endogenous estrogen pose a breast cancer risk. Breast tissue is naturally responsive to this hormone; the normal development of the mammary glands, both at puberty and during pregnancy, is stimulated by estrogen. Women who have no children, who begin to menstruate early, or who continue to have menstrual cycles past the typical age for menopause have a greater chance of developing postmenopausal breast carcinoma. In these situations, the woman undergoes more menstrual cycles over her lifetime and therefore her exposure to estrogen is sustained.

Bernardino Ramazzini in 1713 was the first to notice that women who did not have children, nuns in fact, had a higher incidence of breast cancer than women who had children (Franco, 2001). This observation was statistically confirmed by Janet Lane-Claypon in her 1926 study of breast cancer patients. We now know that estrogen blood levels of women with postmenopausal breast cancer are 15 percent higher than those of healthy postmenopausal women (Lane-Claypon, 1926; Thomas, Reeves, & Key, 1997). More recent epidemiological studies demonstrate that excess weight, low physical activity, and alcohol also contribute to postmenopausal breast cancer risk.

Since the late 1980s, clinical studies monitored by health care providers in controlled settings have been undertaken to determine whether these lifestyle and diet factors were correlated with raised levels of circulating estrogen. To perform these studies, women volunteers participated in detailed weight and body measurements, exercise programs, or alcohol and diet regimens during which blood was drawn periodically. All three risk factors were found to correlate with higher levels of circulating estrogen than control groups (Dorgan et al., 2001; Kaye et al., 1991; McTiernan et al., 2004). The findings that excess adipose tissue and physical inactivity are associated with elevated estrogen levels is not surprising given that in postmenopausal women, adipose or fat cells synthesize estrogen (Clemons & Goss, 2001).

Insulin Epidemiological studies have shown that obesity is a risk factor for colon cancer, especially in men, and physical inactivity is a risk factor for colon cancer in both men and women. Researchers have formulated the hypothesis that these factors mediate tumorigenesis via the hormone insulin and a related molecule called insulin-like growth factor (IGF). Because obesity and physical inactivity lead to increased levels of circulating insulin and IGF, studies were performed to determine whether these hormones were associated with greater risk of colon cancer.

Thousands of study participants answered health questionnaires and donated blood samples periodically over the course of several years so that circulating hormone levels could be assayed. Higher levels of insulin and IGF were found to correlate with an increased risk of colon cancer as well as death from colon cancer (Wolpin et al., 2009). Researchers have also hypothesized that insulin and IGF play a role in mediating breast cancer risk in obese and physically inactive women, separately from effects on estrogen synthesis. To date, data from clinical studies examining the levels of insulin and IGF in women with breast cancer have yielded conflicting results. Hopefully, future studies will resolve this question (Coyle, 2009).

How Irritating   Despite advances in the understanding of carcinogenesis, from the late 1800s until the 1920s, cancer was thought by some to be caused by trauma. This belief was maintained despite the failure to cause cancer in experimental animals by injury. However, inflammation, which is a normal, healthy response to irritation, infection, and injury, may be a cause of cancer. The inflammatory process has the potential to become unregulated, meaning it does not stop when the infectious agents are eliminated or damage from the injury is healed. Chronic inflammation elevates the risk of several types of cancer. Infections with certain bacteria, viruses, or parasites are particularly associated with tumorigenesis. For example, stomach inflammation stemming from infection with the bacteria *Helicobacter pylori* increases the risk of stomach cancer, while chronic liver inflammation caused by the liver fluke parasite elevates the chance of developing hepatic cancer.

The human papillomavirus causes inflammation in the uterine cervix, which contributes to the development of cervical carcinoma. Exposure to the chemical asbestos causes chronic inflammation of the mesothelium, the lining of the lung cavity, raising the chance of developing the rare cancer called mesothelioma. Obesity also can lead to chronic inflammation, contributing to tumorigenesis via the inflammatory pathway as well as altering hormone levels. Chronic inflammation of the intestine caused by autoimmune diseases such as Crohn's disease and ulcerative colitis also predispose the patient to colon cancer. Persistent refluxing of stomach acid up into the esophagus, often referred to as heartburn, may also result in inflammation and increase the risk of esophageal cancer (Aggarwal et al., 2006; Hussain & Harris, 2007).

Asbestos   Asbestos causes a type of lung cancer called mesothelioma, carcinoma of the lining of the lung cavity. Asbestos is the commercial name of a family of silicon-based mineral fibers that are used in construction and manufacturing because they are fire and friction resistant. It must be inhaled to be dangerous, and asbestos fibers have been documented in the lungs of mesothelioma patients. The connection between mesothelioma and the inhalation of asbestos fibers is quite strong, perhaps the strongest cause-effect relationship among all known carcinogens, meaning that almost all mesothelioma cases develop because of asbestos exposure. Mesothelioma is usually fatal. The average survival after diagnosis is 9 to 12 months.

Asbestos is considered an occupational carcinogen because most of the people who develop mesothelioma inhaled asbestos fibers in the workplace. People are exposed because they mine asbestos, or because they work in factories where it is used, or because they work at construction sites with materials containing these fibers. The number of cases of this fatal cancer in men has increased over the past 30 years, although it is still relatively rare in the United States. Researchers connect this development with the fact that asbestos became commonplace in industry about 60 years ago, at a time when most factory workers were men. The rising number of cases also reflects the fact that mesotheliomas seldom appear earlier than 15 years after exposure. After 15 years, the mesothelioma rate begins to rise. In 1986, the United States passed the Asbestos Hazard Emergency Response Act, mandating that asbestos exposure levels in the workplace be kept safe.

Asbestos and mesothelioma have generated a good deal of media attention. One reason is because asbestos was used as a fireproof coating around pipes in many public buildings, including schools. The Asbestos Hazard Emergency Response Act banned its use as a spray-on fireproofing material, but in doing so it brought the dangers of this material to the attention of the public and led to the distorted assumption that the asbestos in schools posed an immediate threat. Asbestos coatings do not shed fibers unless decayed or disturbed by renovation.

A 1989 survey found that even in buildings with damaged asbestos linings, the asbestos fiber content of the air was one-one hundredth of the permissible exposure level. Additionally, the asbestos fibers used for fireproofing were not the most dangerous variety. Scientists believe that those at most risk of contracting mesothelioma from asbestos in public buildings were the workers hired by panicked officials to remove it, and only then if proper precautions were not followed (Mossman et al., 1990; Robinson, Musk, & Lake, 2005).

Sign outside a construction zone warns of the dangers of asbestos. (Bronwyn8/Dreamstime. com)

Radiation Some types of radiation, mainly ultraviolet and ionizing radiation, induce cancer. The most common form of radiation exposure that leads to cancer is ultraviolet rays from the sun, which cause skin cancer, including basal cell carcinoma, squamous cell carcinoma and melanoma (Green et al., 1999). Not surprisingly, given the ubiquity of exposure to sunlight, basal and squamous cell carcinomas are the most common cancers in the United States, but they seldom lead to death. Ionizing radiation, in the form of X-rays and radioactivity, can also be harmful but is considered to contribute to a small portion of total cancers overall.

Radon, a naturally occurring radioactive gas, seeps into buildings from the ground or rocks. Chronic exposure to radon has been linked to lung cancer, with estimates of radon-induced lung cancer deaths ranging between 2 percent and 20 percent of the overall number of annual lung cancer deaths. Most of these deaths arise from the especially dangerous combination of radon exposure and smoking. Home radon levels can be evaluated by detection kits available in hardware stores (Frumkin & Samet, 2001).

You Are What You Eat

Aflatoxin Aflatoxin, a chemical produced by the fungus *Aspergillus flavus oryzae,* has been positively identified as a causative agent of liver cancer and is probably the best-documented carcinogen found in food. It first came to scientific attention when turkeys became poisoned by moldy peanut meal. Next, laboratory rats were found to develop liver cancer after eating moldy feed. Soon, the fungus was identified, and the causative agent, aflatoxin B1 (AFB1) was purified. Epidemiological studies revealed that basic foodstuffs, such as peanuts, are contaminated with *Aspergillus* in countries where liver cancer is prominent. In fact, there is a strong correlation between ingestion of contaminated food, urine levels of AFB1 metabolites, and liver cancer incidence. In the laboratory, scientists found that AFB1 induces mutations in bacteria and human cells. Together, these findings strongly implicate AFB1 as a causative agent of liver cancer (Guengerich, 2001; Wogan et al., 2004).

Red Meat Epidemiological studies have uncovered a small but significant correlation between the consumption of red meat, especially processed red meat, and the incidence of colorectal cancer. One group of known carcinogens, N-nitroso compounds (NOCs) is formed by the digestion of meat in the intestine. Clinical studies in which volunteers were kept on strictly monitored and controlled diets showed that a regimen rich in red meat resulted in higher levels of NOCs in the feces. Fecal analysis determined that the source of the NOCs is heme, or the iron-carrying elements in red meat.

Although NOCs are known carcinogens, scientists were skeptical that NOCs formed from meat digestion are a causative agent in colorectal cancer (Cross, Pollock, & Bingham, 2003). A federal study of more than a half-million people reinforced these findings, however, confirming that eating large amounts of red meat leads to a 20 percent higher risk of dying of cancer (Sinha, Cross, Graubard, Leitzmann, & Schatzkin, 2009).

Playing with Fire Two groups of carcinogens have been discovered in fatty foods subjected to high heat: heterocyclic amines in fried, broiled, and barbecued meats and acrylamide in potato chips and French fries. Both compounds are formed during high-temperature cooking processes. Heterocyclic amines are mutagens and cause cancer in laboratory animals. Acrylamide is weakly mutagenic and weakly carcinogenic to laboratory animals. Experiments to determine if these compounds pose a cancer risk to humans are ongoing. Several considerations pose difficulties in determining this risk. For example, the absorption of acrylamide is different for rodents than humans, making the translation of carcinogenicity from laboratory animals to humans uncertain. Furthermore, it is difficult to assess the relative amounts of consumption of these agents in study populations. One way to address this question is to design questionnaires that inquire about cooking method as an indirect way of gauging cooking temperature (Wogan et al., 2004).

Is DNA Destiny?   Breakthroughs in cell and molecular biology, beginning in the early 19th century, have answered many complex questions about cancer. The recognition of DNA as an instruction manual that outlines the genetic directions for cells has led to some of the biggest advances in cancer research. After learning how to decipher the directions, it became clear that genes were vulnerable to errors in coding, called mutations, which can lead to carcinogenesis. These mutations can be inherited or caused by chemical carcinogens, viruses, or radiation. Inherited, or familial, cancer is not nearly as common as spontaneous cancer and represents less than 15 percent of all cancers. It is important, though, to investigate these cancers because results can identify families at risk and the genes responsible. Genes have been discovered that are associated with familial cancer of the breast, colon, rectum, kidney, ovary, esophagus, lymph nodes, pancreas, and skin.

Six Steps: Tumor Growth and Spread   The development of human cancer is a complex process composed of multiple steps. More than 100 different types of human cancer exist, yet it has been proposed that they share a set of common features and capabilities. The process of transforming normal cells into malignant ones involves at least six major events, summarized here as simply as possible (the reader is directed to a review by Hanahan & Weinberg, 2000, which provides the basis of this discussion). Most importantly, cancer is a disease of individual cells. Tumors bring normal and cancerous cells together and when they interact they spread and grow.

Step One: License to Grow   Most normal human cells require growth signals to proliferate. These signals include growth factors, the extracellular matrix that cells reside in, and signals that come from molecules that keep cells connected to each other. These growth-promoting signals serve as regulators of cell growth and keep the proliferation of normal cells in check. Tumor cells, however, have been shown to grow in a manner that is independent of these outside signals. Cancer cells have circumvented normal growth control mechanisms by using a number of strategies. They can produce their own growth stimulators, change the components of the extracellular matrix that they bind to, and may also even influence their neighboring normal cells to provide growth stimulators that the cancer cells then respond to. Taken together, tumor cells, unlike their normal counterparts, have been shown to grow independent of normal growth factor signals, thereby escaping the restrictive growth control that characterizes normal human cells.

Step Two: No Stop Signs   A second feature of human cancer cells is their lack of response to the signals that inhibit their growth. Under normal circumstances, cell growth is regulated such that the tissue in which cells reside is stably maintained, so that tissue homeostasis is not disrupted. This quiescent state is achieved through the activity of growth inhibitors that are either free to interact with the cells on the surface of interacting cells or housed in the matrix surrounding cells. Normal cells, simply put, respond to these negative growth regulators and stop growing, whereas cancer cells have developed strategies that enable them to circumvent and/or become insensitive to these antigrowth signals and continue to grow without restriction.

Step Three: Forever Young A third feature of successful cancer development is the ability of cancer cells to avoid the natural programmed cell death that controls normal human cells. Programmed cell death is called apoptosis. It represents the counterbalance to cell proliferation and plays a critical role in the regulation of tissue growth and mass. One example of how cancer cells can avoid apoptosis is through the loss of activity of certain tumor suppressors, often by a mutation in that suppressor.

Taken together, the three features described here would not alone result in unrestricted tumor growth unless the tumor cell population could avoid a process called senescence, from the Latin meaning "growing old." Leonard Hayflick, working at the Wistar Institute in Philadelphia, demonstrated in 1965 that normal human cells in vitro have a limited number of doubling times, after which the cell enters senescence (Hayflick, 1965). That number of cell divisions is referred to as the Hayflick number or limit. Once this number of cell divisions is reached, the cell stops dividing, and normal homeostasis is disrupted, ultimately leading to cell death. Cancer cells appear to be exceptions to this limited ability to divide, and most appear to be immortalized with, in some cases, an infinite Hayflick number, thereby resulting in what has been termed a "limitless reproductive potential" (Hanahan & Weinberg, 2000).

Step Four: Arrested Development: Tumor Dormancy Once tumor cells acquire the ability to reproduce with little restriction, small groups of these cells join to form a tiny tumor that will be unable to continue to grow much beyond a few millimeters in diameter (the size of a pinhead) unless it is invaded by new capillaries, a process called angiogenesis (Folkman, 1971). This concept, that tumor growth is dependent on angiogenesis, was first postulated in the early 1970s by the father of the field of angiogenesis research, Judah Folkman.

Folkman described the presence of this small, unvascularized little tumor as a dormant cancer, essentially "cancer without disease" because it is only when the angiogenic program is switched on—and new capillaries invade the dormant cancer lesion, bringing nutrients and removing waste—that the tumor has the capacity to grow exponentially and begin to be "cancer with disease" (Folkman & Kalluri, 2004).

Step Five: Got Blood Simply put, in the absence of a blood supply, tumors are unable to grow, progress, and metastasize. Whether angiogenesis is turned on or not depends on the balance between angiogenic stimulators and inhibitors produced by the tumor cells themselves as well as their associated noncancer cells. A number of angiogenesis inhibitors are now approved for use in the treatment of cancer patients, and many more are currently being tested in clinical trials in the United States and around the world. The critical importance of angiogenesis regulation in human tumor growth and progression was acknowledged in 2004, when Mark McClellan, the commissioner of the U.S. Food and Drug Administration, announced that antiangiogenic therapy had become the fourth major treatment approach for human cancer, joining surgery, radiation, and chemotherapy.

Step Six: Moving On   A sixth and critically important activity of an established tumor is its ability to spread itself, or to metastasize. It is now widely appreciated that the major cause of death from cancer is its metastasis. This level of disease progression is characterized by the seeding of tissues and organs outside of the primary tumor. A multistep process is required for successful tumor metastasis. This process requires participation of the cancer cells themselves, their production of key proteases that facilitate tumor cell migration and invasion, their neighboring stromal and endothelial cells, and the microenvironment of both the primary tumor and the final, distant site where those tumor cells take root.

One of the earliest events in the process of tumor metastasis is the separation of tumor cells from each other and from the extracellular matrix that surrounds them, thereby freeing them to begin the cascade of activities that ends with a distant metastatic growth. Changes in cell-cell adhesion molecules and proteins called integrins liberate the tumor cell from both other tumor cells and their microenvironment. These changes are complemented by the production and activation of a panel of extracellular matrix-degrading enzymes, including the matrix metalloproteinase (MMPs) family of proteases.

MMPs facilitate tumor spread by degrading the escape route of the tumor cell from its parent tumor through the extracellular matrix to the blood vessel that often serves as the conduit for tumor cell spread. This same family of enzymes facilitates the establishment of the secondary site of the tumor along with members of the serine protease family. MMPs are also required for the process of angiogenesis. These proteases and their activities are so inextricably linked to successful solid tumor growth and metastasis that they have recently been the subject of intense research as potential cancer diagnostics and prognostics.

Once tumor cells escape the confines of their parent tumor and invade locally through the extracellular matrix that separates them from the nearest blood vessel, they invade into the blood vessel that will carry them throughout the body via a process called intravasation. After being transported to a distant site, the tumor cells leave the bloodstream via a process called extravasation, and then invade into the secondary metastatic site using some of the same proteolytic machinery. At this point, the tumor cells essentially go through the same processes that characterize the growth of a primary tumor: tumor cell proliferation, invasion, and angiogenesis.

Certain tumor cells can also metastasize through the lymphatic system of vessels, and breast, colon, skin, and prostate cancers commonly use this conduit to spread. The lymphatic system normally plays a key role in the function of the immune system, in regulating body fluids, and in the absorption of fats from the diet. Tumor cells find less resistance to entrance into lymphatic vessels because the latter lack the barrier called the "basement membrane" that protects the capillary system from constant invasion by cells. Once tumor cells enter the lymphatic vessels, they are either trapped in lymph nodes throughout the body, expand and grow in the lymph nodes, or find their way into the capillary system for dissemination.

One long-standing question with respect to tumor metastasis is why certain cancers metastasize preferentially to certain organs, a phenomenon known as "site-specific metastasis" (Hart & Fidler, 1980). It remains unclear, despite significant research efforts to answer this question, why it is that prostate and breast cancer, for example, show preferential metastatic homing to bony sites in the body. Research has focused on the factors that make potential metastatic sites attractive to the disseminated tumor cells, including the nature of the microenvironment or "soil" of the secondary site, the types and roles of the cells that are found at the secondary site, and other factors. It is also true that, for certain types of cancers, the vascular anatomy and blood flow dictate metastatic sites, as is the case for the oft-cited example of gastrointestinal cancer metastasis. In this disease, the tumor cells metastasize into the first local vascular conduit, which results, most often, in metastases to the liver. Bone is another common site for metastasis.

The Statistics   In the early 1900s, it was estimated that there were 80,000 cases of cancer in the United States, causing 5 percent of the annual deaths. In hospital autopsies, cancer was found in 1 case out of 12 (Da Costa, 1910). According to the American Cancer Society (2011), in the United States in 2011, there are expected to be more than 1.5 million new cancer cases for the year and more than 570,000 cancer deaths in the year. The four most common invasive cancers in the United States are breast, colon and rectum, lung and bronchus, and prostate.

In men, cancers of prostate, lung and bronchus, and colon and rectum account for about 50 percent of all newly diagnosed cancers. Prostate cancer alone accounts for about 25 percent of cases in men. For women, the three most commonly diagnosed cancers are breast, lung and bronchus, and colon and rectum, accounting for about 50 percent of cases in women. Breast cancer alone accounts for about 25 percent of all new cancer cases among women. These estimates do not include the common and less threatening in situ cancers as well as squamous and basal cell cancers of the skin (www.seer.cancer.gov).

Cigarette smoking is the single largest cause of cancer in the world. Estimates from the United States, the United Kingdom, and Germany indicate that by the end of the 20th century, smoking was responsible for 30 to 40 percent of all cancers. In the United States, 85 percent of the people who develop lung cancer will die from it, and 80 percent of lung cancer cases are attributable to cigarette smoking (Coyle, 2009; Doll, 1998b; Nelson, 2004).

Keeping Count   Cancer registries collect detailed information about patients with cancer, including the stage at diagnosis, the treatment, and the outcome of each patient's cancer (Hutchinson et al., 2008). This is done by every hospital and then sent on to the state and federal government. This data is then used to provide information for the medical and public health communities.

Two primary agencies maintain websites reporting on cancer trends in the United States: the American Cancer Society (www.cancer.org) and the National Cancer Institute (www.cancer.gov). Hospital cancer registries report to the national registry, SEER (www.seer.cancer.gov). National cancer registries report to the International Agency for Research on Cancer (IARC), a division of the World Health Organization (www.iarc.fr). IARC compiles global cancer statistics, accessed at www-dep.iarc.fr. These gigantic epidemiological efforts pinpoint cancer risk factors, not only saving lives, but also helping direct future research. They also underscore the importance of global communication in the fight against disease.

In the United States, the first cancer registry was established in the early 1920s by Ernest Codman at the Massachusetts General Hospital in Boston for the purpose of tracking bone sarcomas (Hutchinson et al., 2008). Later, registries were established for cancers of the breast, mouth, tongue, colon, and thyroid. In the 1930s, the American College of Surgeons' Commission on Cancer established an approval process for cancer clinics, but at that time there was no requirement for cancer registries, although many hospitals began to develop them. In 1935, a group of interested citizens in New Haven, Connecticut, established the Connecticut Tumor Registry (Haenszel & Curnen, 1986). These individuals were alarmed at the large increase in cancer cases in Connecticut, in which deaths from cancer more than doubled between 1930 and 1934.

These concerned citizens believed that a registry would provide the statistical information needed to determine the cause of the increase. In 1956, cancer registries became a mandatory component of an approved cancer program. Today physicians caring for cancer patients are required to document many details about each patient with a history of cancer. The registries track cancer type, stage, treatment, recurrence, and survival rates.

Analysis of information in registries revealed two major national trends in cancer risk during the 20th century. First, by 1920, cancer mortality (deaths from cancer) began to increase as deaths from tuberculosis decreased. Several reports linked the two trends as cause and effect, suggesting that infection with tuberculosis might protect the patient from cancer. Later it was realized that the decline in deaths from tuberculosis was related to an increase in life span attributable to the development of antibiotics. By reducing the number of deaths due to infectious diseases, such as tuberculosis, antibiotics improved the chances of a longer life. With longevity comes a higher probability that one will develop cancer. The increase in cancer mortality during the first half of the 20th century was especially obvious in urban centers. Researchers related higher cancer rates in cities with lifestyle choices, mainly higher rates of smoking and drinking, as well as exposure to pollutants in urban, industrialized settings.

The second major trend in the study of cancer statistics occurred in the last half of the 20th century. Epidemiologists uncovered an increase in the rate of cancer mortality in suburbs and farm counties, such that the percentage of deaths from cancer in rural areas began to converge with that of cities. Researchers believe that the convergence in mortality was caused by increases in the numbers of suburbanites smoking and drinking, a rise in industrialization in suburban areas, and improved disease reporting in rural districts (Greenberg 1981, 1984).

Registries in Germany and France documented the same trends occurring in Europe. The European studies particularly commented on elevated rates of rectum and colon cancer that they attributed to a change in diet (Mesle, 1983; Norat et al., 2005). In 1950, Ernst L. Wynder and Evarts Graham published an influential epidemiological analysis linking smoking and lung cancer. After scrutinizing the health and habits of 684 lung cancer victims, the pair produced unimpeachable evidence that smoking was a causative agent for lung carcinoma. Wynder first became intrigued by the relationship between smoking and lung cancer as a medical student, after observing an autopsy of a heavy smoker. He convinced Graham, a thoracic surgeon, to sponsor his study. Graham took some convincing, since he was a confirmed cigarette addict! The study persuaded thousands to "kick the habit"—even Graham, but for him it was too late. In 1957, Graham succumbed to lung cancer (Wynder & Graham, 1950).

Focus on Diet, Obesity, and Cancer   One of the first modern epidemiological studies on cancer was performed by Frederick Ludwig Hoffman, a statistician employed by the Prudential Insurance Company (Sypher, 2000). In his prodigious report "The Mortality from Cancer throughout the World," published in 1915, Hoffman made a connection between diet and cancer. He believed that the diet of people in developed nations contributed to the high incidence of cancer. Hoffman recognized that, by contrast, in countries where people followed a simpler diet, there was a much lower cancer rate.

Later, in the 1970s, European epidemiologists particularly noted a rise in colon and rectal cancer that they attributed to a change in traditional European diets. A study conducted in France revealed that the incidence of colorectal cancer doubled between 1950 and 1978. The increase paralleled the increase in the consumption of beef, pork, processed sugar, and flour and a decrease in the consumption of fresh fruits and vegetables (Mesle, 1983).

These studies provoked several related questions. Was the increase in the number of cancers due to decreased consumption of fresh fruits and vegetables? In other words, did fresh produce contain anticarcinogens? Was it the fat per se in the new, Western diet? Was the increase connected to possible carcinogens in meat and processed food? Or was the increase in cancer incidence caused by secondary factors stemming from a fatty diet consisting of animal products and processed foods? In other words, was it obesity and lack of physical activity? Each of these variables could be confounding the others.

Epidemiologists use the word *confounder* to mean possible causes of disease that are entangled with the issue under examination. Lane-Claypon was the first to describe the concept of confounding and to coin the term. Epidemiologists use observation as well as intuition to recognize issues that may be confused with the variable in question. When examining the impact of lifestyle on health, researchers design detailed questionnaires that inquire about possible confounders. Over the last 30 years, epidemiologists have teased apart the contributions to carcinogenesis of obesity, physical inactivity, alcohol consumption, and red meat.

Margaret M. Lotz, Marsha A. Moses, and Susan E. Pories

See also Alcohol; Antioxidants; Cigarettes; Exercise; Nutrition; Obesity.

References

Adams, T. D., A. M. Stroup, , R. E. Gress, et al. "Cancer Incidence and Mortality after Gastric Bypass Surgery." *Obesity* 17 (2009): 796–802.

Aggarwal, B. B., S. Shishodia, S. K. Sandur, et al. "Inflammation and Cancer: How Hot Is the Link?" *Biochemical Pharmacology* 72 (2006): 1605–21.

Allen, N. E., V. Beral, D. Casabonne, et al. "Moderate Alcohol Intake and Cancer Incidence in Women." *Journal of the National Cancer Institute* 101 (2009): 296–305.

American Cancer Society. *Cancer Facts and Figures 2011* (2011), www.cancer.org/acs/groups/content/@epidemiologysurveilance/documents/document/acspc-029771.pdf.

Bastian, H. "Lucy Wills (1888–1964): The Life and Research of an Adventurous Independent Woman." The James Lind Library (2007), www.jameslindlibrary.org.

Boyle, P., and B. Levin. *World Cancer Report.* Lyon, France: World Health Organization International Agency for Research on Cancer Publications, 2008.

Calle, E. E., and M. J. Thun. "Obesity and Cancer." *Oncogene* 23 (2004): 6365–78.

Chao, A., M. J. Thun, C. J. Connell, et al. "Meat Consumption and Risk of Colorectal Cancer." *Journal of the American Medical Association* 293 (2005): 172–82.

"Classics in Oncology. Sir Percivall Pott (1714–1788)." *CA: A Cancer Journal for Clinicians* 24 (1974): 108–16.

Clemons, M., and P. Goss. "Estrogen and the Risk of Breast Cancer." *New England Journal of Medicine* 344 (2001): 276–85.

Coyle, Y. M. "Lifestyle, Genes and Cancer." *Methods of Molecular Biology, Cancer Epidemiology* 472 (2009): 25–56.

Cross, A. J., J. R. A. Pollock, , and S. A. Bingham. "Haem, Not Protein or Inorganic Iron, Is Responsible for Endogenous Intestinal N-nitrosation Arising from Red Meat." *Cancer Research* 63 (2003): 2358–60.

Da Costa, J. C. *Modern Surgery General and Operative.* Philadelphia: W. B. Saunders, 1910.

Delancey, J. O. L., M. J. Thun, A. Jemal, et al. "Recent Trends in Black-White Disparities in Cancer Mortality." *Cancer Epidemiology Biomarkers and Prevention* 17 (2008): 2908–12.

Doll, R. "Epidemiological Evidence of the Effects of Behaviour and the Environment on the Risk of Human Cancer." *Recent Results in Cancer Research* 154 (1998a): 3–21.

Doll, R. "Uncovering the Effects of Smoking: Historical Perspective." *Statistical Methods in Medical Research* 7 (1998b): 87–117.

Doll, R., and R. Peto. "The Causes of Cancer: Quantitative Estimates of Avoidable Risks of Cancer in the United States Today." *Journal of the National Cancer Institute* 66 (1981): 1191–308.

Doll, R., and A.B. Hill. "Smoking and Carcinoma of the Lung." *British Medical Journal* 2, no. 4682 (1950): 739–48.

Dorgan, J.F., D.J. Baer, P.S. Albert, et al. "Serum Hormones and the Alcohol-Breast Cancer Association in Post-menopausal Women." *Journal of the National Cancer Institute* 93 (2001): 710–15.

Duffy, M.J. "Predictive Markers in Breast and Other Cancers: A Review." *Clinical Chemistry* 51 (2005): 494–503.

Edwards, T.M., and J.P. Myers. "Environmental Exposures and Gene Regulation in Disease Etiology." *Environmental Health Perspectives* 115 (2007): 1264–70.

Esteva, F.J., and G.N. Hortobagyi. "Gaining Ground on Breast Cancer." *Scientific American* 298 (2008): 58–65.

Folkman, J. "Tumor Angiogenesis: Therapeutic Implications." *New England Journal of Medicine* 285, no. 21 (1971): 1182–86.

Folkman, J., and R. Kalluri. "Cancer without Disease." *Nature* 427, no. 6977 (2004): 787.

Franco, G. "Bernardo Ramazzini: The Father of Occupational Medicine." *American Journal of Public Health* 91 (2001): 1380–82.

Friedenreich, C., T. Norat, K. Steindorf, et al. "Physical Activity and Risk of Colon and Rectal Cancers: The European Prospective Investigation into Cancer and Nutrition." *Cancer Epidemiology Biomarkers & Prevention* 15 (2006): 2398–407.

Frumkin, H., and J.M. Samet. "Radon." *CA: A Cancer Journal for Clinicians* 51 (2001): 337–44.

Glantz, L.H., and G.J. Annas. "Tobacco, the Food and Drug Administration, and Congress." *New England Journal of Medicine* 343 (2000): 1802–6.

Green, A., G. William, R. Neale, et al. "Daily Sunscreen Application and Betacarotene Supplementation in Prevention of Basal-Cell and Squamous-Cell Carcinomas of the Skin: A Randomized Controlled Trial." *The Lancet* 354 (1999) 723–29.

Greenberg, M.R. "A Note on the Changing Geography of Cancer Mortality within Metropolitan Regions of the United States." *Demography* 18 (1981): 411–20.

Greenberg, M.R. "Changing Cancer Mortality Patterns in the Rural United States." *Rural Sociology* 49 (1984): 143–53.

Guengerich, F.P. "Forging the Links between Metabolism and Carcinogenesis." *Mutation Research* 488 (2001): 195–209.

Haenszel, W., and M.G. Curnen. "The First Fifty Years of the Connecticut Tumor Registry: Reminiscences and Prospects." *Yale Journal of Biology and Medicine* 59 (1986): 475–84.

Hanahan, D., and R.A. Weinberg. "The Hallmarks of Cancer." *Cell* 100, no. 1 (2000): 57–70.

Hart, I.R., and I.J. Fidler. "Role of Organ Selectivity in the Determination of Metastatic Patterns of B16 Melanoma." *Cancer Research* 40 (1980): 2281–87.

Hayflick, L. "The Limited In Vitro Lifetime of Human Diploid Cell Strains." *Experimental Cell Research* 37 (1965): 614–36.

Hecht, S.S. "Tobacco Carcinogens, Their Biomarkers and Tobacco-Induced Cancer." *Nature Reviews Cancer* 3 (2003): 733–44.

Holland, J., and S. Lewis. *The Human Side of Cancer: Living with Hope, Coping with Uncertainty.* New York, NY: Harper Paperbacks.

Hussain, S.P., and C.C. Harris. "Molecular Epidemiology and Carcinogenesis: Endogenous and Exogenous Carcinogens." *Mutation Research* 462 (2000): 311–22.

Hussain, S.P., and C.C. Harris. "Inflammation and Cancer: An Ancient Link with Novel Potentials." *International Journal of Cancer* 121 (2007): 2373–80.

Hutchinson, C.L., H.R. Menck, M. Burch, et al., eds. *National Cancer Registrars Association. Cancer Registry Management: Principles and Practice,* 2nd ed. Dubuque, IA: Kendall Hunt.

Kaye, S.A., A.R. Folsom, J.T. Soler, et al. "Associations of Body Mass and Fat Distribution with Sex Hormone Concentrations in Postmenopausal Women." *International Journal of Epidemiology* 20 (1991): 151–56.

Lane-Claypon, J.E. *A Further Report on Cancer of the Breast: Reports on Public Health and Medical Subjects.* London: British Ministry of Health, 1926.

McTiernan, A., S.S. Tworoger, C.M. Ulrich, et al. "Effect of Exercise on Serum Estrogens in Post-menopausal Women: A 12 Month Randomized Clinical Trial." *Cancer Research* 64 (2004): 2923–28.

Meslé, F. "Cancer et alimenatation: Le cas des cancers de l'intestin et du rectum." *Population* 38 (1983): 733–62.

Mossman, B.T., J. Bignon, M. Corn, et al. "Asbestos: Scientific Developments and Implications for Public Policy." *Science* 247 (1990): 294–301.

Nelson, N. "The Majority of Cancers Are Linked to the Environment." An interview with Aaron Blair, PhD, Chief, Occupational Epidemiology Branch, Division of Cancer Epidemiology and Genetics, NCI (2004), www.cancer.gov/newscenter/benchmarks-vol4-issue3/page1.

Norat, T., S. Bingham, P. Ferrari, et al. "Meat, Fish and Colorectal Cancer Risk: The European Prospective Investigation into Cancer and Nutrition." *Journal of National Cancer Institute* 97 (2005): 906–16.

Olopade, O.I., T.A. Grushko, R. Nanda, and D. Huo. "Advances in Breast Cancer: Pathways to Personalized Medicine." *Clinical Cancer Research* 14 (2008): 7988–99.

Parkin, D.M., F. Bray, J. Ferlay, and P. Pisani. "Global Cancer Statistics, 2002." *CA: A Cancer Journal for Clinicians* 55 (2005): 74–108.

Polednak, A.P. "Estimating the Number of U.S. Incident Cancers Attributable to Obesity and the Impact on Temporal Trends in Incidence Rates for Obesity-Related Cancers." *Cancer Detection & Prevention* 32 (2008): 190–99.

Pott, P. *Chirurgical Observations Relative to the Cataract, the Polypus of the Nose, the Cancer of the Scrotum, the Different Kinds of Ruptures and the Mortification of the Toes and Feet.* London: Hawes, Clarke and Collins, 1775.

Robinson, B.W.S., A.W. Musk, and R.A. Lake. "Malignant Mesothelioma." *The Lancet* 366 (2005): 397–408.

Schiffman, M., and S. Wacholder. "From India to the World—A Better Way to Prevent Cervical Cancer." *New England Journal of Medicine* 360 (2009): 1453–55.

Shaw, J. "Diagnosis and Treatment of Testicular Cancer." *American Family Physician* 77 (2008): 469–74.

Sinha, R., A.J. Cross, B.I. Graubard, M.F. Leitzmann, and A. Schatzkin. "Meat Intake and Mortality: A Prospective Study of over Half a Million People." *Archives of Internal Medicine* 169 (2009): 562–71.

Sypher, F.J. "The Rediscovered Prophet: Frederick L. Hoffman (1865–1946)" *Cosmos Journal 2000.* www.cosmos-club.org.

Thomas, H.V., G.K. Reeves, and T.J. Key. "Endogenous Estrogen and Post-Menopausal Breast Cancer: A Quantitative Review." *Cancer Causes Control* 8 (1997): 922–28.

Wogan, G.N., S.S. Hecht, J.S. Felton, et al. "Environmental and Chemical Carcinogenesis." *Seminars in Cancer Biology* 14 (2004): 473–86.

Wolpin, B.M., J.A. Meyerhardt, A.T. Chan, K. Ng, J.A. Chan, K. Wu, et al. "Insulin, the Insulin-like Growth Factor Axis, and Mortality in Patients with Nonmetastatic Colorectal Cancer." *Journal of Clinical Oncology* 27 (2009): 176–85.

Wynder, E.L., and E. Graham. "Tobacco Smoking as a Possible Etiologic Factor in Bronchiogenic Carcinoma: A Study of 684 Proven Cases." *Journal of the American Medical Association* 143 (1950): 329–36.

CARBOHYDRATES

In all probability, you are already aware that carbohydrates are a category of food. After all, just about all types of foods, except pure vegetable oil, contain some carbohydrates. Even foods that appear to be carbohydrate free—such as meat and fish—have small amounts. Examples of foods with higher amounts of carbohydrates are potatoes, beans, breads, milk, corn, and soft drinks. Carbohydrates come in a variety of forms, such as sugars, starches, and fibers.

People frequently divide carbohydrates into two groups—simple or complex. Simple carbohydrates are those that contain one or two types of sugar. Examples are fruit sugar (fructose), table sugar (sucrose), and corn sugar (dextrose). Complex carbohydrates have three or more types of sugars. Examples of complex carbohydrates are lentils, kidney beans, and yams.

However, it is now known that such differences in carbohydrates are not as precise or significant as people previously believed. Apparently, the digestive system does not differentiate between simple and complex carbohydrates. It breaks down all carbohydrates into single sugar molecules that are sufficiently small to enter the bloodstream. In addition, the digestive system converts most carbohydrates into glucose, which is also known as blood sugar. Glucose is then readily available for the body to use. So the two categories of carbohydrates may no longer be as useful as they were once thought to be, and many people consider the categories to be outdated.

It is important to note that there is one type of carbohydrate that stands apart from the rest—fiber. When fiber passes through the body, it is not broken down and not digested. Why, then, is fiber considered such a crucial component of the diet? While fiber does not provide the body with any nourishment, it does support health. As it passes through the digestive tract, soluble fiber, or the type that dissolves in water, collects fatty substances and eliminates them in stool. This is an important part of cardiovascular (heart and circulatory system) health. Moreover, soluble fiber also helps regulate how the body uses sugars. Insoluble fiber, or fiber that is unable to dissolve in water, passes through the digestive tract and keeps waste moving. Thus, it assists in the removal of waste products. So it is useful in the prevention of constipation.

The Glycemic Index   Carbohydrates such as white flour and white sugar quickly raise the amount of sugar in the blood. This elevation may be quite substantial and take place in a brief period of time. They give a sudden burst of energy. On the other hand, carbohydrates such as brown rice and beans result in more modest rises in blood sugar, and these occur over a longer, extended period of time. Energy levels remain about the same.

In the early 1980s, the glycemic index was created to address the varied ways that the body processes carbohydrates. The glycemic index classifies carbohydrates by

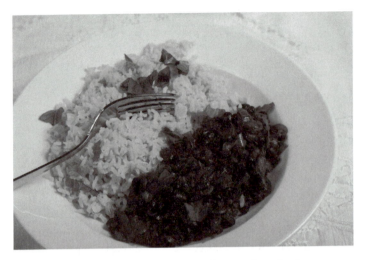

Brown rice and black beans are served on a plate. Both are complex carbohydrates and contribute to a modest but longer-lasting boost in blood sugar. (Paul Cowan/Dreamstime.com)

how high and how quickly they raise blood sugar as compared to pure glucose. Foods that have a high glycemic index—foods with a score of 70 or higher—raise blood sugar very quickly; foods that are lower on the glycemic index—foods with a score of 55 or lower—are digested at a slower pace.

Although the glycemic index provides useful information, it does not provide the amount of digestible carbohydrate found in specific foods and the impact that these carbohydrates have on the blood sugar levels of the body. Thus, a food may have a high glycemic index but actually contain only a small amount of carbohydrates. To address this issue, researchers developed the glycemic load. The glycemic load of a food is calculated by multiplying the glycemic index of a food by the amount of carbohydrates it contains. Normally, a glycemic load of 20 or more is viewed as high; a glycemic load of 11 to 19 is thought to be medium; and a glycemic load of 10 or less is low. The glycemic index and glycemic load values for some common foods are shown in the following table.

Still, there are serious limitations to the glycemic index and glycemic load values. A relatively small number of foods have been tested. Values on the same foods may differ, and similar foods may have dissimilar values. Food preparation methods must also be factored into the mix. Food processing tends to make food easier to digest. Hence, it may raise glycemic index values for certain foods. On the other hand, when food is consumed with another food that has fiber, protein, or fat, it may lower the glycemic index. And, individuals may vary in how they digest carbohydrates. That would create individual variations in glycemic response (Nutrition Data, n.d.).

While acknowledging the limitations of the glycemic index and glycemic load values, it is nevertheless generally believed that a healthier diet should include more foods that are lower on the glycemic index and have lower glycemic loads

Table 1. Glycemic Index and Glycemic Load of Various Foods

	Glycemic Index	Glycemic Load
Peanuts	14	2
Grapefruit	25	3
Potato chips	54	30
Snickers candy bar	55	35
Oatmeal	58	12
White rice	64	33
Watermelon	72	8
Popcorn	72	7
Baked potato	85	28

Source: Nutrition Data, www.nutritiondata.com.

and fewer foods with a high glycemic index and high glycemic loads. In fact, studies have found associations between diets filled with high-glycemic foods and a number of medical problems, such as Type 2 diabetes, heart disease, excess weight, macular degeneration, and colorectal cancer. But the results have not been consistent. For example, in a study published in 2007 in the *Journal of the American College of Cardiology,* Dutch researchers examined the association between dietary glycemic index and dietary glycemic load and risk of cardiovascular disease. The cohort (the group of people they studied) consisted of 15,714 Dutch women between the ages of 49 and 70 who did not have diabetes or cardiovascular disease at the start of the study. During the nine (plus or minus two) years of follow-up, there were 556 cases of coronary heart disease and 243 cases of cerebrovascular accident (stroke). The researchers found that "high dietary glycemic load and glycemic index increased the risk of CVD [cardiovascular disease], particularly for overweight women" (Beulens et al., 2007).

In an Italian study published in 2010 in the *Archives of Internal Medicine,* researchers conducted a similar investigation. Their cohort consisted of 47,749 men and women who were followed, on average, for almost eight years. The researchers determined that eating foods with high glycemic index and a high dietary glycemic load increased the overall risk of coronary heart disease in women but not men (Sieri et al., 2010).

In another study, published in 2009 in *Metabolism,* researchers from Birmingham, Alabama, and Boston fed 24 healthy but overweight or obese African American or white men either a high- or low-glycemic-index or high- or low-glycemic-load diet for four weeks. After a four-week washout period, the men ate the other type of diet for four weeks. The researchers noted that neither diet appeared to have "consistent effects on coronary heart disease" on this group of men. They speculated that the results may have been different if the diets had continued for longer periods of time (Shikany, Phadke, Redden, & Gower 2009), but there is no proof that that would have occurred.

Good Carbohydrates versus Bad Carbohydrates For decades, a number of health care professionals have vilified carbohydrates and blamed them for a host of medical problems, including excess weight and elevated levels of body fat. Generally, proponents of low-carbohydrate diets have maintained that these diets are far more effective for weight loss. One of the first of these diets, the Atkins diet, stressed eating very low amounts of carbohydrates and higher amounts of protein and foods containing saturated fats, such as meat and cheese. And Atkins followers did lose weight. How was this accomplished? There was a serious restriction of caloric intake. Plus, people on a high-protein diet eat lower amounts of all types of carbohydrates, including refined carbohydrates such as jams, jellies, sweets, soda, white rice, and white bread. Lower-carbohydrate diets tend to be controversial. Many health care professionals believe that they are not balanced and that they compromise the overall health and well-being of the people who are dieting. And their arguments are compelling.

When the body has insufficient carbohydrates to burn for fuel, it may be forced to burn its own fat. Though this may sound useful to someone who wants to drop some weight, it may trigger a condition known as ketosis. During ketosis, the body forms ketones, which cause people to feel less hungry and lose weight. But ketosis may harm the body. It is associated with a number of serious health problems such as gout, kidney stones, and kidney failure.

As has been noted, people on high-protein diets often eat meat and dairy products that contain saturated fat. As a result, these diets may have the potential to raise the levels of cholesterol. And, although the topic is debatable, high levels of cholesterol may be associated with an increased risk of heart disease, stroke, and cancer. Furthermore, high-protein diets foster the excretion of more calcium from the bones, thus increasing the risk for loss of bone mass. Such loss may result in conditions of low bone mineralization such as osteopenia and osteoporosis, which place people at increased risk for bone fractures. In some parts of the world—including the United States, Europe, and Japan—rates of osteopenia and osteoporosis are already at record levels.

With all the problems that may occur with low-carbohydrate/high-protein diets, you might think people would shy away from them, but that is not true. Many people follow one or more of the seemingly endless varieties. A number of the books on these diets have been best-sellers. If you decide that your road to weight loss is a low-carbohydrate/high-protein diet, try to remain on the diet for a relatively short period of time—no more than a few months. Also, consume proteins that are lower in saturated (animal) fats, such as fish, lean beef, lean pork, skinless chicken or turkey, and low- or no-fat dairy products. Avoid eating large amounts of higher-fat foods such as marbleized steaks and whole-fat dairy products. Be certain to consume carbohydrates that are high in fiber, such as brown rice, beans, vegetables, and fruits. And if you are already dealing with a medical problem, such as kidney or liver disease, do not begin a low-carbohydrate/high-protein diet without consulting your health care provider. You have the potential to create a serious or even life-threatening medical problem for yourself.

Carbohydrates and Diabetes-Related Illness As noted, when a person eats a food that contains carbohydrates, the digestive system breaks the food down into sugar. The sugar then enters the bloodstream. When the increased amounts of sugar enter the bloodstream, the pancreas, an organ in the middle of the body, releases more insulin, a hormone that directs the cells to absorb the blood sugar. As the cells absorb the sugar, the levels of sugar in the blood start to fall. At that point, the pancreas releases the hormone glucagon, which signals the liver, a large organ in the upper abdomen, to release stored sugar. These interactions between insulin and glucagon enable the cells in the body, and particularly in the brain, to have an ongoing supply of blood sugar.

In some people, this system does not work as well as it should. People who have Type 1 diabetes do not produce a sufficient amount of insulin. As a result, their cells may not absorb all of the sugar. People with the far more common condition known as Type 2 diabetes tend to begin with a different medical problem known as insulin resistance. With insulin resistance, the cells fail to respond when insulin signals that they should absorb more sugar. As a result, insulin levels remain high for extended periods of time. Eventually, the production of insulin slows, and then it stops. Insulin resistance is linked to other medical problems, such as low levels of HDL ("good") cholesterol, excess weight, high blood pressure (hypertension), and high levels of triglycerides (a type of fat) in the blood. When insulin resistance occurs with these medical problems, it is known as metabolic syndrome. It is not uncommon for metabolic syndrome to lead to cardiovascular disease, colorectal cancer, and, as has been noted, Type 2 diabetes. While people may have a genetic predisposition to these health problems, they are frequently associated with a sedentary lifestyle, obesity, and the consumption of large amounts of processed carbohydrates, which play havoc with blood sugars, and too few whole grains, which help to maintain a steadier level of blood sugars.

Refined or Processed Carbohydrates Refined or processed carbohydrates seem to be just about everywhere—from that loaf of white bread to that box of white lasagna noodles—but why are they considered so detrimental? The problem is really what they do not contain. When carbohydrates are refined or processed, their beneficial nutrients—such as the bran, fiber, germ, vitamins, and minerals—are removed. What is left is primarily bland starch. For example, when wheat kernel is processed, the resulting white flour has only 20 percent of the original vitamins and minerals and 25 percent of the original fiber. Hence, manufacturers tend to enrich these products. That is the only way to give these depleted foods some substance. There is no doubt that whole-grain carbohydrates are better for you than refined or processed carbohydrates, and a good deal of research supports this contention.

In a study published in 2009 in *Metabolism,* Indian researchers examined the association between the consumption of refined grains and insulin resistance and metabolic syndrome in 2,042 people from urban south India. When the researchers compared the participants who consumed the least amount of refined grains with those who consumed the most, they found that the higher consumers were significantly more likely to have metabolic syndrome. The researchers noted that "higher intake of refined grains was associated with insulin resistance and the metabolic syndrome in this population of Asian Indians who habitually consume high-carbohydrate diets" (Radhika et al., 2009).

Researchers from Milan, Italy, investigated the association between dietary glycemic index and glycemic load and pancreatic cancer. Their findings were published in 2010 in the *Annals of Epidemiology*. The study included 326 people with pancreatic cancer, a rare but exceedingly deadly disease, and 652 people who served as controls. While the researchers found a positive association between the consumption of foods high on the glycemic index and pancreatic cancer, no such association was found between glycemic load and pancreatic cancer. They noted that the "consumption of sugar, candy, honey, and jam was positively associated with pancreatic cancer, whereas consumption of fruit was inversely associated" (Rossi et al., 2010).

In a study published in 2010 in the *Archives of Internal Medicine*, Harvard School of Public Health researchers examined the association between the consumption of white rice and brown rice and the risk of developing Type 2 diabetes in 39,765 men and 157,463 women. They found that an increased intake of white rice "was associated with a higher risk of type 2 diabetes." At the same time, "higher brown rice intake . . . was associated with a lower risk of type 2 diabetes." Why is this important? The researchers wrote that "Substitution of whole grains, including brown rice, for white rice may lower risk of type 2 diabetes." Moreover, "these data support the recommendation that most carbohydrate intake should come from whole grains rather than refined grains to help prevent diabetes" (Sun et al., 2010).

In a study published in 2010 in *Nutrition and Cancer*, Pennsylvania researchers reviewed the results of different studies that examined the association between dietary patterns and colorectal cancer or adenoma (benign tumor). Although the studies differed markedly in "population characteristics, study design and methods used for characterizing dietary patterns across the different studies," two patterns did emerge. A diet consisting of higher intakes of fruits and vegetables and a reduced intake of red and processed meat "appeared protective against colorectal adenoma and cancer incidence." A less healthful pattern "characterized by higher intakes of red and processed meat, as well as potatoes and refined carbohydrates, may increase risk" (Miller et al., 2010).

In a hospital-based case-control study published in 2009 in the *Asian Pacific Journal of Cancer Prevention*, researchers from Kolkata, India, recruited 108 people treated for colorectal cancer and 324 controls. All of the participants were from the Malabar region of Kerala, India. The researchers found "that intake of beef, refined carbohydrates, and tobacco promote colorectal cancer" (Nayak, Sasi, Sreejayan, & Mandal, 2009).

Consumption of Sugar-Sweetened Drinks   There are a wide variety of sugar-sweetened beverages. Of course, there are the many types of sodas, such as

Coke and Pepsi. But there are also energy drinks such as Red Bull and Monster, fruit drinks such as Kool-Aid and Hi-C, and fruit ades, such as Gatorade and lemonade. They all contain large amounts of sugar. And, according to an article published in 2009 in the *Archives of Pediatrics and Adolescent Medicine,* "sugary drinks are the main source of added sugar in the daily diet of children." A 12-ounce serving of soda has "the equivalent of 10 teaspoons of sugar." Moreover, "between 56% and 85% of children in school have at least one can of soda every day." Clearly, the high levels of sugar in these drinks "provide a lot of calories very quickly" (Moreno, Furtner, & Rivara, 2009).

An 2008 article in *Pediatrics* presented a stunning finding. Researchers from New York City, Boston, and Baltimore noted that "per-capita daily caloric contribution from sugar-sweetened beverages and 100% fruit juice increased from 242 Kcal/day . . . in 1988–1994 to 270 Kcal/day in 1999–2004." Moreover, "sugar-sweetened beverage intake increased from 204 to 224 kcal/day and 100% fruit juice increased from 38 to 48 kcal/day." The researchers said that the greatest increases—about 20 percent—were seen among children between the ages of 6 and 11. While there were no changes in per capita consumption among white adolescents, significant increases were found among black and Mexican American youths. Preschool-age children tended to consume fruit drinks; adolescents were more likely to drink soda. The researchers concluded that "children and adolescents today derive 10% to 15% of total calories from sugar-sweetened beverages and 100% fruit juice." The researchers noted that such high levels of sugar-sweetened beverage consumption contribute to the alarming and ever-growing rates of children who are overweight or obese (Wang, Bleich, & Gortmaker, 2008). In fact, it is now very common for children to be overweight or obese. And children who are overweight and obese are at increased risk for high cholesterol, Type 2 diabetes, high blood pressure, and psychiatric and social problems.

A study conducted at the New York City Department of Health and Mental Hygiene and published in 2009 in *Obesity* examined the association between excess weight and obesity and the consumption of sugar-sweetened beverages by 365 low-income African American preschool children between the ages of 3 and 5three and five. The children were examined at a dental clinic between 2002 and 2003; the examination was repeated two years later. During the first visit, the researchers found that 12.9 percent of the children were overweight; two years later, that figure had increased to 18.7 percent. During the first visit, the children had an obesity rate of 10.3 percent; two years later, that had increased to 20.4 percent. The researchers determined that "high consumption of sugar-sweetened beverages was significantly associated with an increased risk for obesity" (Lim et al., 2009).

And, it appears that children who drink sugar-sweetened carbonated beverages are likely to grow into adolescents who have less-than-ideal diets. In a study published in 2010 in the *Journal of the American Dietetic Association,* Pennsylvania researchers found that, compared to children who did not consume soda at the age of five years, children who did consume soda at the age of five years "had higher subsequent soda intake, lower milk intake, higher intake of added sugars, lower protein, fiber, vitamin D, calcium, magnesium, phosphorous, and potassium from ages 5 to 15 years" (Fiorito et al., 2010).

In another study from New York City, Boston, and Baltimore that was published in 2009 in the *American Journal of Clinical Nutrition,* researchers reviewed trends in the consumption of sugar-sweetened beverages by U.S. adults. The researchers learned that between the periods 1988 to 1994 and 1999 to 2004, the percentage of adults who drank sugar-sweetened beverages increased from 58 percent to 63 percent. On average, the daily consumption increased by six ounces. Consumption was highest among young adults, especially young blacks, and lowest among the elderly. The researchers noted that the consumption of sugar-sweetened beverages "comprises a considerable source of total daily intake and is the largest source of beverage calories." Why is this important? The consumption of sugar-sweetened beverages "is highest among subgroups also at greatest risk of obesity and type 2 diabetes" (Bleich, Wang, Wang, & Gortmaker, 2009). It should therefore surprise no one that the Dietary Guidelines for Americans prepared by the United States Department of Agriculture (2011) advise Americans to reduce their intake of sugar-sweetened beverages.

Whole-Grain Carbohydrates   It is important to underscore that there is a huge difference between refined or processed carbohydrates and whole-grain carbohydrates. While refined or processed carbohydrates are primarily empty calories, whole-grain carbohydrates comprise an integral part of a healthful diet. Whole-grain carbohydrates consist of three main edible components: the endosperm, germ, and bran. The endosperm, which is the inner part of the grain, is all starch. It has very little nutritional value. However, the germ and bran have incredible amounts of nutrients. The germ contains B vitamins, vitamin E, selenium, magnesium, iron, copper, zinc, and trace minerals. In addition, it has phytochemicals. The consumption of phytochemicals has been associated with improving cardiovascular health and reductions in levels of cancer. The bran is filled with fiber, which is associated with lowering levels of cholesterol, reducing heart disease, and supporting digestive health. There is plenty of research supporting these claims.

In a randomized controlled trial published in 2010 in the *Journal of the American Dietetic Association,* Illinois researchers investigated whether a whole grain, ready-to-eat (RTE) oat cereal could improve the health of overweight and obese adults. At the beginning of the study, all of the participants had elevated levels of LDL ("bad") cholesterol. The participants were divided into two groups. One group ate two daily portions of a whole-grain RTE oat cereal that contained fiber; the other ate energy-matched low-fiber foods. At the end of 12 weeks, 144 participants had completed the study. The researchers found that the group of people eating RTE oat cereal had significantly lowered levels of LDL cholesterol. While there was no difference in weight loss between the two groups, the group eating RTE oat cereal had greater decreases in waist circumference (Maki et al., 2010).

In a study published in 2010 in *Circulation,* researchers from the Harvard School of Public Health attempted to determine whether a diet that includes whole-grain carbohydrates (and its components cereal fiber, bran, and germ) could lower the risk of cardiovascular disease in women who had Type 2 diabetes. The researchers chronicled the diets of 7,822 women with Type 2 diabetes for up to 26 years. During this time, there were 852 documented deaths from all causes and 295 deaths from cardiovascular disease. The researchers found a significant association between consumption of whole grains and bran and reduction in death from all causes and from cardiovascular disease. Their findings, according to the researchers, "suggest a potential benefit of whole-grain intake in reducing mortality and cardiovascular risk in diabetic patients" (He et al., 2010).

Another study from the Harvard School of Public Health was published in 2009 in the *American Journal of Clinical Nutrition.* This time, researchers reviewed the association between the intake of whole grains and the onset of high blood pressure (hypertension) in men. The researchers studied of group of 31,684 men ranging in age from 40 to 75. When originally enrolled in the study, none of the men had high blood pressure. Over the 18 years of follow-up, a total of 9,227 cases of hypertension were reported. The men who ate the highest amounts of whole grains were 19 percent less likely to develop high blood pressure than the men who ate the lowest amounts of whole grains. Furthermore, the men who ate the most bran were 15 percent less likely to develop high blood pressure than the men who ate the least amount of bran. The researchers observed that "whole-grain intake was inversely associated with risk of hypertension" in men. Moreover, they added that "bran may play an important role in this association" (Flint et al., 2009).

In a study published in 2007 in the *American Journal of Clinical Nutrition,* researchers from the National Cancer Institute, National Institutes of Health in Bethesda, Maryland, reviewed the relationship between the intake of dietary fiber and whole-grain foods and invasive colorectal cancer. The cohort consisted of almost half a million men and women between the ages of 50 and 71. During the five years of follow-up, there were 2,974 cases of colorectal cancer. Though the researchers found no relationship between total dietary fiber and colorectal cancer, "whole-grain consumption was associated with a modest reduced risk" of colorectal cancer (Schatzkin et al., 2007).

On the other hand, in a randomized, crossover study published in 2010 in *Nutrition Journal,* researchers from the University of Minnesota compared differences in levels of antioxidants (which protect cells from free radical, unstable molecules that cause cellular damage) in subjects who consumed either refined-grain or whole-grain diets for 14 days and then ate the other diet for 14 days. The researchers found "no differences in antioxidant measures . . . when subjects consumed whole grain diets compared to refined grain diets" (Enright & Slavin, 2010).

Nevertheless, the overall evidence is overwhelming. Whole grains have multiple benefits. And, as has been advised by the federal government, Americans should increase their consumption of high fiber whole grain carbohydrates and lower their intake of refined grains (United States Department of Agriculture, 2011).

Myrna Chandler Goldstein

See also Antioxidants; Atkins, Robert C.; Cholesterol; Diabetes; Fats; Fiber.

References

Beulens, Joline W.J., Leonie M. de Bruijne, Ronald P. Stolk, et al. "High Dietary Glycemic Load and Glycemic Index Increase Risk of Cardiovascular Disease among Middle-Aged Women: A Population-Based Follow-Up Study." *Journal of the American College of Cardiology* 50 (2007): 14–21.

Bleich, Sara N., Y. Claire Wang, Youfa Wang, and Steven L. Gortmaker. "Increasing Consumption of Sugar-Sweetened Beverages among US Adults: 1988–1994 to 1999–2004." *American Journal of Clinical Nutrition* 89, no. 1 (January 2009): 372–81.

Enright, L., and J. Slavin. "No Effect of 14 Day Consumption of Whole Grain Diet Compared to Refined Grain Diet on Antioxidant Measures in Healthy, Young Subjects: A Pilot Study." *Nutrition Journal* 9 (March 19, 2010): 12.

Fiorito, L.M., M. Marini, D.C. Mitchell, et al. "Girls' Early Sweetened Carbonated Beverage Intake Predicts Different Patterns of Beverage and Nutrient Intake across Childhood and Adolescence." *Journal of the American Dietetic Association* 110, no. 4 (April 2010): 543–50.

Flint, Alan J., Frank B. Hu, Robert J. Glynn, et al. "Whole Grains and Incident Hypertension in Men." *American Journal of Clinical Nutrition* 90, no. 3 (September 2009): 493–98.

He, M., R.M. van Dam, E. Rimm, et al. "Whole-Grain, Cereal Fiber, Bran, and Germ Intake and the Risks of All-Cause and Cardiovascular Disease-Specific Mortality among Women with Type 2 Diabetes Mellitus." *Circulation* 121, no. 20 (May 25, 2010): 2162–68.

Lim, S., J.M. Zoellner, J.M. Lee, et al. "Obesity and Sugar-Sweetened Beverages in African-American Preschool Children: A Longitudinal Study." *Obesity* 17, no. 6 (June 2009): 1262–68.

Maki, K.C., J.M. Beiseigel, S.S. Jonnalagadda, et al. "Whole-Grain Ready-to-Eat Oat Cereal, As Part of a Dietary Program for Weight Loss, Reduces Low-Density Lipoprotein Cholesterol in Adults with Overweight and Obesity More than a Dietary Program Including Low-Fiber Control Foods." *Journal of the American Dietetic Association* 110, no. 2 (February 2010): 205–14.

Miller, P.E., S.M. Lesko, J.E. Muscat, et al. "Dietary Patterns and Colorectal Adenoma and Cancer Risk: A Review of the Epidemiological Evidence." *Nutrition and Cancer* 62, no. 4 (May 2010): 413–24.

Moreno, Megan A., Fred Furtner, and Frederick P. Rivara. "Sugary Drinks and Childhood Obesity." *Archives of Pediatrics and Adolescent Medicine* 163, no. 4 (April 2009): 400.

Nayak, S.P., M.P. Sasi, M.P. Sreejayan, and S. Mandal. "A Case-Control Study of Roles of Diet in Colorectal Carcinoma in a South Indian Population." *Asian Pacific Journal of Cancer Prevention* 10, no. 4 (October–December 2009): 565–68.

Nutrition Data (n.d.), www.nutritiondata.com.

Radhika, G., R.M. van Dam, V. Sudha, et al. "Refined Grain Consumption and the Metabolic Syndrome in Urban Asian Indians (Chennai Urban Rural Epidemiology Study 57)." *Metabolism* 58, no. 5 (May 2009): 675–81.

Rossi, M., L. Lipworth, J. Polesel, et al. "Dietary Glycemic Index and Glycemic Load and Risk of Pancreatic Cancer: A Case-Control Study." *Annals of Epidemiology* 20, no. 6 (June 2010): 460–65.

Schatzkin, A., T. Mouw, Y. Park, et al. "Dietary Fiber and Whole-Grain Consumption in Relation to Colorectal Cancer in the NIH-AARP Diet and Health Study." *American Journal of Clinical Nutrition* 85, no. 5 (May 2007): 1353–60.

Shikany, James M., Radhika P. Phadke, David T. Redden, and Barbara A. Gower. "Effects of Low- and High-Glycemic Load Diets on Coronary Heart Disease Risk Factors in Overweight/Obese Men." *Metabolism* 58, no. 12 (December 2009): 1793–801.

Sieri, Sabina, Vittorio Krogh, Franco Berrino, et al. "Dietary Glycemic Load and Index and Risk of Coronary Heart Disease in a Large Italian Cohort: The EPICOR Study." *Archives of Internal Medicine* 170, no. 7 (April 12, 2010): 640–47.

Sun, Q., D. Spiegelman, R. M. van Dam, et al. "White Rice, Brown Rice, and Risk of Type 2 Diabetes in US Men and Women." *Archives of Internal Medicine* 170, no. 11 (June 14, 2010): 961–69.

United States Department of Agriculture, Center for Nutrition Policy and Promotion. *Dietary Guidelines for Americans, 2010* (January 31, 2011), www.cnpp.usda.gov/dietaryguidelines.htm.

Wang, Y. Claire, Sara N. Bleich, and Steven L. Gortmaker. "Increasing Caloric Contribution from Sugar-Sweetened Beverages and 100% Fruit Juices among US Children and Adolescents, 1998–2004." *Pediatrics* 121, no. 6 (June 2008): e1604–e1614.

CARDIOPULMONARY RESUSCITATION (CPR)

Approximately 92 percent of people in cardiac arrest die before reaching the hospital (American Heart Association, 2011). That statistic prompted important changes in the American Heart Association's guidelines for cardiopulmonary resuscitation (CPR). If more people could administer CPR, more victims would have better odds of surviving. CPR can also saves lives in cases of drug overdose, alcohol intoxication, carbon monoxide poisoning, a severe asthma attack, drowning, or choking.

Two significant changes were made to the CPR guidelines in 2010 and 2011. The first was to encourage bystanders and CPR-trained laypeople to bypass checking an unconscious person for a pulse before administering chest compressions. According to research, at least 35 percent of both trained and untrained rescuers were wrong when checking for a pulse ("New CPR Guidelines," 2010). Checking for a pulse wastes valuable time that could be spent giving chest compressions, which are vital to survival if an individual has had a heart attack.

The second change in policy released by the American Heart Association in early 2011 called for trained and untrained rescuers to skip rescue breathing or mouth-to-mouth resuscitation and perform only chest compressions on victims of cardiac arrest. Individuals who suffer cardiac arrest are likely to have been breathing normally before their collapse and have enough oxygen in their lungs and blood. In that case, studies show there is no benefit in rescue breathing. Instead, continuous chest compressions are needed to generate blood flow throughout the body until medical help arrives (Ewy, 2007). This change is expected to double the victim survival rate if performed quickly and correctly (Ashford, 2011).

CPR has a long history dating back to the 1700s. Starting in 1740, the Paris Academy of Sciences endorsed mouth-to-mouth resuscitation for drowning victims. Almost 30 years later, the Society for Recovery of Drowned Persons became the first organization devoted to sudden and unexpected death. The first documented chest compressions were administered in 1891 by Friedrich Maass. In the 1960s, cardiopulmonary resuscitation was born. In 1972, the world's first mass CPR class was held for citizens in Seattle, Washington (American Heart Association, 2011).

CPR classes teach individuals how to keep blood circulating through the body until medical help arrives on the scene. Compression-only CPR is when a person delivers quick, firm compressions in the middle of the chest without giving mouth-to-mouth. Continuous chest compressions of at least two inches each time, performed without interruption, generate the needed blood flow, at a rate of 100 compressions per minute. The songs "Staying Alive" by the Bee Gees or "Hey Mama" by the Black Eyed Peas are the right pace for hands-only CPR.

One does not have to be a first-responder or clinician to successfully administer CPR in an emergency. Before the recent guideline changes, CPR traditionally combined rescue breathing with chest compressions to help in several situations, including a person who has stopped breathing and is in respiratory arrest; someone whose heart has stopped, called cardiac arrest; or who anyone who is having a heart attack, otherwise known as a myocardial infarction.

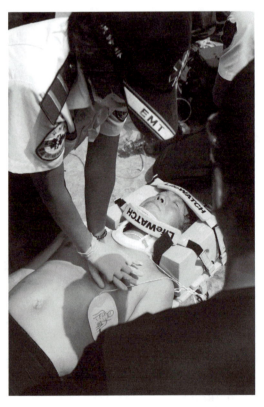

Emergency medics perform cardiopulmonary resuscitation (CPR). (Fang Chun Che/Dreamstime.com)

However, research shows that bystander CPR is more likely to happen if mouth-to-mouth is not necessary. The success of compression-only CPR was dramatically demonstrated in Goodhue, Minnesota, in early 2011, when 20 strangers joined together and performed CPR on a man for 96 minutes (Metz, Dacy, & Harris, 2011). The man, Howard Snitzer, 54, collapsed with a massive heart attack while buying groceries. An off-duty corrections officer in the store was the first person to start CPR. She was eventually joined by some two dozen people who all lined up, then took turns giving chest compressions. When the Mayo Clinic emergency helicopter arrived, paramedics were astonished to see the line of people waiting their turn to perform CPR. Snitzer was airlifted to the Mayo Clinic and released 10 days later. He later met with everyone who worked to save his life at the town's fire station and thanked them for their efforts.

Unfortunately, in some cases of cardiac arrest, compressions alone will not restart a heart. If a device called an automated external defibrillator (AED) is available, it should be used to get a heart beating again. The device comes with audible instructions that can be understood by most adults. The AED sends electrical charges to the heart to get it beating again. Likewise, in the event of a heart attack, a defibrillator is an integral part of rescuing a victim. While preparing the device, the chest compressions should be maintained (Ewy, 2007).

Cardiac arrest differs from a heart attack in that the victim suddenly experiences a change in heart rhythm, which can cause the heart to stop beating. During a heart attack, an artery has become blocked, preventing blood, oxygen, and nutrients from reaching the heart. A heart attack can cause cardiac arrest, but cardiac arrest does not always mean a heart attack is occurring (American Heart Association, 2011).

In the event of respiratory arrest, mouth-to-mouth is still recommended. In these cases, it is not the heart that has caused a person to collapse but a lack of oxygen that could later bring on cardiac arrest. Examples of these types of cases include drug overdose or drowning. Given the circumstances, the victim's collapse is neither unexpected nor sudden (Ewy, 2007). So how can a bystander know which type of arrest a victim may be experiencing?

It is recommended that bystanders who witness a collapse call out to the victim and shake them to see if they respond. If unresponsive, the bystander should assess breathing. If breathing is abnormal or nonexistent and the person appeared to have collapsed for no reason, cardiac arrest can be assumed. The bystander should then call 9-1-1 and begin chest compressions. Often, a 9-1-1 dispatcher can offer instructions over the phone after asking a few questions (Ewy, 2007).

To learn CPR and how to use an AED, there are a host of classes one can take. The American Heart Association's website lists ways adults can connect with an instructor to learn the lifesaving skills needed to help someone who has collapsed suddenly or stopped breathing. There is also a smart phone application called iRescU, designed to offer CPR training, emergency use, and AED location all in one. The app is about one megabyte in size and is designed to work on multiple mobile platforms. Pilot testing is ongoing.

Abena Foreman-Trice

See also Heart Health; Mayo Clinic; Target Heart Rate.

References

American Heart Association. (February 2011), www.heart.org.
Ashford, Molika. "New CPR Saves Lives." *Science World* 67, no. 10 (March 7, 2011): 5.

Erich, John. "What an AED Is and Where to Find One." *EMS Magazine* 40, no. 2 (February 2011): 53.

Ewy, Gordon A. "New Concepts of Cardiopulmonary Resuscitation for the Lay Public." *AHA Journals* (2007): 566–68.

Metz, Jennifer, Glen Dacy, and Dan Harris. "CPR Marathon: More Than Two Dozen Responders Resuscitate Neighbor for 96 Minutes." *ABC News* (March 3, 2011), http://abcnews.go.com.

"New CPR Guidelines May Save More Lives." *ABC News* (August 15, 2010), www.abcnews.go.com.

CARDIOVASCULAR HEALTH. *See* HEART HEALTH

CARPAL TUNNEL SYNDROME

Carpal tunnel syndrome and computers are forever linked in the public perception. The explosion of personal computer use coincided with an increase in repetitive motion injuries, sending many Americans looking for medical relief from this painful condition. Now health care providers say the newest source for carpal tunnel, the painful, progressive condition that affects the median nerve and runs from the forearm into the hand, may be texting.

Americans, especially young adults and teens, are texting all day, every day, using their thumbs to quickly type short messages to friends. However, that repetitive motion with the thumb puts a great deal of stress on the thumb joint, stress that would not be caused by other motions. The end result is a jump in carpal tunnel type injuries occurring with younger and younger patients (Wilkerson, 2011).

Although symptoms can begin gradually, they can progress from light tingling and occasional numbness to pain and weakness until it may be hard to pick up small objects or do other routine tasks with the affected hand or arm.

Interestingly, carpal tunnel syndrome occurs more often in women than in men, due in part to the fact that in women, the carpal tunnel passageway may be narrower than it is for most men. The tunnel protects the main nerve of the hand and the nine tendons that work the individual fingers. Any compression of the nerve causes numbness, pain, and the tingling that is indicative of the condition.

Other factors hasten carpal tunnel syndrome, including some chronic illnesses such as diabetes or alcoholism, which also increase the risk of nerve damage, especially to the median nerve. Inflammatory illnesses such as rheumatoid arthritis or an infection can also put pressure on the main nerve and lead to pain. The prolonged use of vibrating tools or work in the same position such as on an assembly line may also play a role in worsening any nerve inflammation, especially if those tasks are repeated over many years. In general, anything that crowds, injures, or repeatedly presses on the median nerve can be a factor in the development of carpal tunnel syndrome.

Individuals with persistent symptoms should see their doctor. If the symptoms are not too severe, the doctor will ask patients to make changes in home or work activities, practice additional stretching and strengthening exercises, use ice to

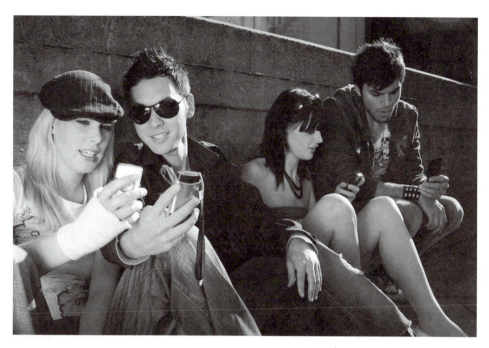

Teenagers send an increasing number of text messages, making texting a new source of carpal tunnel syndrome. (iStockPhoto)

reduce the inflammation, and recommend nonsteroidal anti-inflammatory drugs such as ibuprofen. One issue with this treatment is that people cannot always change the action that is creating their injury if it is part of their daily employment.

A doctor may also recommend an X-ray of the wrist to check for other causes of wrist pain such as a broken bone. Other tests include an electromyogram, which measures the small electrical discharges given off by the muscles. In this test a, thin, needlelike electrode is inserted into the area the doctor wishes to examine. The electromyogram then measures electrical activity in that muscle while it is still and when it is in movement. In a variation of that test, a nerve conduction study uses a small shock that is passed through the nerve and then measured to see if the electrical impulse is slowed by inflammation in the carpal tunnel area.

Corticosteroids, also known as steroids, may also be prescribed to decrease inflammation and swelling, which would then relieve the median nerve pain. If the symptoms are very severe or do not improve, surgery is also an option. Carpal tunnel surgery works to ease pressure on the median nerve by cutting the ligament that presses on the nerve. Recuperation takes anywhere from a couple of weeks to several months, depending on the severity of the situation. During the recuperation, the ligament tissue grows back together, and this provides more room for the nerve than before.

There are two choices for surgery: endoscopic surgery and open surgery. The endoscopic surgery uses a tiny camera attached to a telescope device so the surgeon can see inside the carpal tunnel. This option requires a small incision in the hand or wrist. Open surgery involves a larger incision and requires more recuperation time because the procedure is more invasive.

Health care professionals recommend taking precautions to try and prevent carpal tunnel syndrome, such as taking breaks when possible from repetitive tasks, especially if they involve twisting or bending the wrist. Do not rest wrists on hard surfaces or hold your arms too close or too far from your body when doing tasks. Make sure the keyboard is level with your forearms, and, if possible, switch hands during work tasks.

Sharon Zoumbaris

See also Diabetes; Steroids.

References

Chang, C.W., and Y.C. Wang. "A Practical Electrophysiological Guide for Nonsurgical and Surgical Treatment of Carpal Tunnel Syndrome." *Journal of Hand Surgery* 33 (2008): 32–37.

Goodyear-Smith, F., and B. Arroll. "What Can Family Physicians Offer Patients with Carpal Tunnel Syndrome Other Than Surgery? A Systematic Review of Nonsurgical Management." *Annals of Family Medicine* 2, no. 3 (2004): 267–73.

Mayo Foundation for Medical Education and Research. "Carpal Tunnel Syndrome." *Mayo Clinic Health Manager,* www.mayoclinic.com.

National Institutes of Health, National Institute of Neurological Disorders and Stroke. "Carpal Tunnel Syndrome Fact Sheet," www.ninds.nih.gov/disorders/carpal_tunnel/detail_crpal_tunnel.htm.

Wilkerson, April. "Trouble at Hand: Texting Creates New Generation of Carpal Tunnel Sufferers." *Oklahoma City Journal Record* (January 17, 2011), http://journalrecord.com/2011/01/17/carpal-punishment-smartphone-use-can-hurt-hands.

"Workout for Aching Hands." *Harvard Women's Health Watch* (October 1, 2010), www.health.harvard.edu/healthbeat/HEALTHbeat_061908.htm.

CELL PHONES

In less than two decades, the cell phone has become one of the world's most popular innovations, and for 5 billion people it is now a part of everyday life (Engeler, 2010). For many, it is difficult to conceive of a time before cell phones existed. And along with their extensive use comes questions about their safety, especially in regard to cancer.

Does cell phone use cause brain tumors or cancer? The answer depends on whom you ask and who conducts the study, and even then the experts continue to disagree. For example, one study published in the *Journal of the American Medical Association* in February 2011 indicated that people who cradle their cell phones next to their heads could be altering their brain activity (Volkow et al., 2011). This was the first investigation into cell phone use and glucose metabolism in the brain.

Researchers found that the majority of the radiofrequency energy from the cell phone is absorbed by the hand and head of the user. The authors were uncertain whether the brain changes they measured, which included an increase in glucose metabolism, have any negative impact on health. This left cell phone users wondering, once again, what they should do to protect themselves or if they even need to change their cell phone behavior.

It isn't difficult to find those who say cell phones are safe. The Federal Communications Commission (FCC) continues to maintain that the standard it sets for radiation emissions by the phones is safe. That standard, known as the specific absorption rate (SAR) indicates how much radiation is absorbed by the body when using the phone at maximum power. U.S. cell phones must have an SAR below 1.6 watts per kilogram; in Europe, the maximum is 2 watts per kilogram.

The SAR is not always easy to find when comparing phones for purchase, but organizations such as the Environmental Working Group offer a list of SAR values for most cell phones on its website. In fact, the FCC suggests that the SAR value is misleading since most phones rarely operate at maximum power. However, it is important to note that cell phones emit less radiation when the user is stationary rather than in a car. When the phone is moving, there are repeated bursts of radiation emitted as the phone moves in and out of range of various towers. Plus, when the cell phone shows a weak signal, it must work harder and consequently emit more radiation than if it is in range of a tower and shows a strong signal.

The debate about cell phones and cancer caught the attention of consumers in 1993, when Florida businessman David Reynard filed a lawsuit against the cell phone industry after his wife died of brain cancer. Although the suit was dismissed for lack of evidence, the fear factor was lodged in the public consciousness and has not been laid to rest yet. When researchers in Europe, where cell phone use was strong a decade before it was in the United States, released some

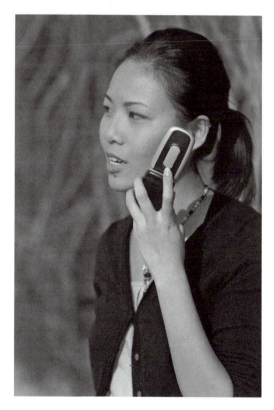

Chinese girl talks on cell phone. Even though the Internet has been credited with major advances in the telecommunication revolution in China, earlier devices such as mobile phones, faxes, and pagers predate the Internet by nearly two decades and are popular with consumers. (iStockPhoto.com)

studies that showed links between forms of tumors and heavy cell phone usage, concerns were raised even higher.

Those findings led to another study, Interphone, that involved participants from over a dozen countries who were evaluated from 2000 to 2004. The results, published in May 2010 in the *International Journal of Epidemiology,* suggested no increased risk of the most common types of brain tumors from average cell phone use (Cardis, 2010). However, the researchers concluded that "the possible effects of long-term heavy use of mobile phones on risk of brain tumors require further investigations, given increasing mobile phone use, its extension to children and its penetration worldwide." The United States Food and Drug Administration added its opinion on the available scientific evidence following the release of the World Health Organization (WHO) Interphone study results, saying there is no increased health risk due to radiofrequency energy.

Still, due to the concerns raised by the $14 million WHO Interphone study, international researchers have launched a longer-term study, named the Cohort Study on Mobile Communications (COSMOS), that will involve more than 250,000 cell phone users from the United Kingdom, Finland, the Netherlands, Sweden, and Denmark over the course of 30 years. COSMOS researchers will also study the use of hands-free devices, how and where people carry their phones, and whether there are links to neurological diseases such as Parkinson's or Alzheimer's from cell phone use.

Cell phones have been in widespread use since the 1990s. However, their development dates back to mobile radio usage in vehicles. As early as 1921, the Detroit, Michigan, Police Department was the first organization to officially use the radios in their patrol cars. Police and emergency use then pushed early development of the technology. Still, researchers saw little use for mobile phones at that time.

In the 1940s, especially following World War II, radio communications increased in popularity, which led to more advances in the technology, and once again scientists turned to mobile phones. By 1977, AT&T had built a model cell system of broadcast towers to accommodate a cellular system. However, the FCC did not see the commercial need for increasing the airwaves to accommodate cell phones until 1981, following positive results from cell phone system tests. By the time the FCC opened an additional communications band in the late 1980s, the demand by consumers had exploded.

Even though it took decades for the cellular phone industry to develop before the FCC met its demands, consumers around the world accepted cell phones immediately. According to statistics from the Cellular Telecommunications and Internet Association (CTIA), by 1999 there were more than 80 million subscribers in the United States generating over $37 billion in revenue. In 2009, the CTIA survey indicated that 276 million U.S. subscribers generated more than $76 billion for the cell phone industry for just the first half of that year (CTIA, 2009).

The debate over cell phones and brain cancer ebbs and flows depending on the studies published; however, all experts agree on the importance of exercising caution with regard to cell phone use by children. Since children have thinner skulls, they can absorb more radio energy from a cell phone than an adult. Cell phone use among children under the age of 12 has increased rapidly since the early 2000s. To lessen any potential problems, a number of standard safety tips have been developed. Those include using a headset as one way to decrease any risk of exposure to radiation. Another suggestion is to keep the phone away from the body, protecting sensitive areas such as the eyes, testes, and hips, where 80 percent of red blood cells are formed. Using the speakerphone feature also keeps the phone away from the head. Texting—which is now extremely popular, especially among young cell phone users—might be safer than talking with the phone resting against the head. Another suggestion is to put the phone in off-line mode when carrying, storing, or charging it, a change that stops the electromagnetic emissions.

Governments at every level have tried to protect consumers from potential problems. In December 2000, the British government handed out pamphlets that recommended reducing the amount of time children spend on a cell phone. In the United States, the city of San Francisco approved an ordinance in 2010 that would require retailers to display the SAR of cell phones. While the bottom line is there is still no conclusive evidence to connect the use of cell phones with an increased risk of tumors or cancer, the research will continue as scientists work to answer the question definitively. In the meantime, researchers such as Devra Davis, director of the Center for Environmental Oncology at the University of Pittsburg Cancer Institute, suggests that people practice a better-safe-than-sorry approach (Davis, 2010).

Sharon Zoumbaris

See also Cancer; Environmental Health; Food and Drug Administration (FDA); World Health Organization (WHO).

References

Agar, Jon. *Constant Touch: A Global History of the Mobile Phone. Revolutions in Science.* Cambridge, MA: Icon, 2004.

Cardis, Elisabeth. "Brain Tumour Risk in Relation to Mobile Telephone Use: Results of the Interphone International Case-Control Study." *International Journal of Epidemiology* (2010): 1–20.

Cellular Telecommunications and Internet Association. "CTIA-The Wireless Association Announces Semi-annual Wireless Industry Survey Results" (April 1, 2009), www.ctia.org/media/press/body.cfm/prid/1811.

Cohort Study of Mobile Phone Use and Health, www.ukcosmos.org/index.html.

Davis, Devra. *Disconnect: The Truth about Cell Phone Radiation, What the Industry Has Done to Hide It, and How to Protect Your Family.* New York, NY: Dutton, 2010.

Engeler, Elaine. "Cell Phone Use Surging in Developing Countries." *Associated Press* (February 23, 2010).

Goggin, Gerard. *Cell Phone Culture: Mobile Technology in Everyday Life.* London: Routledge, 2006.

Jacobson, Joy. "Do Cell Phones Cause Cancer? Caution Is Advised Until Better Research Is Available." *American Journal of Nursing* 110, no. 9 (September 2010): 14.

Marchese, Marianne. "Cell Phones and Brain Cancer Risk." *Townsend Letter* 325–326 (August–September 2010): 42–44.

Murphy, Kate. "Cellphone Radiation May Alter Your Brain, Let's Talk." *New York Times* (March 31, 2011): B9.

Raloff, Janet. "Cell Phone-Cancer Study an Enigma: Researchers Remain Uncertain about Safety of Mobile Devices." *Science News* 177, no. 13 (June 19, 2010): 13.

"State Weighs Cell Phone Cancer Warnings." *Harvard Reviews of Health News* (December 22, 2009).

Volkow, Nora D., et al. "Effects of Cell Phone Radiofrequency Signal Exposure on Brain Glucose Metabolism." *Journal of the American Medical Association* 305, no. 8 (February 23, 2011): 808–13.

World Health Organization. "Cancer: Interphone Study on Mobile Phone Use and Brain Cancer Risk" (August 6, 2010), www.who.org.

CENTER FOR FOOD SAFETY AND APPLIED NUTRITION (CFSAN)

The Center for Food Safety and Applied Nutrition (CFSAN) is a branch of the United States Food and Drug Administration (FDA). The center is responsible for protecting and promoting the public health by keeping the nation's food supply safe and honestly labeled. It is also responsible for the safety and labeling of cosmetic products.

Among its food safety duties, the center is responsible for making sure things like food additives—including radiation, color additives, ingredients developed through biotechnology or genetic engineering—are safe, sanitary, wholesome, and carry accurate labels. In addition it maintains seafood and juice Hazard Analysis and Critical Control Point (HACCP) regulations; it reviews health risks associated with food-borne, chemical, and biological contaminants; and it reviews regulations and activities dealing with the proper labeling of foods, including their ingredients and the nutritional health claims on the packaging. The FDA adopted the HACCP system in 1995 for seafood and in 2002 for juice. The HACCP system attempts to find potential food safety problems and early solutions rather than waiting for problems to develop before they take action.

The center works closely with the FDA, which is the scientific regulatory agency responsible for overall safety of the nation's domestically produced and imported foods, drugs, medical devices, cosmetics, and radiological products. CFSAN and the FDA share a small amount of responsibility for food safety with the U.S. Department of Agriculture and that agency's Food Safety and Inspection Service, which oversees the safety of meat, poultry, and eggs. That leaves the center to protect and monitor $417 billion worth of sales in domestic food, $49 billion worth of sales in imported foods, and the over $60 billion worth of cosmetics sold in the United States.

While many consider the U.S. food supply among the safest in the world, there has been a huge increase in items available from outside the country, bringing with them increased public health concerns. Since sources of food contamination are as varied as the contaminants and can occur anytime during processing, packaging, transportation, or preparation, the CFSAN must increase its understanding of international food safety standards to better protect U.S. consumers. Among domestic concerns, the staff continues to research the "four Ws" of food safety: workers, water, wildlife, and waste—all of which have been linked to outbreaks of food-borne illness.

Along with the increased complexity in food safety, changes in the cosmetic industry and its technologies and ingredients also bring additional challenges. Cosmetic products and ingredients are entering the United States from a growing number of countries, each with different regulatory and safety standards. CFSAN's current areas of focus for cosmetic health concerns include microbiological contaminants, chemical contaminants, botanical ingredients and their safety, and alternatives to animal testing.

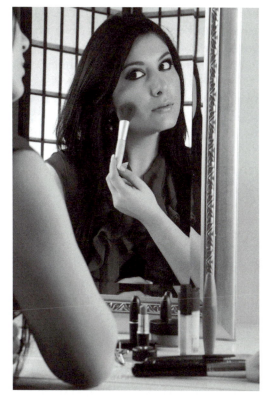

The Center for Food Safety and Applied Nutrition (CFSAN) regulates the overall safety of the nation's cosmetics, as well as food, drugs, medical devices, and radiological products. (Imagesolution/Dreamstime.com)

CFSAN also partners with other international organizations, including the World Health Organization, the Food and Agriculture Organization (FAO) of the United Nations, the Codex Alimentarius Commission (the international food standard setting organization of the FAO), and some foreign governments. On the national front, the center collaborates with several academic institutions through a program called Centers of Excellence (COE). The four COEs in operation are the National Center for Food Safety and Technology in conjunction with the Illinois Institute of Technology; the Joint Institute of Food Safety and Applied Nutrition in collaboration with the University of Maryland; the FDA COE for Botanical Dietary Supplement Research at the National Center for Natural Products Research in cooperation with the University of Mississippi; and the Western Center for Food Safety with the University of California, Davis.

As part of its role in educating U.S. consumers, the center conducted a question-and-answer webinar on nutrition facts. This webinar was the seventh in a series of monthly online sessions hosted by different FDA centers and offices. The webinars allow the CFSAN to showcase various food scientists, something both government and the food industry have in short supply, according to an August 2010 subcommittee meeting of the FDA Science Board.

At that meeting, the board announced its review of CFSAN's strengths and weaknesses and suggested the agency could improve its program by hiring more scientists who understand food processing, food technology, and nutritional science. However, according to food industry and government officials, budget dollars for research and staffing have been shrinking, and they don't anticipate receiving financial support for new positions.

Sharon Zoumbaris

See also Food and Drug Administration (FDA); Food Safety; U.S. Department of Agriculture (USDA).

References

"Federal Food Safety Oversight, A Fragmented Picture." *Journal of Environmental Health* 71, no. 8 (2009): 41.

"The Four W's." *Food Chemical News* (June 7, 2010): 3.

Murphy, Joan. "CFSAN's Thomas Maps Out Enforcement Priorities." *Food Chemical News* 52, no. 31 (October 18, 2010): 11.

Murphy, Joan. "FDA Science Board Discusses Response to Shortage of Food Safety Scientists." *Food Chemical News* 38, no. 52 (November 19, 2010): 8.

United States Food and Drug Administration. "About the Center for Food Safety and Applied Nutrition," www.fda.gov.aboutfda/centersoffices/cfsan/default.htm.

CENTERS FOR DISEASE CONTROL AND PREVENTION (CDC)

The Centers for Disease Control and Prevention (CDC) is the premier agency in the world working to prevent illness and, when illness occurs, to conduct disease surveillance and outbreak investigation. Under the umbrella of the U.S. Department of Health and Human Services, this public health agency has been in existence for over 50 years and began as a small branch of the Public Health Service. Originally named the Communicable Disease Center, founder Joseph W. Mountin set up shop on one floor of the Volunteer Building on Peachtree Street in Atlanta, Georgia, on July 1, 1946. At that time, he and some 400 employees were responsible for any communicable disease except for tuberculosis and venereal disease, which had separate units in Washington, D.C. At first the agency worked to control malaria and typhus fever, but Mountin pushed the staff to expand their focus to include epidemiology.

Although epidemiologists were scarce at that time, in 1949 Alexander Langmuir joined the office to head the epidemiology branch. With the start of the Korean War in 1950, the CDC created its Epidemic Intelligence Service, which focused on the threat of biological warfare, something Langmuir was knowledge-able about from his time in the Public Health Service.

The CDC achieved its first notable successes due to two major health crises in the mid-1950s. The first occurred in 1955, when polio shots were halted because polio was appearing in children who had received the Salk vaccine. The CDC traced the problem to the laboratory where the vaccine was initially developed and discovered that some of the vaccine was contaminated. Once the problem was corrected, the national inoculation program continued. Two years later, the agency used this same style of surveillance to trace the course of a huge flu epi-demic. From the data gathered at that time and in following years, the agency was able to establish national guidelines for influenza vaccines.

Once the agency established credibility, it grew through acquisition as pro-grams on nutrition, venereal disease, tuberculosis, immunization practices, fam-ily planning, surveillance of chronic diseases, and foreign quarantine were added to its growing mission. The CDC, through its work in disease surveillance and immunizations, played a crucial role in what has been called the greatest ac-complishment of public health: the eradication of smallpox. The agency set up a smallpox surveillance unit in 1962 and a year later began testing a vaccine and jet gun delivery system. The original vaccination program reached people in the Pacific island region, Brazil, and central and west Africa. At that time, the World Health Organization applauded the CDC's use of surveillance and used what it called this "eradication escalation" technique around the world. By 1977, small-pox was considered eradicated throughout the world.

Other disease triumphs for the CDC included tracking and finding the cause of Legionnaires disease and toxic shock syndrome in the mid-1970s and early 1980s. In 1981 the agency's newsletter made its first mention of a fatal disease later named acquired immune deficiency syndrome (AIDS). Since then, the news-letter continues to focus on AIDS, and a large portion of today's CDC budget is assigned to address this disease.

While the CDC has received international praise for its accomplishments, the agency is not without criticism. In 1972 the agency came under protest after news reports uncovered troubling information about the Tuskegee study on long-term effects of untreated syphilis. Although the study had been initiated by Public Health Service and other organizations in 1932, it was transferred to the CDC in 1957, and the continued practice of not treating the African American men in the study brought with it a storm of protest when it was finally brought to public attention in 1972. The CDC also came under fire in 1976 for its effort to vacci-nate Americans against swine flu. That program was criticized when individuals who received the vaccines developed Guillain-Barre syndrome. The program was quickly stopped, especially since the epidemic had not materialized.

As the scope of the agency's activities grew, its name was changed in 1970 to Center for Disease Control. After reorganization, the word *Center* was changed to *Centers* in 1981, and finally the words *and Prevention* were added in 1992. However, the organization remains known by its three-letter acronym. The CDC joins sev-eral other smaller agencies in the Department of Health and Human Services that deal with food and nutrition, including the Food and Drug Administration and the National Institutes of Health. Although the CDC focuses on national issues of illness and health, its response to global problems has increased in the past decade. The CDC's contributions to world health include its work combating the Ebola virus and plague as well as efforts to eradicate polio and the international prevention of neural tube defects.

Sharon Zoumbaris

See also Food and Drug Administration (FDA); Influenza; U.S. Department of Health and Human Services (HHS).

References

Gerding, Justin, and Jansen Kunz. "Putting Theory into Practice, CDC's Summer Program." *Journal of Environmental Health* 73, no. 6 (January–February 2011): 96.
"Historical Perspectives: History of the CDC." *Morbidity and Mortality Weekly Report MMWR,* June 28, 1996, www.cdc.gov.
"Regulatory Agencies." In *Nutrition and Well-being A–Z,* edited by Delores C. S. James. 2 vols. New York: Macmillan Reference USA, 2004.

CHEESEBURGER BILL

The Personal Responsibility in Food Consumption Act, commonly known as the Cheeseburger Bill, is federal legislation that was introduced in the summer of 2004 in the U.S. House of Representatives to ban obese customers from suing fast-food chains for making them fat. It was an attempt by some lawmakers to put the responsibility where they believe it belonged—on the individual rather than on the manufacturer or restaurant. Even though the bill passed in the House that year, it was not brought to a vote in the Senate.

Critics of the bill suggest the problem lies in the American desire for convenience food. From the 1950s, the U.S. diet has become composed of more foods that are fried, processed, and pumped full of salt, fat, sweeteners, and additives. The nation became obsessed with cheap, easy food. Fast-food restaurants multiplied across the landscape until America had homogenized itself with golden arches, pizza restaurants, taco stands, and burger joints.

Americans are now seeing the unintended results of their desire for low-priced convenience in the unprecedented numbers of people with obesity, diabetes, and other diseases, brought on at least in part by the classic American diet, which is high in fat, sweeteners, salt, and additives. Food technologists know that fat, high-fructose corn syrup, and sodium are the cheapest ingredients to add flavor to processed food, but their use, especially in fast food, has created an economic paradox.

Decades after reshaping how American families eat, what they eat, and even where they eat it, the food industry is being asked to improve consumer

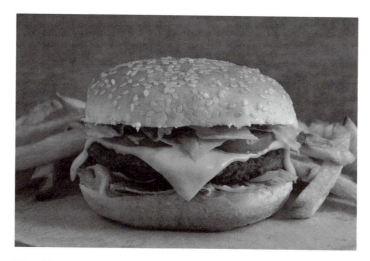

The Cheeseburger Bill was an attempt by some lawmakers to put the responsibility where they believe it belonged, on the individual rather than on the manufacturer or restaurant. (Christian Draghici/Dreamstime.com)

awareness of nutrition and to offer healthier products. The problem for the manufacturers and fast-food restaurants is simple: if they are to stay profitable, they cannot afford to have consumers eat any less of their food. On the other hand, to keep the customers happy, manufacturers and restaurants must hold down prices even as government officials now mandate the use of healthier and costlier ingredients.

The Cheeseburger Bill was reintroduced in the Senate in 2005. It still failed to pass, but between 2003 and 2006, some 24 states enacted similar legislation shielding fast-food restaurants from liability. Critics of those bills say their success has at least partially been linked to lobbying efforts by the food industry in those individual states. According to a 2005 report from the Montana-based Institute on Money in State Politics, the restaurant industry donated some $5.5 million to legislators in the states that have passed their own cheeseburger bills (Francis-Smith, 2007).

Critics of the bill argue that it disregards the reality of economic disparities and an increasingly toxic food environment, especially in areas referred to as "food deserts"—a description adopted by social policy planners in the 1990s that describes a growing number of low-income areas with little or no access to affordable, healthy food. Instead critics suggest that states would be better served by focusing on the prevention or treatment of obesity rather than using their time and energy to close off potential legal recourse.

The Commonsense Consumption Act was reintroduced once again in May 2007 in both the House and Senate. All of these attempts to pass a national cheeseburger bill stem from a lawsuit filed in 2002, in which families of several

New York teenagers accused McDonald's of making the teens fat by serving them highly processed food. U.S. District Court Judge Robert Sweet said in his final ruling for the lawsuit that "if consumers know or reasonably should know the potential ill health effects of eating at McDonald's, they cannot blame McDonald's if they, nonetheless, choose to satiate their appetite with a surfeit of supersized McDonald's products" (Collins, 2003). However, Sweet left open the possibility that other cases could be filed if those fast-food establishments failed to properly disclose the nutritional content of their menu choices. While current U.S. citizens may be the most informed generation of Americans, with 24-hour media saturation, many U.S. consumers remain confused about nutrition and healthy food choices. Opponents of cheeseburger legislation argue that, even though the federal government has a nutrition education program, the idea that people will change their habits (such as eating an apple instead of French fries) without changing the food environment is not realistic. They suggest that Americans are more influenced by advertising than by hard facts and point to earlier attempts to change national tobacco health habits through education as an example of how education alone falls short and why the industry cannot be counted on to offer what is best for consumers. They also suggest that the threat of lawsuits and regulation can encourage the fast-food industry to offer healthy selections on their menus.

What Next?   If federal legislation fails to materialize, state and local governments appear ready to address food policy from both sides of the issue, illustrated by state-sponsored versions of the Cheeseburger Bill, as well as by state regulations banning fast-food restaurants in certain geographic areas and requiring calorie counts on menus. For example, the Los Angeles City Council passed a fast-food moratorium in the summer of 2008, which stopped any new fast-food or freestanding quick-service restaurants from opening within a 32-square-mile area in the southern part of the city. The moratorium was extended a second year and expired in April 2010. Other California cities, such as San Jose, are now looking to follow the Los Angeles example.

In fact, California for years has taken the lead in pushing the public health envelope with food legislation. The state recently passed a law that will require thousands of restaurants in California to post calorie counts on their menus as of 2011. In 2004, both the Los Angeles Unified School District and the San Francisco Unified School District implemented bans on soft drinks, candy, and other high-fat snack foods from school vending machines. School districts across the country have now followed their lead.

These local regulatory initiatives gained momentum because of rising rates of obesity, diabetes, and heart disease. Still, critics of any government intervention that tells people what to eat argue that, while the government may have good intentions, the laws are a form of "nanny government" and send the message, especially in low-income areas such as in Los Angeles, that residents are not capable of making up their own minds about what they eat. While lawmakers continue to debate the pros and cons of various food-related legislation, such regulation, whether it is in production, preparation, or consumption on the local or national level, will remain controversial.

Sharon Zoumbaris

See also High-Fructose Corn Syrup; Obesity.

References

Burnett, David. "Fast-Food Lawsuits and the Cheeseburger Bill: Critiquing Congress's Response to the Obesity Epidemic." *Virginia Journal of Social Policy and Law* 14 (2007): 357–58.

Collins, Dan. "McDonald's Wins Fat Fight," CBSnews.com (January 22, 2003), www.cbsnews.com/stories/2003/health/main537520.shtml.

Fletcher, Anthony. "Food Industry Still Wary after 'Cheeseburger Bill' Victory." FoodNavigator.com (October 21, 2005), www.foodnavigator.com.

Francis-Smith, Janice. "Oklahoma House Bill Would Protect Agriculture Industry from Obesity Lawsuits." *Journal Record* (Oklahoma City) (February 7, 2007).

Hirsch, Jerry. "Fast-Food Ban Is No Fat Cure: Barring New Eateries in South L.A. Is Unlikely to Curb Obesity." *Los Angeles Times* (October 6, 2009): B1.

Kingston, Anne, and Nicholas Kohler. "L.A.'s Fast-Food Drive-By: A City Council's Ban on Fast-Food Chains Is a Provocative Social Experiment." *Macleans* 121, no. 33 (August 25, 2008).

Kish, Matthew. "Banning 'McLawsuits': State Bill Outlawing Fast-Food Litigation Nears Passage." *Indianapolis Business Journal* 26, no. 52 (February 27, 2006): 29.

MacVean, Mary. "Food Concerns Are Finding a Place on Local Politicians' Agendas." *Los Angeles Times* (February 18, 2010): E1.

Myers, Jim. "Cheeseburger Bill on Menu in House: U.S. Rep. Dan Boren Introduces a Measure That Would Take Fast-Food Obesity Lawsuits off the Table." *Tulsa World* (May 10, 2007).

Pomeranz, Jennifer L. "A Historical Analysis of Public Health, the Law and Stigmatized Social Groups: The Need for Both Obesity and Weight Bias Legislation." *Obesity* 16, no. 2 (November 2008).

CHELATION

Chelation therapy is a form of treatment that uses chelating agents to remove heavy metals from the body by binding the molecules and holding them so they can be removed. In the United States, chelation has been scientifically proven to rid the body of toxic metals such as lead, iron, copper, arsenic, mercury, and calcium and is approved by the United States Food and Drug Administration (FDA) for that use. Current uses for chelation therapy range from cancer treatments to arthritis, Alzheimer's disease, and heart disease as well as limited use in the treatment of autism, kidney dysfunction, and ovarian cancer. However, the usefulness and safety of these alternative practices remain controversial.

Chelation (pronounced key-Lay-shun) comes from the Greek root word *chele,* meaning claw. Chelating agents were originally designed for industrial applications in the early 1900s and became more widely used in the 1940s with the advent of the chelating agent ethylenediamine tetraacetic acid (EDTA), a manufactured amino acid. The medical use of EDTA followed World War II and focused on workers from factories who suffered from lead poisoning as a result of their work with lead-based paint and other factory workers who had overexposure to lead.

How Treatment Works Treatments involve intravenous injection of EDTA, which binds with metals in the bloodstream, allowing those metals to be excreted in the urine. Blood pressure, blood sugar, and kidney function are monitored during a treatment, and vitamin and mineral supplements and antioxidants are often added to an EDTA infusion. The treatments last between three and four hours, and doctors recommend anywhere from 20 to 50 treatments for metal poisoning depending on the severity of the poisoning and the overall health of the patient.

Patients with preexisting conditions such as poor kidney function, congestive heart failure, clotting problems, or hypoglycemia are at more risk for complications from chelation treatment. Evaluation and treatment of these individuals should be done only after a thorough physical examination, lifestyle evaluation, medical history, and necessary laboratory tests are performed by medical professionals experienced in the use of chelation treatments. Although the EDTA binds harmful toxic metals, it also binds important nutrients such as copper, iron, calcium, zinc, and magnesium, which makes the vitamin and mineral supplements necessary to treatment success.

Controversial Treatment Choices Chelation therapy has also been used to treat other illnesses, including heart disease, Alzheimer's disease, multiple sclerosis, stroke, arthritis, and cancer. Many doctors warn against these treatments and warn of side effects such as anemia, blood clots, bone marrow damage, low blood pressure, and severe inflammation of the area where the intravenous needle was inserted.

However, based on case studies and other reports, the government began a study of the effectiveness of chelation therapy in the treatment of heart disease. The National Center for Complementary and Alternative Medicine and the National Heart, Lung, and Blood Institute components of the National Institutes of Health have launched the first large-scale clinical trial to determine the safety and efficacy of EDTA chelation therapy for victims of coronary heart disease. The $30 million federal study began in 2002 and now involves more than 2,300 patients at more than 100 research sites across the country. The study will continue through 2011 with the results to be analyzed in 2012.

More controversial than the use of chelation therapy for heart disease has been the use of chelation therapy for the treatment of cancer and autism. Its use in cancer treatment stems from the belief by some that heavy metal toxicity is a contributing cause of cancer. It is suggested by advocates of the treatment that heavy metals propagate free-radical reactions, which suppress the human immune system. Supporters of chelation therapy for cancer patients believe that by reducing the body's free-radical situation, chelation therapy can then allow that person's immune system to better fight the cancer. The American Cancer Society, the FDA, and the American Medical Association do not endorse the use of chelation therapy for any treatment except for heavy metal poisoning.

The use of chelation therapy in the treatment of autism is based on speculation that mercury poisoning may trigger the onset of autism. A study released in 2003 received attention when it showed that the baby hair of children who were later diagnosed with autism had lower levels of mercury than other infants, leading to speculation that autistic children do not absorb mercury or cannot excrete it (Lathe & LePage, 2003). While the study findings support the theory that some children have a genetic fault that makes them more susceptible to mercury poisoning, scientists say the results do not support the speculation that mercury triggers the onset of autism. The theory that the measles, mumps, and rubella vaccine, which contains a mercury-based preservative, may contribute to the onset of autism in some children has been around for years, and scientists say there is no scientific evidence that the vaccine has any relationship to autism.

According to the study authors, in this instance, most of the mercury came from the mothers with the main sources of exposure being mercury amalgam fillings, immunoglobulin injections given to Rhesus-negative mothers, and heavy consumption of fish. The study also found that even when the mothers' exposure was high, the baby hair of autistic children still had consistently low mercury levels.

According to the latest figures, the incidence of autism in the United States is increasing dramatically. Approximately 1 in every 91 children ages 3 to 17 was on the autism spectrum according to an American Academy of Pediatrics report issued in 2009 (Kogan et al., 2009). These latest figures make autism the most prevalent childhood developmental disorder. Along with the growing rate in autism diagnosis has come a growing number of theories about its causes, including genetics, vaccinations, pesticides, industrial contaminants, and the United States' increasing reliance on prescription drugs as well as an increase in chelation therapy for autistic children.

Training and Certification The medical establishment continues to strongly challenge the safety and theory behind chelation treatments for anything except heavy metal toxicity. For information about chelation therapy and its accepted uses, patients should contact the American College for Advancement in Medicine (ACAM) for its directory of U.S. doctors who are members and who follow the accepted guidelines for chelation therapy. In 2009, ACAM completed the process for developing a certification program for chelation therapy. This is the first such program offered by ACAM, and its CCT designation exam allows physicians to apply the highest standard of care and training when administering chelation treatments. The ACAM recommends that patients look for the CCT designation when selecting a health care provider for diagnosis or chelation therapy. Also, the American Board of Chelation Therapy offers minimum standards for its members as well as oral and written tests to receive certification.

Sharon Zoumbaris

See also Autism; Cancer; Minerals (Food); Vitamins.

References

American Heart Association. "Chelation Therapy: Questions and Answers" www.ameri canheart.org/presenter.jhtml?identifiere=3000843.

Green, Saul. "Quackwatch: Chelation Therapy" (July 24, 2007), www.quackwatch. com/01QuackeryRelatedTOpics/chelation.html.

Hawken, C.M. *Chelation Therapy for Cardiovascular Health*. Chapmanville, WV: Woodland Press, 2007.

Kogan, Michael D., et al. "Prevalence of Parent-Reported Diagnosis of Autism Spectrum Disorder among Children in the US, 2007." *Pediatrics* 10, no. 1542 (2009): 1522.

Lathe, Richard, and Michael LePage. "Toxic Metal Clue to Autism: A Study Has Revealed Startling Differences in Mercury Levels in the Hair of Autistic and Normal Children." *New Scientist* 178, no. 2400 (June 21, 2003): 4.

"Pharmacy Update: Continuing Professional Development in Use of Chelating Agents." *Chemist and Druggist* (September 9, 2006): 33.

Turner, Judith, Teresa G. Odle, and David Edward Newton. *The Gale Encyclopedia of Alternative Medicine*, 3rd ed., 4 vols. Detroit: Gale, 2009.

Whaley, George. "Preservative Properties of EDTA." *Manufacturing Chemist* 62, no. 9 (September 1991): 22.

CHOLESTEROL

Cholesterol is a soft waxy substance that is a steroidal alcohol or sterol. It is the most abundant steroid in the human body and is a component of every cell. Cholesterol is essential to life, and most animals and many plants contain this compound. Cholesterol biosynthesis occurs primarily in the liver, but it may be produced in other organs. A number of other substances are synthesized from cholesterol, including vitamin D, steroid hormones (including the sex hormones), and bile salts. Cholesterol resides mainly in cell membranes.

Cholesterol was discovered in 1769 by Poulletier de la Salle (1719–1787), who isolated the compound from bile and gallstones. It was rediscovered by Michel Eugène Chevreul (1786–1889) in 1815 and named cholesterine. The name comes from the Greek words *khole* meaning bile and *steros* meaning solid or stiff. The *ine* ending was later changed to *ol* to designate it as an alcohol.

Humans produce about one gram of cholesterol daily in the liver. Dietary cholesterol is consumed through food. High-cholesterol foods are associated with saturated fats and trans-fatty acids (commonly called trans fats). Dietary cholesterol comes from animal products (plants contain minute amounts of cholesterol) such as meats and dairy products. Table 1 shows the amount of cholesterol in common foods.

Cholesterol is commonly associated with cardiovascular disease, and its routine measurement is used to determine its potential health risk. High blood serum cholesterol levels are often correlated with excessive plaque deposits in the arteries, a condition known as atherosclerosis or hardening of the arteries.

Cholesterol in Common Foods Although high total blood cholesterol levels are associated with heart disease, it is important to distinguish between types

Table 1. Cholesterol in Common Foods

Item	Quantity	Cholesterol in mg.
Butter	1 tablespoon	30
Mozzarella cheese	1 oz.	22
Cheddar cheese	1 oz	30
Egg	1	200
Chicken	4 oz.	70
Liver	4 oz.	340
Ham	4 oz.	80
Skim milk	1 cup	5
Whole milk	1 cup	35
Ice cream	½ cup	30
Low-fat ice cream	½ cup	10

Source: Myers, Richard L. *The 100 Most Important Chemical Compounds: A Reference Guide*. Santa Barbara, CA: Greenwood, 2007.

of cholesterol when interpreting cholesterol levels. Cholesterol has been labeled as "good" and "bad" depending on its physiological role.

Forms of cholesterol depend on the lipoproteins that are associated with it. Low-density lipoprotein (LDL) cholesterol is often referred to as bad cholesterol, and high-density lipoprotein (HDL) is identified as "good" cholesterol. An understanding of the difference between LDL and HDL cholesterol requires an understanding of substances associated with cholesterol in the body. Cholesterol is a lipid, so it has very low solubility in water and blood. For the cholesterol synthesized in the liver to be delivered by the bloodstream to the rest of the body, the liver manufactures lipoproteins that can be viewed as carriers for cholesterol (and triglycerides).

Lipoproteins, as the name implies, are biochemical assemblages of fat and protein molecules. Several types of lipoproteins are found in human blood. A lipoprotein can be viewed as a globular structure with an outer shell of protein, phospholipid, and cholesterol surrounding a mass of triglycerides and cholesterol esters. The proteins in lipoproteins are called apolipoproteins, with different apolipoproteins associated with different lipoproteins.

Cholesterol leaves the liver in the form of very-low-density lipoprotein (VLDL). VLDL has a high percentage (50–65%) of triglycerides and relatively low protein composition of 10 percent or less. The percentage of fat and protein in different forms of lipoproteins dictates their density; a greater proportion of protein gives a higher density. As the VLDL moves through the bloodstream, it encounters an enzyme called lipoprotein lipase in the body organs' capillaries, which causes the triglycerides to be delivered to cells. Triglycerides are used for energy or stored as fat.

As the triglycerides are depleted from the lipoprotein, it becomes intermediate density lipoprotein (IDL). As IDL circulates in the blood, cell structures called LDL receptors bind to the apolipoprotein called Apo B-100 with its enclosed cholesterol and in the process converts IDL to LDL. This delivers cholesterol to the cell. Apo B-100 allows LDL cholesterol to be delivered to the tissues, but it has a tendency to attach to blood vessel walls. The accumulation impedes blood flow and can build up as plaque and lead to atherosclerosis.

Atherosclerosis is a type of arteriosclerosis (the latter being a more general term to include normal aging processes) that occurs when excess cholesterol combines with other substances such as other fats, lignin, and calcium to form a hard deposit on the inner lining of the blood vessels. Because of the problems associated with Apo B and LDL, LDL cholesterol is labeled as bad cholesterol. HDL is produced in the liver, intestines, and other tissues. It has a low level of triglycerides but a high protein content of approximately 50 percent. HDL cholesterol, or good cholesterol, transports cholesterol in the bloodstream back to the liver, where it is broken down and excreted. Although HDL cholesterol has been labeled as good, it has not been demonstrated definitively that high levels of HDL reduce heart disease, but there is an inverse relation between HDL and heart disease.

A proper balance of cholesterol in the bloodstream requires having an adequate balance of receptors to process the amount of cholesterol in the blood. Receptors are continually regenerated, produced, and disappear in the cell in response to blood biochemistry. The liver contains the greatest concentration of receptors. Too few receptors or excess dietary cholesterol intake can lead to elevated blood cholesterol. A genetic disorder called familial hypercholesterolemia results when a person inherits a defective gene from one parent resulting in the inability to produce sufficient receptors. A diet with too much cholesterol represses the production of LDL receptors and leads to high blood cholesterol and Apo B.

Standard lipid screening to obtain a cholesterol profile for the risk of cardiovascular disease routinely reports total cholesterol, LDL cholesterol, HDL cholesterol, and triglycerides. Cholesterol values are reported in milligrams per deciliter of blood (mg/dL). Different organizations have made recommendations for normal cholesterol levels, but these must be interpreted carefully, because they are contingent on other risk conditions. For example, the recommendations for smokers or those with a family history of heart disease are lower for someone without these conditions.

The National Center for Cholesterol Education (NCEP), endorsed by the American Heart Association, believes that LDL is the primary cholesterol component to determine therapy. LDL cholesterol accounts for 60 percent to 70 percent of blood serum cholesterol. An LDL of less than 160 mg/dL is recommended for individuals with no more than one risk factor and less than 100 mg/dL for individuals with coronary heart disease. The NCEP classifies HDL, which comprises between 20 percent and 30 percent of blood cholesterol, below 40 mg/dL as low. Triglycerides are an indirect measure of VLDL cholesterol. The NCEP considers a normal triglyceride level as less than 150 mg/dL.

Heart disease is the leading cause of death in adults over 35 years old in the United States, responsible for more than 1 million deaths annually. Cholesterol's role in contributing to heart disease has led to several broad strategies to lower blood cholesterol. Major treatment strategies to control cholesterol include changes in diet, lifestyle changes, and drug therapy. Dietary changes for lowering cholesterol primarily involve reducing fat intake, especially saturated fats and trans fats. Trans fats are made when liquid oils are hydrogenated (or more likely partially hydrogenated) to solidify them. During this process, the hydrogens bonded to carbons are reconfigured from being on the same side of the double bond (cis position) to a cross or trans position. Saturated and trans fats raise the LDL cholesterol, but trans fats also lower HDL. Starting on January 1, 2006, the United States Food and Drug Administration (FDA) required trans fat content to be included on nutritional labels of foods sold in the United States. Another dietary strategy is to eat foods high in soluble fiber, such as oatmeal, oat bran, citrus fruits, and strawberries. Soluble fiber binds to cholesterol and eliminates it in the feces. Eating foods and taking supplements containing omega-3 fatty acids are another strategy for lowering cholesterol. In addition to changes in the diet, other lifestyle changes include exercise, smoking cessation, and losing weight.

In the last 20 years, the use of statin drugs has revolutionized the treatment of heart disease. Statins work by inhibiting the enzyme HMG-CoA reductase, which is required to produce cholesterol in the liver. During cholesterol biosynthesis, HMG-CoA (3-hydroxy-3-methylglutaryl-CoA) is converted to mevalonate. All statin drugs contain a structure similar to mevalonate. Generic names of statins are sold under specific brand names. For example, lovastatin, which was the first FDA-approved statin in 1987, was marketed as Mevacor by Merck. Atorvastatin is sold as Lipitor by Pfizer, and Merck sells simvastatin as Zocor. Several of the top-selling drugs worldwide are statins. Lipitor has been the top-selling drug for several years, with annual sales in 2005 of approximately $13 billion and Zocor bringing in more than $5 billion.

Having high cholesterol increases the risk of heart disease, which continues to be the leading cause of death in the United States according to the Centers for Disease Control and Prevention (CDC). However, there is good news in the latest CDC statistics: fewer adults now have high cholesterol compared to earlier decades. According to the CDC, the proportion of the population ages 20 to 74 with high cholesterol has dropped by half, from 33 percent in a 1960–1962 study down to just over 16 percent in 2003–2006. Still, one in every six adults has high total cholesterol, and women with high cholesterol outnumber men, 30 percent to 16 percent in the 55 to 64 age range (Centers for Disease Control and Prevention, 2010).

Richard L. Myers

See also Fats; Heart Health; Trans Fats.

References

Aftalion, Fred. *A History of the International Chemistry Industry,* 2nd ed. Philadelphia: Chemical Heritage Foundation, 2001.

Baird, Colin, and Michael Cann. *Environmental Chemistry,* 3rd ed. New York: W.H. Freeman, 2004.

Centers for Disease Control and Prevention. "America's Cholesterol Burden" (February 9, 2010), www.cdc.gov/cholesterol/facts.htm.

"Chemical and Engineering News." *Top Pharmaceuticals* 83, no. 25 (June 20, 2005): 44–139. Special issue devoted to reports on 46 of the most important drugs for human society.

Kent, James A. *Riegel's Handbook of Industrial Chemistry,* 10th ed. New York: Kluwer Academic/Plenum, 2003.

May, Paul. *The Molecule of the Month,* www.chm.bris.ac,uk/motm/motm.htm.

Mayo Clinic, www.mayoclinic.com/health/site-map/smindex.

The Merck Index, 12th ed. Whitehouse Station, NJ: Merck, 1996.

Myers, Richard L. *The Basics of Chemistry.* Westport, CT: Greenwood Press, 2003.

National Institutes of Health. *Third Report of the National Cholesterol Education Program* (September 2002), http://circ.ahajournals.org/cgi/reprint/106/25/3143.

Snyder, Carl H. *The Extraordinary Chemistry of Ordinary Things,* 3rd ed. New York: John Wiley, 1998.

Tobin, Allan J., and Jennie Dusheck. *Asking About Life.* Fort Worth, TX: Saunders College Publishing, 1998.

Walsh, Christopher. *Antibiotics: Actions, Origins, Resistance.* Herndon, VA: ASM Press, 2003.

CHRONIC FATIGUE SYNDROME (CFS)

In the July 2003 issue of the *New Yorker* magazine, author Laura Hillenbrand described her encounter with chronic fatigue syndrome (CFS) (Hillenbrand, 2003). As she tells it, she was a healthy 19-year-old college student one minute and chronically, deathly ill the next. She was confined to bed for months at a time, suffering from strange fevers, swollen glands, vertigo, and the inability to eat. She also reported strange disruptions of her thoughts and senses. Her weight plummeted, and she became too weak to leave her home. Hillenbrand visited several doctors, some of whom concluded her disease was psychiatric. Her psychiatrist sent her back to the doctors. Although Hillenbrand's condition has waxed and waned many times since her college days, she has never truly been well. Her experience describes a case of one of the most puzzling and misunderstood illnesses of modern times.

Chronic fatigue syndrome is an incapacitating illness affecting approximately 800,000 Americans. The annual total value of lost productivity in the United States due to this illness has been estimated at $9.1 billion. The chronic fatigue that patients with CFS experience can be accompanied by a combination of other serious symptoms, including feeling sick after exercising, memory and concentration problems, unrefreshing sleep, muscle or joint pain, headache, sore throat, and tender lymph nodes.

Some researchers think that CFS had its origins in the 19th century, with the condition known as neurasthenia. At that time, this disorder was thought to be a neurological disease, and its symptoms included weakness or fatigue. By the late 1800s, neurasthenia was one of the most frequently diagnosed illnesses. However, by World War I, the diagnosis of neurasthenia almost disappeared. At the beginning of the 20th century, medical skepticism concerning this illness increased, and neurasthenia began to be viewed as a psychiatric disorder rather than a neurological illness. In addition, neurasthenia patients were increasingly held in low esteem by medical personnel. The debate that occurred about 100 years ago concerning whether neurasthenia was a disease of the body or mind has reappeared with CFS.

Throughout the 20th century, several outbreaks of fatigue illnesses of unknown origin were reported. Chief among these were an outbreak of a severe fatigue illness at the Los Angeles County Hospital in 1934 and another outbreak at the Royal Free Hospital in England in 1955. Finally, in Lake Tahoe, Nevada, and surrounding communities, an outbreak of cases of a severe fatigue illness occurred between 1984 and 1986. The symptoms of the Lake Tahoe outbreak included prolonged fatigue, abrupt onset of symptoms, severe pain, and prominent cognitive disorder. It was after the Lake Tahoe outbreak that national attention began to focus on this illness.

Interest in this illness increased in the late 1980s, and it was later renamed chronic fatigue syndrome (CFS). The criteria for CFS were developed in 1988 and later refined in 1994. To meet the 1994 criteria for CFS, an individual must exhibit severe, disabling fatigue that lasts six months or more. An individual also needs to report four or more of eight additional symptoms: sore throat, headaches, lymph node tenderness or pain, joint pain, muscle pain, unrefreshing sleep, feeling sick after minimal exercise, and memory or concentration difficulties. Finally, to appropriately diagnose CFS, a comprehensive medical and psychiatric evaluation must be conducted to ensure that the fatigue and related symptoms cannot be better explained by another medical illness or condition or by a psychiatric condition.

Recently, a new clinical case definition has been developed in Canada. The Canadian clinical case definition specifies that the illness needs to persist for at least six months. In addition, an individual must report feeling sick after minimal exercise, unrefreshing sleep, and a significant degree of joint pain or muscle pain. An individual must also report two or more symptoms such as confusion and impairment of concentration and short term-memory. Finally, there needs to be at least one symptom from two of the following categories involving the circulatory, nervous, and immune systems (e.g., recurrent sore throats). Many within the patient community feel that this Canadian case definition is more appropriate, because two of the central symptoms of this illness (feeling sick after minimal exercise and cognitive problems) are required for this case definition.

Most patient advocacy groups believe that the term *chronic fatigue syndrome* trivializes the seriousness of the illness and has contributed to health care providers having negative attitudes toward those who suffer from it. In reality, CFS is typified by many severe symptoms in addition to fatigue. The negative stigma associated with CFS could be due in part to its name. The word *fatigue* implies garden-variety tiredness, which is difficult for many people to accept as illness; to many, it sounds more like laziness. The term selected to characterize an illness such as chronic fatigue syndrome can influence how patients are perceived and ultimately treated by medical personnel, family members, and work associates. In fact, the term may actually influence the type and quality of medical care that a patient receives. Many patient advocacy groups prefer the names myalgic encephalomyelitis or myalgic encephalopathy. Variations of these names are currently being used by many patient advocacy groups throughout the world.

The cause (or causes) of this illness is still unclear. Some researchers think that persons with CFS have internal systems that are overstimulated. Over a long period of time this lack of internal regulation can lead to changes in immune response, which could affect the body's defense against viral or bacterial infections. Poor immunity sets up a host of smaller problems as microbes gain a foothold: fevers, sore throat, and so on. Although no virus has been identified as the primary cause of CFS, the immune system may be fighting a type of virus or viruses in some persons with CFS. As we learn more about the immune system, there may be other links to CFS that will help us to better understand its causes. There is also some evidence that CFS may be caused by deficient hormones in the adrenal gland. Brain dysfunction is also a possibility. Last, researchers are beginning to look into the genetic makeup of those with this illness in the hope that this may reveal important clues about its origins.

Leonard Jason

See also Fibromyalgia; Immune System/Lymphatic System.

References

Bharadvaj, Daivati. *Natural Treatments for Chronic Fatigue Syndrome.* Santa Barbara, CA: Praeger, 2007.

Hillenbrand, Laura. "A Sudden Illness." *The New Yorker*, July 7, 2003, 56.

Jason, Leonard A., P. Fennell, and R.R. Taylor, eds. *Handbook of Chronic Fatigue Syndrome.* New York: John Wiley, 2003.

Johnson, Hillary. *Osler's Web: Inside the Labyrinth of the Chronic Fatigue Syndrome Epidemic.* New York: Crown, 1996.

Taylor, R.R., F. Friedberg, and L.A. Jason. *A Clinician's Guide to Controversial Illnesses: Chronic Fatigue Syndrome, Fibromyalgia, and Multiple Chemical Sensitivities.* Sarasota, FL: Professional Resource Press, 2001.

CIGARETTES

A cigarette usually refers to a slim, paper-wrapped cylinder containing an addictive mixture of tobacco and other ingredients, but it may also refer to other products such as marijuana that have been rolled into cigarette paper for smoking. Although they are significantly different from cigars, early European cigarettes may have been modeled on the crude product that the poor created out of discarded cigar butts that the wealthy tossed into the streets. Well before that, probably as early as the 9th century, indigenous cultures in the Americas were smoking a harsh form of tobacco in reeds or other crude forms of smoking tubes.

Records show that in the 1600s, colonial settlers smoked a type of cigar as well as pipes, first consuming the harsh tobacco to which the Indians had introduced them before learning to cultivate a milder form that proved to be very addicting. Cigarette smoking quickly caught on during the 1800s, after the British, who were exposed to the practice during the Crimean War during the mid-1800s, introduced it to the United States. As a newly developed machine able to produce 200 cigarettes per minute made them more affordable, cigarettes quickly began to outstrip the use of chewing tobacco, pipes and cigars, and snuff.

Although most people purchased tobacco and papers to roll their own cigarettes well into the 1940s and 1950s, mass production made manufactured cigarettes accessible everywhere. Cigarette companies spent lavishly to sell their product through print and radio ads and the newly developed medium known as television.

By the late 1950s, when nearly every household had at least one smoker living in it, disquieting news about the ill effects of smoking had become more widespread. In 1964, the U.S. Surgeon General issued a report detailing the harmful effects smoking could have on health. Almost immediately, cigarette consumption dropped by 20 percent, then rebounded quickly. Despite subsequent legislation restricting advertising and U.S. government–funded reports that verified and strengthened earlier concerns about the dangers of cigarettes and other tobacco products, high consumption has continued. The tobacco industry is now a powerful lobby that has successfully obscured the obvious dangers of its product with aggressive marketing campaigns. Nevertheless, the message has gotten through to many, and so, with fewer consumers choosing to smoke cigarettes and

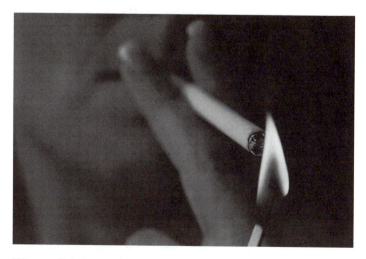

Woman lighting a cigarette. Smoking just one cigarette leaves a noticeable amount of tar in the lungs. (PhotoDisc, Inc.)

aware that the sooner people start smoking in life the more likely they are to be addicted for life, cigarette companies are marketing mini cigars and smokeless tobacco products more aggressively to appeal to adolescents, according to the U.S. Department of Health and Human Services Substance Abuse and Mental Health Services Administration.

Kathryn H. Hollen

See also Addiction; Cancer; Comprehensive Smoking Education Act; Smoking.

References

Federal Trade Commission. "FTC Releases Reports on Cigarettes and Smokeless Tobacco" (April 26, 2007), www.ftc.gov/opa/2007/04/cigaretterpt.shtm.

U.S. Department of Health and Human Services. *Nicotine Addiction: A Report of the Surgeon General.* Centers for Disease Control and Prevention, Public Health Service, Center for Health Promotion and Education, Office on Smoking and Health, Atlanta, GA, 1988.

U.S. Department of Health and Human Services. *Results from the 2006 National Survey on Drug Use and Health: National Findings.* Substance Abuse and Mental Health Services Administration, Office of Applied Studies. DHHS Publication No. SMA 07-4293, Rockville, MD, 2007.

U.S. Department of Health and Human Services, Centers for Disease Control and Prevention. "Smoking and Tobacco Use" (November 2007), www.cdc.gov/tobacco.

U.S. Department of Health and Human Services, National Cancer Institute "Smoking" (December 2007), www.cancer.gov/cancertopics/tobacco.

U.S. Department of Health and Human Services, National Institute on Drug Abuse. *Research Report Series: Tobacco Addiction.* NIH Publication No. 06-4342, Bethesda, MD, July 2006.

COMMON COLD (UPPER RESPIRATORY VIRUSES)

According to the National Institute of Allergy and Infectious Diseases, as many as 1 billion upper respiratory infections may occur each year in the United States. More widely known as the common cold, these infections can be caused by more than 200 different viruses. The primary viruses responsible for the common cold are called rhinoviruses (from the Greek word *rhin,* for nose), which cause an estimated 25 to 35 percent of all colds. (Rhinoviruses may be the main cause of colds because they grow best at 91.4 degrees Fahrenheit or 33 degrees Celsius, which is the temperature of human nasal mucosa.) Other viruses that can cause colds include the myxoviruses (such as the influenza and parainfluenza viruses), coronaviruses, and adenoviruses. Bacterial agents cause approximately 10 percent of colds.

Viruses are transmitted or spread from person to person in several ways. Studies have shown that cold viruses reach their highest concentration in the nasal secretions three to four days after infection, which means this is when the infected person is most contagious and likely to pass on the virus. One common way of

Viruses and Bacteria

Because bacteria and viruses cause many familiar diseases, especially in the respiratory system, people often get them confused or think that they are the same type of microbes. In fact, viruses are as different from bacteria as plants are from animals.

Bacteria have a rigid cell wall and a rubbery cell membrane that surround the cytoplasm inside the cell. Within the cytoplasm is all the genetic information that a bacterium needs to grow and to duplicate or reproduce, such as deoxyribonucleic acid (DNA), ribonucleic acid (RNA), and ribosomes. A bacterium also has flagella so that it can move.

Despite the minute size of bacteria, viruses are much smaller. Viruses are surrounded by a spiky layer called the envelope and a protein coat. They also have a core of genetic material, either in the form of DNA or RNA. Unlike bacteria, viruses do not have all the materials needed to reproduce on their own. As a result, they invade cells, either by attaching to a cell and injecting their genes or by being enveloped by the cell. Once inside the cell, they harness the host cell's machinery to reproduce. Viruses eventually multiply and cause the cell to burst, releasing more of the virus to invade other cells.

catching a cold, or most viral or bacterial infections, is to touch almost anything that an infected person has also touched, sneezed on, or coughed on—from a doorknob to a telephone to their hands. (Some viruses, such as the human immunodeficiency virus, or HIV, cannot be caught in this manner.) After touching the surface, the virus can be transmitted to the body when the person then touches their nose or eyes, which have ducts that drain into the nasal cavity. Inhaling droplets in the air resulting from someone sneezing or coughing close to you is also a common way to catch a cold. Viruses cause colds when they penetrate the nasal mucosa, after which they enter cells lining the nasal region and the pharynx. Rhinoviruses, for example, bind to a molecule much like a docking system in a space station. Specifically, they contain depressions on their protein shell, sometimes referred to as canyons, that fit onto surface protein receptors on the nasal cells known as the intercellular adhesion molecules. This provides the portal for the virus to enter into the cell and begin replicating. It ultimately reproduces thousands of copies of itself, leading to cell disruption and release into the nose, where the infection is further spread to nearby nasal epithelial cells.

U.S. consumers spend billions of dollars every year on cold remedies, and while many people swear by their choices, they may or may not actually shorten the duration of the cold. However, doctors all agree that antibiotics have no effect on the common cold. The reason is simple: colds are viruses; they are not influenced by antibiotics, which attack only bacteria, and bacteria are very infrequently involved with respiratory infections. A very common misconception about colds is if nasal

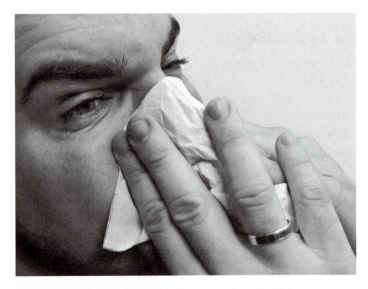

Studies have shown that cold viruses reach their highest concentration in the nasal secretions three to four days after infection. (Agnieszka Guzowska/Dreamstime.com)

discharge is green in color, it is a sign of a bacterial infection and a sign that antibiotics are needed. According to doctors, nasal secretion color is not indicative of any particular kind of illness or of bacterial infection. Of course, if the cold eventually leads to a secondary bacterial infection, antibiotics may be needed. Cold sufferers who suspect a secondary infection should visit their primary care physician for a diagnosis.

What are the most common cold remedies? Vitamin C, echinacea, and zinc supplements have become popular in recent years, but researchers say any benefit in curing a common cold is minimal at best. Over-the-counter cold medicines with several ingredients such as acetaminophen, a decongestant, or antihistamine may also have minor benefits and they do relieve some symptoms. Still, doctors caution that with the multiple ingredients it is important to read labels carefully to avoid problems. Homeopathic remedies are gaining in popularity, but researchers say there is not enough evidence to determine whether these therapies work. It may be that the timeless advice of drinking lots of fluids and eating chicken soup is still the best medicine for the common cold.

David Petechuk

References

Ackeman, Jennifer. *Ah-choo!: The Uncommon Life of Your Common Cold.* New York: Twelve, 2010.

Alderman, Lesley. "Money Tips for When the Sniffles Start." *New York Times* (January 2, 2010), www.nytimes.com/2010/02/health/02patient.html.

Janse, Allison. *The Germ Freak's Guide to Outwitting Colds and Flu: Guerilla Tactics to Keep Yourself Healthy at Home, at Work, and in the World*. Deerfield Beach, FL: Health Communications, 2005.

Petechuk, David. *The Respiratory System*. Westport, CT: Greenwood, 2004.

Sahelian, Ray. *The Common Cold Cure: Natural Remedies for Colds and Flu*. Garden City Park, NY: Avery, 1999.

COMPREHENSIVE SMOKING EDUCATION ACT

In October 1984, an act "to establish a national program to increase the availability of information on the health consequences of smoking, to amend the Federal Cigarette Labeling and Advertising Act, to change the label requirements for cigarettes, and for other purposes" (Public Law, 1984) was enacted by the joint houses of the U.S. Congress. Known as the Comprehensive Smoking Education Act of 1984, this relatively short piece of legislation of a mere five and a half pages was part of a continuing attempt to make health information on smoking and nicotine available to the U.S. public, so that they might make better decisions about the consequences of smoking on their health.

This act stipulated a number of factors, including items that are familiar to nearly every person living in the United States For example, the "SURGEON GENERAL'S WARNING" was mandated to appear on all cigarette packaging and advertisements (Hanson, Venturelli, & Fleckenstein, 2006). A list of cigarette ingredients was also duly provided to the Secretary of Health and Human Services by the manufacturers, so no "secret" ingredients were allowed in cigarettes after this act was passed (Cummings, 2002).

Smoking, or the inhalation of smoke from burnt tobacco leaves, allows for the reinforcing activity of nicotine. Nicotine is the psychoactive drug in tobacco, and most smokers use tobacco on a regular basis because they feel the need or craving for nicotine (American Society of Addiction Medicine [ASAM], 2010). Nicotine produces "an intense effect on the central nervous system . . . [and] activates the brain circuitry in regions responsible for regulating feelings of pleasure" (Hanson et al., 2006). This liquid alkaloid increases the release of dopamine, an internal, chemical brain transmitter, located in the brain's reward center. So nicotine is a substance that contributes greatly to the abuse and addiction potential of smoking.

Smokers often and habitually seek out their preferred method of nicotine delivery: many of these individuals are "characterized by compulsive drug seeking and abuse, even in the face of negative health consequences" (National Institute on Drug Abuse [NIDA], 2009). As seen by the numerous research studies, articles, public service announcements, and federal and local laws that have been published over the past several decades, the medical facts about smoking have been made clear. Almost 35 million smokers in the United States wish to stop smoking each year but relapse because of the addictive quality of nicotine (NIDA, 2009).

Another clear statement comes from a report from the American Academy of Pediatrics: "The use of tobacco, in any form, can lead to addiction, significant morbidity, and premature death. . . . There is no safe method, level, frequency, or duration of tobacco use or exposure" (Sims, 2009). (Smokeless tobacco use—including smokeless chewing tobacco and snuff—is also widespread, especially among younger users today [ASAM, 2010].)

But why was such an act of Congress necessary? To understand that, we need to look more closely at the history of the health risks of smoking during the time before its negative effects were well known.

From the earliest days of the American colonies in the 1700s, tobacco was a cash crop for large parts of the southern region of the country. Growing and exporting tobacco was economically beneficial for the region (Cummings, 2002). By the late 1800s, tobacco use was widespread. Up until that time, most people used pipes, cigars, chewing tobacco, or snuff. This radically changed with the development of the automated cigarette rolling machine in 1883 (Hanson et al., 2006). The machine made the cost per cigarette affordable to the average American. Cigarettes later gained prominence during World War I, when soldiers received them in their military-issued K rations. Cigarettes eventually replaced pipes, cigars, and chewing tobacco as a primary source of tobacco and nicotine (Hanson et al., 2006).

At the beginning of the 1900s, antismoking sentiment came primarily from moral and religious beliefs, but medical objections were beginning to be raised as well. By the end of World War I, various groups had joined forces to stop the sale of both tobacco and alcohol during what is known as the Prohibition era. "However, the negative backlash against the federal prohibition on alcohol coupled with the more pragmatic approach of allowing governments to tax tobacco as a way of controlling its use resulted in the rescinding of most state and local prohibitions against tobacco" (Hanson et al., 2006).

Throughout the 1920s and 1930s, negative medical and scientific data were increasingly seen in Germany. There was a high-profile campaign to limit and tax smoking and cigarettes in Germany through the 1940s. This included the implementation of a strong public education program. However, the scientific and medical evidence from Germany was largely ignored by the U.S. and British scientific communities until the 1950s and 1960s (Hanson et al., 2006).

In January 1964, the first report of the United States Surgeon General's Advisory Committee on Smoking and Health was released. The U.S. government's action "emphasized the need for smokers to make decisions about their habit on the basis of 'informed choice'" (Bailey, 2004). According to that report (Centers for Disease Control and Prevention [CDC], 2009), the Advisory Committee concluded that cigarette smoking is:

- A cause of lung cancer and laryngeal cancer in men
- A probable cause of lung cancer in women
- The most important cause of chronic bronchitis

As a result of this report's publication, cigarette sales fell substantially. The *New York Times* reported an 18 percent decline in the state of New York's cigarette tax revenue for February 1964 compared to the year before (Bailey, 2004).

This report was the first in a number of attempts "to diminish the impact of tobacco use on the health of the American people" (CDC, 2009). Subsequent reports and studies prompted Congress to adopt the Federal Cigarette Labeling and Advertising Act of 1965 and the Public Health Cigarette Smoking Act of 1969. These laws required the following (CDC, 2009):

- A health warning on cigarette packages
- A ban on cigarette advertising in the broadcast media
- A call for an annual report on the health consequences of smoking

The Public Health Cigarette Smoking Act of 1970 was another attempt by the U.S. government to provide information to the general public (Bailey, 2004). This act prohibited cigarette advertising from appearing in the broadcast media after January 1971. The ban was put in place to counteract ads that stated "the relative safety of smoking" and failed to mention various health risks and hazards (Bailey, 2004).

The 1970 act was eventually strengthened by the Comprehensive Smoking Education Act of 1984, which was an attempt to establish an overarching federal response to the issue of cigarette labeling and advertising. This additional warning requirement counterbalanced the attractive and glamorous packaging and presentation that cigarette manufacturers tried to present (Kees, Burton, Andrews, & Kozup, 2006). Moreover, the 1984 act affected smokers, smoking, and even general tobacco use by discouraging consumers with brief, clear, unambiguous information and specific warnings about health hazards (Cummings, 2002).

An overwhelming amount of information on the negative aspects of smoking and wider tobacco use is now available for consumers as well as a number of options for those who wish to stop smoking.

Nicotine addiction remains one of the more difficult addictions to overcome. However, if a smoker really decides to quit, there are possible choices. Nicotine gum and nicotine patches have both been used with some degree of success. Other effective treatments include cognitive-behavioral interventions coupled with changing the smoker's thinking, expectations, and behavior related to their smoking behavior. Support groups are available, as are self-help materials. In addition, research shows that the more individual therapy is tailored to a person's unique situation, the more likely it is that the individual will have success at quitting (NIDA, 2009).

Additional resources can be found in the recovery movement. Alcoholics Anonymous and Narcotics Anonymous are both 12-step programs. The 12 steps address nicotine addiction in much the same way they address drug and alcohol addiction and have been successful for some individuals who wish to stop smoking.

The U.S. Department of Health and Human Services (HHS) has established a national toll-free number, 800-QUIT-NOW (800-784-8669), for smokers seeking information and assistance in quitting. Callers to this number are routed to their state's smoking cessation quit line or, in states that have not established quit lines, to an assistance desk maintained by the National Cancer Institute.

HHS also offers a website—www.smokefree.gov—with online advice and downloadable information to make stopping smoking easier.

The American Lung Association has a website: www.lungusa.org/stop-smoking. This organization works to help people quit smoking and improve lung health throughout the United States.

The American Cancer Society has several helpful web pages, including: www.cancer.org/Healthy/StayAwayfromTobacco/GuidetoQuittingSmoking/index and www.cancer.org/Cancer/CancerCauses/TobaccoCancer/Questionsabout SmokingTobaccoandHealth/index.

Elizabeth Jones

See also Addiction; Cancer; Cigarettes; Secondhand Smoke; Smoking.

References

American Society of Addiction Medicine. *Public Policy Statement on Nicotine Dependence and Tobacco.* Chevy Chase, MD: ASAM, 2010.

Bailey, C.J. "From 'Informed Choice' to 'Social Hygiene': Government Control of Cigarette Smoking in the US." *Journal of American Studies* 38, no. 1 (2004): 41–65.

Centers for Disease Control and Prevention. "History of the Surgeon General's Reports on Smoking and Health," Office on Smoking and Health, National Center for Chronic Disease Prevention and Health Promotion (July 6, 2009), www.cdc.gov/tobacco/data_statistics/sgr/history/index.htm.

Cummings, K.M. "Programs and Policies to Discourage the Use of Tobacco Products." *Oncogene* 21 (2002): 7349–64.

Hanson, G.R., P.J. Venturelli, and A.E. Fleckenstein. *Drugs and Society,* 9th ed. Sudbury, MA: Jones and Bartlett, 2006.

Kees, J., S. Burton, J.C. Andrews, and J. Kozup. "Tests of Graphic Visuals and Cigarette Package Warning Combinations: Implications for the Framework Convention on Tobacco Control." *Journal of Public Policy and Marketing* 25, no. 2 (Fall 2006): 212–23.

National Institute on Drug Abuse. "Tobacco Addiction." NIDA Research Report Series (June 2009). National Institutes of Health, U.S. Department of Health and Human Services.

Public Law 98-474-Oct.12, 1984 Comprehensive Smoking Education Act (October 12, 1984), www2.tobaccodocuments.org/ti/TIMN0050203-0206.html.

Sims, TH, MD, MS and the Committee on Substance Abuse. "Technical Report—Tobacco as a Substance of Abuse." *Pediatrics* 124, no. 5 (November 2009).

D

DAILY VALUE OF NUTRIENTS

Americans are greeted in grocery stores with a huge selection of items to purchase, and on the packaged items they now find detailed information known as the Nutrition Facts Label. The label, required by law, can vary with each product, but it must contain some specific information, including the daily value (DV) of nutrients, which covers the important nutrients in that particular food such as the fats, sodium, and fiber content. What can be misleading for consumers is the Percent Daily Values (% DV) also listed on the food labels. The % DV is simply a percentage corresponding to the total daily value of nutrients government-recommended requirement, based on a hypothetical 2,000-calorie diet.

In other words, the label lists the DV so consumers can see how much of a certain nutrient they need to eat. The % DV listed on the label lets them know how much of each nutrient is contained in one serving of the food and how that compares to what they should be eating daily of that nutrient. If a serving has 5 percent or less of the daily value, it is thought to be on the low side. If the label indicates the food has 20 percent of the daily value in just one serving, that food is considered to have a high percentage of the needed nutrient.

The DV of each nutrient is based on daily reference values and the reference daily intake (RDI). The RDI, renamed from the recommended daily allowance, established recommended levels for vitamins and minerals. The daily reference values set the rates for other nutrients that have an important impact on health, including fat, saturated fat, sodium, cholesterol, and so forth.

The DV for total fat consumption is 65 grams, saturated fat is 20 grams, and there is no DV for trans fats, although health experts recommend consumers eat as little as possible to avoid health risks associated with them. There is no DV for sugar as well. The DV for cholesterol is 300 milligrams, and the total carbohydrate DV is 300 grams. There is a DV for fiber of 25 grams, sodium is 2,400 milligrams, and potassium is 3,500 milligrams. The DV for protein depends on individual characteristics such as age and if the individual is pregnant or nursing.

The DV for vitamin A is 5,000 IU (international units), vitamin C is 60 milligrams, vitamin D is 400 IU, vitamin E is 30 IU, thiamin's DV is 1.5 milligrams, and riboflavin is 1.7 milligrams. The DV for other vitamins and minerals are 20 milligrams for niacin, 2 milligrams for vitamin B6, 6 micrograms for vitamin B12, 18 milligrams for iron, 15 milligrams for zinc, and 1,000 milligrams for calcium. The DV for phosphorus is also 1,000 milligrams, 10 milligrams for pantothenic acid, 150 micrograms for iodine, and 400 milligrams for magnesium.

Sharon Zoumbaris

See also Dietary Reference Intakes; Nutrition Facts Label; Trans Fats.

References

Anderson, Jean, and Barbara Deskins. *The Nutrition Bible: A Comprehensive, No-Nonsense Guide to Foods, Nutrients, Additives, Preservatives, Pollutants and Everything Else We Eat and Drink.* New York: Morrow, 1995.

Taub-Dix, Bonnie. *Read It before You Eat It: How to Decode Food Labels and Make the Healthiest Choice Every Time.* New York: Penguin Group, 2010.

U.S. Department of Health and Human Services. "Calculate the Percent Daily Value for Appropriate Nutrients." U.S. Food and Drug Administration (May 23, 2011), www.fda.gov.

Zeratsky, Katherine. "What Does Percent Daily Value Mean on Food Labels?" Mayo Clinic (November 5, 2010), www.mayoclinic.com/health/food-and-nutrition/AN00284.

DANCE THERAPY

Dance is more than a creative expression of telling stories through movement of the body to music; it can also be therapeutic and can shape the quality of a person's health. Dance can be aerobic, and based on some extremely vigorous styles of dance, it can be anaerobic. In addition to its benefits as a moderate to intense physical activity, when done slowly dance can also provide benefits similar to the ancient form of movement called tai chi. Those measured and purposeful movements can be meditative and beneficial for an individual's mental health. For cancer patients, specifically women with breast cancer, dance therapy is said to reduce pain and discomfort in the underarm region and help women experience improved range of motion during and after treatment. Increasingly, the medical community is learning what the holistic health community has known for a long time: dance can be healing.

The use of dance as therapy dates back to the 1940s. The woman who sat at the precipice of the movement was Marian Chace. Participants in her dance classes demonstrated measurable improvements to their mental health. Chace's approach was especially useful for patients who had trouble verbalizing their feelings. Dance and movement approaches were found to provide the nonverbal therapy needed for certain types of clients to express themselves (National Coalition of Creative Arts Therapies [NCCATA], 2011).

Chace's success with her dance students was noticed by the psychiatrists who worked with these dance class participants. They reached out to Chace, who began working at St. Elizabeth's Hospital in Washington, D.C. At the same time on the West Coast, Trudi Schoop, a dancer and mime, began working with patients in a California hospital. This was when the concept of dance as therapy really began to take shape, and by the 1970s and 1980s, dance therapy had officially become recognized as a therapeutic approach (American Cancer Society, 2011).

According to the American Dance Therapy Association (ADTA), dance therapy, also known as dance movement therapy, is "the psychotherapeutic use of movement to promote emotional, social, cognitive and physical integration of the individual" (ADTA, 2009). Established in 1966, the ADTA has grown from 73 members in 15 states to almost 1,200 members in 46 states and more than a dozen countries. The group keeps a registry of dance therapy providers or Dance Therapist Registered (DTR), who are qualified to help people through this healing art form. Those with extended clinical practice time and experience are given the title of Academy of Dance Therapists Registered (ADTR). These practitioners are often dancers with an added layer of expertise.

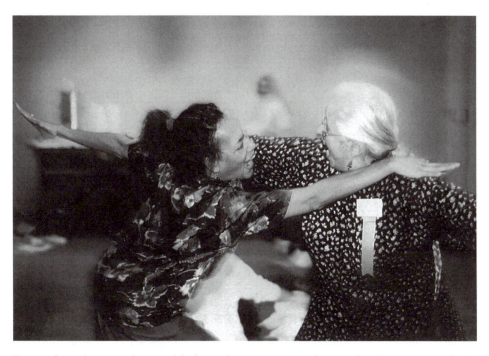

Dance therapists experiment with dynamic movement as they work with patients to find a healthy balance physically and emotionally. (American Dance Therapy Association)

Dance therapists are trained in dance movement therapy or psychotherapy, which requires a master's degree. Beginning-level therapists (DTRs) may begin practicing with at least 700 hours of supervised, clinical experience. More advanced dance therapists (ADTRs) have logged more than 3,000 hours. Once established as an ADTR, dance therapists may go into private practice and even teach others entering into the profession (ADTA, 2009). These practitioners may also work in institutional settings.

The ADTA has established a code of ethics for its therapists to follow as well as a way to evaluate the effectiveness and ability of dance therapy programs to meet the organization's guidelines. These codes inform practitioners of the standards and rules for professional behavior and for protecting clients. For research and scholarly works in the area of dance movement therapy, the *American Journal of Dance Therapy* is the preeminent publication on the subject (ADTA, 2009). The journal reports on the latest study findings and best practices in the clinical realm. Studies discussed in the journal examine dance therapy among different populations, including prisons, homeless shelters, substance abuse centers, and people with chronic illnesses.

Dance therapy sessions include a variety of techniques that take into consideration an individual's needs and level of dance ability. Emphasis is placed on the formation of relationships between instructors and patients by use of nonverbal communication and movement interactions. The dance relationship grows, starting with a range of subtle movements up through improvisational dancing (American Cancer Society, 2011).

The array of different techniques available allow participants at various skill levels to experience what is called the healing relationship between the mind and the body through dance and movement. There may or may not be talking during a session. Therapists may offer couples, family, and group sessions. The therapists also lead the classes and help their clients create goals and develop treatment plans. They document these plans and often collaborate with professionals from other disciplines to help provide counsel (ADTA, 2009).

The main facets of dance therapy are described as the joining of the mind, body and soul; controlling the body's response to stress through activities such as relaxation and breath work, touch and body empathy; developing physical and emotional techniques for coping with stressors; and promoting emotional wellness (Goodill, 2005). Other conditions for which dance therapy is useful include developmental conditions such as autism, learning disabilities, mental and emotional trauma, and impaired hearing and sight.

Dance therapy is considered beneficial for older adults and pregnant women. As with recreational dance, there is value in combining dance therapy movement with music. One study suggests that depressed teen girls experienced lower levels of the hormone cortisol in their blood when they listened to music (Goodill, 2005). Cortisol is a hormone released in the body during moments of stress. In addition to relaxation, the use of energy is also integrated into dance therapy. These activities have been shown to improve immune response and reduce sensitivity to certain allergens, respectively (Goodill, 2005).

An emerging area of specialization for the use of dance therapy is in disease prevention and health promotion. Some of these innovative programs provide dance therapy to those with cardiovascular disease, hypertension, and chronic pain (NCCATA, 2011). According to information provided by the American Cancer Society, a small number of studies have been conducted to examine the effectiveness of dance therapy in improving health. A few of these publications have reported some success in helping patients following breast cancer treatment. A recent trial called for breast cancer survivors to take a 12-week dance therapy and movement class. The class participants showed an improvement in the range of motion in their limbs, more so than the group who did not participate in the class. The patients also had an improved image of their bodies, something that can suffer when a patient has one or more breasts removed due to cancer (American Cancer Society, 2011).

The benefits of dance and movement can sometimes mimic the benefits of exercise, which is known to increase brain chemicals known as endorphins. These heighten feelings of happiness and welfare. In addition, dance and movement are thought to boost other body processes involving circulation, respiration, and musculoskeletal functions.

However, patients with chronic conditions such as arthritis and heart disease should talk with their physician before taking on a regimen that involves dance therapy or any other type of exercise. The American Cancer Society also cautions against relying on these types of therapies alone without seeking traditional medical care for cancer. Further study with well-controlled protocols are needed to confirm the true benefits of dance therapy in the healing of certain illnesses, including cancer (American Cancer Society, 2011).

There are many supporters of dance therapy, according to the ADTA. Several arms of the U.S. government recognize the benefits of dance therapy, including the Healthcare Financing Administration (HCFA), which is part of the Department of Health and Human Services (HHS). HCFA offers some coverage for dance therapy in Medicare facilities. The Administration on Aging, also under the HHS, recognizes research findings that suggest dance or movement therapy improves functions such as balancing, detecting changes in rhythmic patterns, increasing social interaction, and having an improved mood in people with neurological injury. In the early 1990s, dance therapy was represented in the Older American Act Reauthorization Amendments. The office of alternative medicine at the National Institutes of Health was among the first groups to receive funding to study the effects of dance therapy on various illnesses.

How does an individual become a certified dance movement therapist? The ADTA has six approved graduate programs across the country: Antioch New England Graduate School (New Hampshire); Columbia College (Chicago); Drexel University (Philadelphia); Lesley University (Cambridge, Massachusetts); Naropa University (Boulder, Colorado); and Pratt Institute (Brooklyn, New York). Other approved programs can be found on the ADTA website. It can take up to three years to complete the required academic coursework to become a dance therapist. Internships, which provide the necessary hours of clinical training and practice, can vary. Board certification is available after a significant number of years of experience.

To prepare for a career in the field, individuals should receive a broad dance education including instruction in modern, ethnic, folk, and social dance styles. Successful applicants enrolled in dance therapy education programs should learn how to choreograph, perform, and teach. An understanding of physiology and psychology is also recommended as well as volunteer experience (ADTA, 2009).

For those with a love of dance, work as a dance therapist offers the opportunity to use that passion to help others. Practitioners maintain their dance skills and ability to express emotions and tell stories through movement. The dance therapist also spends time verbally teaching and explaining the craft and its benefits, acting as an advocate for the field in professional circles as well as a teacher to clients and their families. More information about dance therapy can be found on the ADTA website (www.adta.org). Those interested can follow the group on Facebook, the social networking website. Information about dance therapy resources is listed by state. Some states may have local chapters with members devoted to the field. There are also online forums where experts and students of dance discuss questions and share advice. Each year, the ADTA hosts devotees at a national conference held in different locations. The conference is a great way to become familiar with dance therapy and network with experts in the field.

Abena Foreman-Trice

See also Cancer; Exercise; U.S. Department of Health and Human Services (HHS).

References

American Dance Therapy Association. *Healing Through Movement* (2009), www.adta.org/.

American Cancer Society. *Dance Therapy* (2011), www.cancer.org/Treatment/Treatmentsand SideEffects/ComplementaryandAlternativeMedicine/MindBodyandSpirit/dance-therapy.

Burroughs, Hugh, and Mark Kastner. *Alternative Healing: The Complete A–Z Guide to Over 160 Different Alternative Therapies.* La Mesa, CA: Halcyon, 1993.

Chodorow, Joan. *Dance Therapy and Depth Psychology: The Moving Imagination.* London and New York: Routledge, 1991.

Field, Shelly. *Career Opportunities in Health Care.* New York: Checkmarks Books, 2007.

Goodill, Sherry. *An Introduction to Medical Dance/Movement Therapy Health Care in Motion.* Philadelphia, PA: Jessica Kingsley, 2005.

Halprin, Anna, and Rachel Kaplan. *Moving Toward Life: Five Decades of Transformational Dance.* Hanover, NH: Wesleyan University Press, 1995.

Hanna, Judith Lynne. *Dancing for Health: Conquering and Preventing Stress.* Lanham, MD: AltaMira Press, 2006.

National Coalition of Creative Arts Therapies. "Dance Movement Therapy" (2011), www.nccata.org/dance_therapy.htm.

Schoop, Trudi. "Motion and Emotion." *American Journal of Dance Therapy* 22, no. 2 (Fall/Winter 2000): 91–101.

DENTAL HEALTH

The term *oral* refers to the mouth. Not merely comprised of the teeth and the gums, the mouth also includes the hard and soft palate, the mucous lining of the mouth and throat, the tongue, the lips, the salivary glands, the chewing muscles, and the upper and lower jaws. Furthermore, these are all set within a series of skull and face components referred to as craniofacial structures.

As one may guess given the complexity of the system, oral health means much more than healthy teeth. It means being free of all oral-facial diseases, lesions, cancers, defects, and pain. As the Surgeon General emphasized in his seminal report *Oral Health in America* in 2000, the mouth and all of its associated parts "represent the very essence of our humanity" (U.S. Department of Health and Human Services, 2000, p. 1). "They allow us to speak and smile; sigh and kiss; taste, chew, and swallow; cry out in passion and convey a world of feelings and emotions through facial expressions" (U.S. Department of Health and Human Services, 2000, p. 1).

Furthermore, it is often said the mouth is a mirror. Examining oral tissues can reveal a wealth of information about the rest of the body. A thorough oral assessment can detect signs of nutritional deficiencies and systemic diseases such as microbial infections, immune disorders, and some cancers. Beyond simply indicating the presence of other conditions, though, poor oral health has been linked to heart and lung disease, stroke, diabetes, and premature births. As is apparent, oral health, reaching far beyond healthy teeth, plays a major role in and is inextricably linked to overall health and general well-being.

Consequences of Poor Dental Health   Again, "the health of the mouth and surrounding tissues affects us physically, emotionally, mentally and socially and is integral to overall health status" (U.S. Bureau of Health Professions, 2004, p. 5). The effects of poor oral health are systemic, so far reaching that they impact fundamental elements of a person's identity such as the foods they choose, how they look, and how they communicate. Left untreated, simple dental caries can result in cavities, pain, infection, diminished quality of life, missed school and work days, the delivery of low-weight, preterm babies, aggravated respiratory diseases, increased prevalence of heart disease, heart attacks, and strokes and sometimes even death, as was the case for 12-year-old Deamonte Driver from Prince George's County, Maryland, in February 2007. Deamonte had an infection in an abscessed tooth, which, left untreated, spread to his brain, causing his death. Furthermore, poor oral health is a cycle: "poor oral health begins with children suffering in pain and ultimately developing low self-esteem due to an unattractive appearance and problems with speech that persist into adulthood. These adults may have difficulty securing well-paid jobs and most likely will not be able to access and value oral health care throughout life for themselves or their children" (American Dental Hygienists' Association, 2004).

Diseases of the Mouth   Poor oral health can lead to numerous diseases in the mouth. Oral diseases are progressive and cumulative and become more complex over time. The two leading dental diseases are dental caries, also known as tooth decay, and periodontal or gum diseases such as gingivitis and periodontitis.

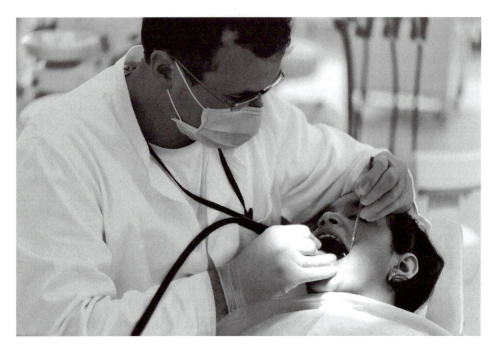

Good oral hygiene practices should start at an early age. Children should be introduced to dental exams through regular check-ups. (Zurijeta/Dreamstime.com)

Other major diseases include oral and pharyngeal cancer—cancer of the lip, tongue, pharynx, and mouth.

Dental Caries Dental caries is a type of bacterial infection. Colonies of bacteria, commonly referred to as dental plaque, adhere to the surface of teeth. These bacteria produce acids, which in turn dissolve minerals in the tooth enamel and form opaque white or brown spots under the enamel. These spots are called caries or cavities. If the caries go unchecked, the infection can extend through the entire tooth (dentin and pulp tissue). Such a cavity typically results in a severe toothache often accompanied by sensitivity to temperature and sweets. If treatment is still not obtained, the infection can lead to the formation of an abscess (a localized collection of pus often surrounded by inflammation) and the destruction of bone and can spread via the bloodstream.

Dental caries can occur at any age after teeth erupt. Early in development, primary teeth are vulnerable to a particularly damaging type of caries called early childhood caries. These often appear in children who are given bottles of juice, milk, or formula to drink during the day or overnight. Other risk factors for early childhood caries include arrested development of tooth enamel, altered salivary composition, mouth breathing, and blockage of saliva flow (U.S. Department of Health and Human Services, 2000, p. 38).

Periodontal Diseases Like dental caries, periodontal diseases are infections caused by the bacteria of dental plaque. There are two main classifications of periodontal disease: gingivitis and periodontitis. Gingivitis affects the gums, whereas periodontitis may involve both the soft tissue and bone of the mouth. Gingivitis and milder forms of periodontitis are common in adults. Moderate to severe periodontitis, where the destruction of tissue causes teeth to fall out, becomes more common with increasing age. More specifically, gingivitis is an inflammation of the gums. The gums typically become red, sensitive, and tender and may swell and bleed. These changes are due to the immune system's response to bacteria-containing dental plaque that accumulates along the edges of the gums. The early stages of gingivitis are reversible by brushing the teeth and flossing to reduce plaque. However, without adequate oral hygiene, early changes can become more severe as chronic infection takes hold. Such gum infections can persist for months or years. Gingival inflammation may be influenced by steroid hormones, which encourage the growth of certain bacteria and trigger an exaggerated response to plaque buildup (U.S. Department of Health and Human Services, 2000, p. 39). There are two common forms of adult periodontitis: general/moderately progressing and severe/rapidly progressing, the latter of which is often resistant to treatment. With moderately progressing periodontitis, the periodontal ligament gradually detaches from the gums and bone. Supportive bone structures of the jaw also begin to deteriorate. The destruction of periodontal ligament and bone results in the formation of a pocket between the tooth and the adjacent tissues, which harbors plaque beneath the gums. General periodontitis is often accompanied by gingivitis. It typically begins in adolescence but is not clinically significant until the mid-30s. Prevalence and severity increase, but do not accelerate, with age (U.S. Department of Health and Human Services, 2000, p. 40). Certain behavioral and demographic variables and comorbidities increase susceptibility to general periodontitis. One of the strongest behavioral associations is tobacco use. The risk of bone loss for heavy smokers is seven times greater than for those who have not smoked (U.S. Department of Health and Human Services, 2000, p. 41). Smoking also impairs the body's ability to neutralize infection, which results in the destruction of healthy tissues surrounding an infection site, and to combat the infection itself. Increased prevalence of periodontitis is also associated with increasing age, infrequent dental visits, low education level, and low income. Men often have higher levels of periodontitis than women. Some systemic diseases such as diabetes (Types 1 and 2) and osteoporosis also increase risk. Severe, rapidly progressing periodontitis is much less common than the mildly progressing form. Typically affecting people in their early 20s and 30s, it is characterized by severe inflammation of the gums and rapid loss of connective tissue and bone. Several systemic diseases have been associated with this form of periodontal disease, including type 1 diabetes, Down syndrome, and HIV infection (U.S. Department of Health and Human Services, 2000, p. 41).

Oral and Pharyngeal Cancer   Oral and pharyngeal cancer affects approximately 30,000 people annually and claims 8,000 lives in the same period. With only 52 percent of people diagnosed surviving five years, oral and pharyngeal cancer, has one of the worst five-year survival rates of any cancer. Moreover, men have twice the risk of women of being diagnosed with oral cancer and African American men suffer disproportionately. While oral cancer is the sixth leading cancer in U.S. men, it is the fourth leading cancer in African American men. Approximately 95 percent of cases of oral cancer occur in people over the age of 40, and the average age of diagnosis is 60. Oral cancer treatment—including surgery and radiation—can be painful, disfiguring, and costly, both monetarily and psychologically.

Tobacco and alcohol use are the major risk factors for oral and pharyngeal cancer. Risk increases with greater consumption. For instance, heavy drinkers who smoke more than one pack of cigarettes a day are 24 times more likely to develop oral cancer. Warning signs of oral cancer include a sore in the mouth that does not heal, a white or red patch on the gums, tongue, tonsil, or lining of the mouth, a lump or thickening in the cheek, and difficulty chewing and swallowing. Early detection of oral and pharyngeal cancers is critical and greatly increases survivals rates, but unfortunately only 35 percent of oral cancer is detected at its earliest stage (U.S. Department of Health and Human Services, 2000, p. 45).

Beyond the Mouth   Impacting more than simply the teeth and mouth, poor oral health has consequences throughout the body. Associations between chronic oral infections and diabetes, heart disease, stroke, and low-birth-weight, premature births have been noted.

Diabetes   There is an increased prevalence of gum disease among people with diabetes. This association between gum disease and diabetes is a two-way street. Diabetes increases the risk of serious gum disease, but serious gum disease also increases the risk of diabetes. This is because gum disease can impact blood glucose control, which can fuel the development of diabetes. On the other hand, individuals with diabetes have an increased risk for serious gum disease because they are generally more susceptible to bacterial infection and have a decreased ability to fight bacteria that invade the gums (diabetes.org). Furthermore, diabetes causes elevated levels of glucose in the blood. High blood glucose fosters the growth of the bacteria that form dental plaque. If diabetes patients have difficulty controlling their blood glucose levels and have levels that are consistently high, they develop periodontal disease more often and more severely (National Diabetes Information Clearinghouse, 2011).

Heart Disease   Connections between periodontal disease and heart disease have also been made. Researchers have found that people with gum diseases are almost twice as likely to suffer from coronary artery disease (American Academy of Periodontology, 2011). Several theories exist to explain this link. To begin, recall that periodontitis is the erosion of tissue and bone that support the teeth. It is posited that chewing and tooth brushing in people with periodontitis releases bacteria into the bloodstream. Some of these bacteria attach to fatty plaque in the arteries of the heart. This plaque, in turn, contributes to clot formation and the thickening of the walls of the arteries. Blood clots can obstruct normal blood flow, restricting the amount of nutrients and oxygen required for the heart to function properly (American Academy of Periodontology, 2011). This may lead to heart attack. It is also believed that oral bacteria could harm blood vessels or cause blood clots by releasing toxins that resemble components found in artery walls and the bloodstream. The immune system's response to these toxins could harm vessel walls or make blood clot more easily. Finally, inflammation in the mouth due to gingivitis may increase inflammation and swelling throughout the body, including in the arteries, where it can lead to heart attack and stroke (Harvard Medical School, 2007).

Pregnancy Oral health and pregnancy also have a reciprocal relationship. Pregnancy is associated with diet and hormonal changes that can increase the risk of tooth decay and gum disease. Vice versa, infections from tooth decay and gum disease can affect the health of a mother and her baby. More specifically, pregnant women are more susceptible to cavities. Vomiting caused by morning sickness can allow stomach acid to weaken a woman's tooth enamel. The loss of this protective covering increases the risk of cavities. Eating more frequently during pregnancy also increases the risk for cavities, especially if sugary or starchy foods are eaten. Finally, many pregnant women experience dry mouth. Having less saliva or spit again leaves the teeth vulnerable to the development of cavities (Columbia University College of Dental Medicine, 2010).

Pregnancy also heightens the risk of gingivitis. It can appear as early as the second month and tends to peak around the eighth month. This increased likelihood of gingivitis may be due to hormonal changes. During pregnancy, the level of progesterone (a hormone) in the body can be 10 times higher than normal. This can enhance the growth of bacteria that cause gingivitis. Also, pregnancy causes changes in the function of the immune system, which can impact how the body reacts to the bacteria responsible for gingivitis. Another common manifestation in pregnant women is pregnancy granulomas. These growths on the gum occur in approximately 2 percent to 10 percent of pregnant women. Typically developing in the second trimester, they are red nodules often found attached to the upper gum line by stalks of tissue. These growths bleed easily and can form an ulcer or crust over. While granulomas cause discomfort, they are not dangerous; they are essentially a type of benign (noncancerous) tumor. However, if one does interfere with the ability to eat or speak, it can be surgically removed, although there is the possibility it will grow back. Potential causes of granulomas include poor oral hygiene, trauma, hormones, viruses, and malformed blood vessels.

As previously mentioned, though, this relationship is two-way. If a woman has gum disease, germs from her mouth can spread throughout the body, which in turn can cause delivery of a preterm, low-birth-weight baby and can increase the risk for diabetes and high blood pressure during pregnancy. In addition, after the birth of the baby, germs that cause tooth decay can be passed from the mother to the baby's mouth through kissing, sharing utensils, or putting the baby's pacifier or hands in the mother's mouth (Iowa Department of Public Health, 2011).

Understanding Oral Health A confluence of health behaviors can contribute to oral infection and decay. These include poor dietary choices, tobacco use, and excessive alcohol use.

Poor Dietary Choices The adage "an apple a day keeps the doctor away" is applicable to the dentist as well. A nutritious diet helps to prevent tooth decay and other oral diseases. What an individual eats has a large impact on the health of his or her mouth. Starches and foods high in sugar greatly increase the likelihood of tooth decay. As previously mentioned, plaque bacteria in the mouth convert sugars and starches into waste in the form of acid. The longer the sugar and starch sit on the teeth (i.e., are not brushed off), the longer the bacteria produce the acid. The acid then erodes the enamel on the teeth and eventually causes tooth decay. Moreover, poor nutrition, by failing to supply the body with necessary nutrients, weakens the entire immune system and thereby leaves people at a higher risk for gum disease. With a suppressed immune system, gum disease can progress faster and become more severe. Adults should avoid snacks full of sugars and starches.

Tobacco Use   Smoking increases the risk of many oral diseases. Tobacco use in any form increases the risk of gum disease, oral, pharyngeal and throat cancers, and oral fungal infection. Chewing tobacco containing sugar increases the risk of tooth decay. Smokers are four times more likely than people who have never smoked to have gum disease. Researchers have been able to correlate level of smoking with likelihood of periodontitis. "Cigarette smokers who smoked less than half a pack per day were almost three times more likely than nonsmokers to have periodontitis. Those who smoked more than a pack and a half per day had almost six times the risk" (Health News, 2011, p. 9). Pipe and cigar smoking have an equally adverse effect on gum disease risk as cigarette smoking. Beyond periodontitis, smoking also increases the risk of bone loss and depresses healing and defense mechanisms by reducing the delivery of oxygen and nutrients to gingival tissue (Health News, 2011, p. 9). This means that smokers are more likely to lose teeth, not respond to treatment, and develop infections, such as periodontitis. Yet another risk of smoking is oral cancer. Approximately 90 percent of those diagnosed with any form of oral cancer are tobacco users. All forms of tobacco increase the risk of oral cancer. Those who smoke cigarettes, pipes, or cigars are six times more likely than nonsmokers to get oral cancer. Finally, in addition to seriously threatening oral and overall health, smoking also causes bad breath and stained teeth. Stopping the use of tobacco seems to gradually erase the harmful effects of tobacco on periodontal health.

Excessive Alcohol Use   Heavy use of alcohol can cause a host of oral health problems. Those who use alcohol in excess have a higher risk of periodontal disease and of tooth decay from the increased exposure to sugars and acids within drinks. Perhaps most threatening, though, is the greater incidence of oral and throat cancers among people who drink heavily. One study assessed the oral health of patients in a rehabilitation center for alcohol abuse. Patients were asked to describe their dental hygiene behaviors and general lifestyles. They also underwent oral health assessments that looked for the presence of plaque, missing teeth, and periodontal inflammation, among other symptoms of poor oral health. ("Alcohol Abuse, Higher Incidence," 2003) Upon assessment, it was discovered that 82 percent had moderate-to-severe gingival inflammation, and more than two-thirds had a heavy accumulation of dental plaque. Fifteen percent of the subjects had missing teeth, with 41 percent of the remaining teeth showing signs of enamel erosion. In addition, 79 percent of those studied had at least one carious tooth, with an average of 3.2 carious teeth per subject, while more than one-third had potentially precancerous oral lesions ("Alcohol Abuse, Higher Incidence,"

2003). The incidence rates of these conditions are all significantly higher than they are in the general population.

Social Determinants The social determinants of health are "the conditions in which people are born, grow, live, work and age, including the system. These circumstances are shaped by the distribution of money, power, and resources and they influence people's health" (World Health Organization, 2011). Several social determinants affect oral health. People with lower levels of education and income and people from specific racial/ethnic groups experience higher rates of disease. Other barriers limiting people from achieving good oral health include limited access to and availability of dental services, lack of awareness of the need for care, cost, and fear of dental procedures.

Dental History At the start of the 20th century, most Americans were likely to be toothless by the age of 45. This status quo no longer holds true. Most people now expect they will maintain their teeth over their lifetime and they take steps to do so. However, oral health conditions such as dental caries, periodontitis, and oral cancer are still very much real problems for many people in the United States.

Children Dental caries is the most common chronic childhood disease. It is five times more common than asthma and seven times more common than hay fever (Office of the Surgeon General, 2011). Over 50 percent of 5- to 9-year-olds have at least one cavity or filling, and that proportion increases to 78 percent of 17-year-olds. Children can also experience birth defects that impact the mouth, such as cleft lip/palate and hereditary ectodermal dysplasias, where all or most teeth are missing or misshapen. The social impact of oral disease in children is substantial. Nationally, "more than 51 million school hours are lost each year to dental related illnesses" (Office of the Surgeon General, 2011). Furthermore, if left untreated, children's dental problems can progress to unbearable levels. What "begins small, with plaque buildup a dental hygienist would attack with a stern lecture . . . swells to nasty abscesses and infections that threaten their whole bodies. They're in so much pain they have trouble concentrating in school, sleeping at night, eating, and speaking" (Auer, 2005).

Adults Most adults show signs of periodontal or gingival (gum) disease. Severe periodontal disease affects about 14 percent of adults aged 45 to 54 and 23 percent of adults aged 65 to 74. Many adults must deal with the common symptom of pain from their craniofacial disorders. According to the Surgeon General, 22 percent of adults reported some form of oral facial pain in the past six months. This pain is typically so severe that it interferes with vital functions such as eating, swallowing, and speech. Furthermore, employed adults lose more than 164 million hours of work each year due to dental disease. Many adults are also not taking the necessary steps to achieve good oral health. A little less than two-thirds of adults report having visited a dentist in the last 12 months. For elderly adults, many (approximately 5 percent of Americans aged 65 and older) live in long-term care facilities where obtaining dental care is problematic. Approximately 30 percent of adults aged 65 and older are edentulous, meaning they have no teeth. While this is an improvement from the 46 percent 20 years ago, it is still a significant portion of the population. As mentioned, approximately 30,000 Americans are diagnosed with oral and pharyngeal cancer each year, and they are primarily the elderly. Finally, most older Americans take both prescription and over-the-counter drugs. In all probability, at least one of the medications used will have an oral side effect such as dry mouth. The inhibition of salivary flow increases the risk for oral disease, because saliva contains antimicrobial components as well as minerals that can help rebuild tooth enamel after attack by acid-producing, decay-causing bacteria (Office of the Surgeon General, 2011).

Disparities In the last 50 years, vast improvement has been made in the understanding of common oral diseases such as tooth decay and gum diseases and in the nation's oral health. However, not all segments of the population have received the benefits of or have experienced these improvements equally. In 2000, the Surgeon General described it as "a silent epidemic of dental and oral diseases affecting some population groups—a burden of disease that restricts activities in school, work, and home, and often significantly diminishes quality of life" (U.S. Department of Health and Human Services, 2000, p. vii). The literature on dental health seems to unanimously agree that it is usually the poor, less educated, minorities, and rural residents who bear a disproportionate burden of oral diseases and have problems with access to dental care.

Socioeconomic status is a major determinant of oral health. Among both children and adults, the poor have less favorable oral health outcomes and are less likely to receive dental care and to have dental insurance. More specifically, poor children experience twice as many dental caries as their more affluent peers, and these caries are more likely to be untreated (Office of the Surgeon General, 2011). More than one-third (36.8 percent) of poor children aged two to nine have one or more untreated decayed primary teeth, compared to 17.3 percent of nonpoor children (U.S. Department of Health and Human Services, 2000, p. 63). This poor-affluent difference continues into adolescence. The social impact of untreated dental decay is immense. Poor children suffer nearly 12 times more restricted-activity school days than children from higher-income families. Furthermore, professional care is necessary for maintaining oral health, yet 25 percent of poor children have not seen a dentist before entering kindergarten. Beyond children, adults with income at or above the poverty level are twice as likely to report a dental visit in the past 12 months as those who are below the poverty line. Finally, a higher percentage of individuals living below the poverty level are edentulous than are those living above. Individuals with incomes equal to or above twice the poverty level have a rate of edentulism of 6.9 percent. This rate is less than half the rate for those with incomes below twice the poverty level (14.3 percent) (U.S. Department of Health and Human Services, 2000, p. 66).

Insurance is a strong predictor of access to dental care. Uninsured children are two and a half times less likely than insured children to receive dental care and thus are three times more likely to have dental needs. Currently, over 108 million children and adults lack dental insurance, which is more than double the number of people who lack medical insurance. Furthermore, public insurance (Medicaid) has not been able to fill the gap in providing dental care to poor children.

Less than one in five Medicaid-covered children received a single dental visit in a study completed around 2000. This is in part because many dentists refuse to accept Medicaid patients. Beyond children and adults, many elderly individuals lose their dental insurance when they retire. Although Medicaid will fund dental care for the low-income and disabled elderly in some states, the reimbursements are low such that few dentists accept it. Furthermore, Medicare does not reimburse for dental care at all.

People living in rural areas also typically have worse oral health outcomes. Every summer for the past 10 years, the Remote Area Medicine (RAM) Clinic has traveled to Wise County in southwest Virginia to conduct what is the largest free clinic in the Western Hemisphere. The people who attend the RAM Clinic will literally walk in from East Tennessee, Kentucky, and the surrounding counties in Virginia and will wait for hours overnight to receive treatment. During this three-day event, it is the dentists who see the most people. At the end of the weekend, over 4,000 teeth will have been extracted, all done in horse stalls and without the use of pain medication. A two-year-old whose teeth are abscessed and literally crumbling out of his head due to a loss of enamel (which in turn has made him unable to drink milk and thus has caused his calcium deficiency) will have all of his teeth removed. The lack of access to dental services in rural areas is a major contributing factor to the poor oral health in these regions. In large metropolitan areas, the dentist-to-population ratio was 61 per 100,000 as compared to 29 dentists per 100,000 in rural areas of the United States (American Dental Hygienists' Association, 2008).

Preventive Care   The irony of dental caries, periodontal disease, and oral cancer is that, while they are the most widespread and common oral diseases, they are also the most preventable. And it is prevention which is the most efficient and effective way to limit their prevalence. Poor dental health is expensive—biologically and monetarily. In 2000, the nation's dental bill was $60 billion, and this does not include indirect costs for corollary health issues or productivity lost (U.S. Department of Health and Human Services, 2000, p. 4). The Coalition on Oral Health has determined that "every dollar invested in preventative oral health care saves between $8 and $50 in restorative care" (Sharon, Connolly, & Murphee, 2005). There are numerous ways that people can achieve good oral health and prevent the development of dental caries, periodontal disease, and other oral maladies.

Fluoride   It was in the 1930s that researchers first discovered that people living in communities with naturally fluoridated water supplies had fewer dental caries. However, official investigations and clinical trials to confirm the connection between fluoride and decreased caries did not take place until after World War II. Once the link was scientifically founded, adjusting the fluoride content of community water supplies was pursued to prevent dental caries, becoming one of the largest and most successful public health initiatives in history. In the 1950s, dental caries began to decline among children who grew up in fluoridated cities, and by the 1970s declines in decay were present for many Americans across the country. Today, fluoridated water reaches approximately 144 million people in the United States, of which 10 million receive water that is fluoridated naturally (Centers for Disease Control and Prevention, 2011).

As mentioned, dental caries form when acid dissolves minerals in tooth enamel. Fluoride concentrated in plaque and saliva inhibits the demineralization of enamel and enhances the remineralization (in other words, recovery) of demineralized enamel. Remineralization increases tooth hardness and mineral content, rendering the tooth surface more resistant to subsequent acid attacks. Fluoride's protection against tooth decay works at all ages. It has been shown to decrease tooth decay by 18 to 40 percent. For most people, the low levels of fluoride found in water coupled with the use of a fluoride-containing toothpaste twice a day provides a sufficient dosage to protect their teeth. However, people at high risk for dental caries might require more frequent or more concentrated exposure to fluoride and might benefit from use of other fluoride products.

Some people are reticent to use fluoride because it can cause enamel fluorosis. Enamel fluorosis is when fluoride ingested during tooth development results in a range of, often noticeable, changes in enamel opacity. Concerns regarding the risk for enamel fluorosis are limited to children under the age of eight. Beyond this age, the enamel is no longer susceptible to this effect. The occurrence of enamel fluorosis is reported to be most strongly associated with cumulative fluoride intake during enamel development, but the severity of the condition depends on the dose, duration, and timing of fluoride intake. With that said, fluoride has proven itself invaluable to preventing and controlling dental caries, and most fluorosis today is of the mildest form, which affects neither cosmetic appearance nor dental function. Consequently, a low prevalence of the milder forms of enamel fluorosis has been accepted as a reasonable and minor consequence balanced against the substantial protection from dental caries drinking water containing fluoride provides (Centers for Disease Control and Prevention, 2011).

Following the success of water fluoridation, many other fluoride-containing products, such as toothpastes, mouth rinses, and dietary supplements, have been developed. In addition, processed beverages and even some food can contain small amounts of fluoride. Thus, U.S. residents have many more sources of fluoride available now than they did 50 years ago. Recognizing that it is now possible to receive enough fluoride with slightly lower levels of fluoride in water because of the existence of so many other fluoride-containing products, the U.S. Department of Health and Human Services (HHS) has recently proposed an adjustment to the ideal fluoride level in drinking water. In September 2010, the HHS convened a panel of scientists to review new information related to fluoride intake and to develop new recommendations. After reviewing information, including the prevalence and trends in dental caries and water intake in children, the HHS has suggested changing the recommended fluoride level for community water systems from a range of 0.7 to 1.2 milligrams per liter to 0.7 milligrams per liter (U.S. Department of Health and Human Services, 2011).

Tooth Brushing Thorough tooth brushing at least twice a day with a fluoride toothpaste is a simple, widely recommended method of maintaining good oral health. Brushing reduces bacteria-containing dental plaque, thus preventing tooth decay and gingivitis. The use of a fluoride toothpaste also helps to prevent cavities. There are several recommendations about appropriate brushing. To begin, the toothbrush should be rinsed in water after use to remove bacteria, saliva, and other particles from the mouth that collect on it. For the same reason, toothbrushes should not be covered for long periods of time, should not be shared between individuals, and should be replaced every three to four months. Finally, tooth brushing should begin as soon as a child's first tooth is erupted. At this point, rather than a brush, a cloth can be used. This can then be transitioned to a soft-bristle brush and then eventually a regular toothbrush (Centers for Disease Control and Prevention, 2011).

Dental Sealants   Dental sealants complement the use of fluoride in preventing dental caries. Dental sealants are thin plastic coatings that are applied to the grooves on the chewing surfaces of the back teeth to protect them from tooth decay. The films prevent decay from developing in the grooves, which are hard to reach with brushing and where fluoride may be less effective (U.S. Department of Health and Human Services, 2000, p. 38). Sealants tend to work most effectively on permanent molars, which come in at 6 years and 12 years of age. It is best if the sealant is applied soon after the teeth have erupted, before they have a chance to decay. They typically last 5 to 10 years and can be reapplied if they are no longer in place. Dental sealants have proven so effective that school-based dental sealant delivery programs have been designed to provide sealants to children unlikely to receive them otherwise (such as those who are low income). Findings from scientific studies clearly show that school dental sealant programs are working to stop tooth decay among children (Centers for Disease Control and Prevention, 2011).

Visits to the Dentist and Dental Hygienist   Having regular visits (typically every six months) to a dentist or dental hygienist is critical to maintaining good oral health. Check-ups can detect early signs of oral health problems and can lead to treatments that will prevent further damage—and, in some cases, reverse the problem. Also, professional tooth cleaning (prophylaxis) is important for preventing oral problems, especially when self-care is difficult. Unfortunately, in many regions of the country, there is a shortage of available dentists, especially for those who are low income and/or living in rural areas. Consequently, many states are attempting to increase the independence and expand the use of dental hygienists. Dental hygienists can provide the same prophylactic cleanings as a dentist, but typically for less money as their overhead costs are not as great.

Laura McLaughlin

See also Alcohol; Cancer; Diabetes; Heart Health; Immune System/Lymphatic System; Smoking.

References

"Alcohol Abuse, Higher Incidence of Oral Health Problems Linked." *Journal of the American Dental Association* 134 (2003): 554.

American Academy of Periodontology. "Gum Disease Links to Heart Disease and Stroke" (February 23, 2011), www.perio.org/consumer/mbc.heart.htm.

American Dental Hygienists' Association. "American Dental Hygienists' Association Adopts Official Policy to Address U.S. Oral Health Disparities," www.adha.org.

American Dental Hygienists' Association. "Competencies for the Advanced Dental Hygiene Practitioner (ADHP)" (2004).

American Diabetes Association. "Living with Diabetes" (2008), www.diabetes.org/living-with-diabetes/treatment-and-care/oral-health-and-hygiene/diabetes-and-oral.

Auer, Holly. "Dental Woes Threaten Kids' Health AH: Many Johns Island Children Seldom, If Ever, See a Dentist." *Post and Courier* (April 11, 2005).

Centers for Disease Control and Prevention. "Dental Fluorosis" (2011), www.cdc.gov/fluoridation/safety/dental_ fluorosis.htm.

Centers for Disease Control and Prevention. "Dental Sealants" (2011)www.cdc.gov/Oral Health/ publications/factsheets/sealants_faq.htm.

Centers for Disease Control and Prevention. "FAQs on Use and Handling of Toothbrushes" (2011), www.cdc.gov/OralHealth/infectioncontrol/factsheets/toothbrushes.

Centers for Disease Control and Prevention. "Recommendations for Using Fluoride to Prevent and Control Dental Caries in the United States" (2011), www.cdc.gov/mmwr/preview/ mmwrhtml/rr5014a1.

Columbia University College of Dental Medicine. "How Pregnancy Affects Your Oral Health" (June 28, 2010), www.simplestepsdental.com/SS/ihtSS/r.==/st.31848/t.35020/pr.3.

Harvard Medical School. "Heart Disease and Oral Health: Role of Oral Bacteria in Heart Plaque" (February 2007), www.health.harvard.edu/press_releases/heart-disease-oral-health.

Health News. "The Effects of Smoking on Oral Health" (2011), www.healthnews.com/dental-health/effects-smoking-oral-health-370.html.

Healthy People 2020. "2020 Topics and Objectives: Oral Health" (2011), www.healthypeople.gov /2020/topicsobjectives2020/overview.aspx?topicid=32.

Iowa Department of Public Health. "Oral Health and Pregnancy" (2011), www.idph.state.ia.us/ hpcdp/common/pdf/oral_health/ oral_health_pregnancy.pdf.

National Diabetes Information Clearinghouse. "Prevent Diabetes Problems: Keep Your Teeth and Gums Healthy" (2011), http://diabetes.niddk.nih.gov/dm/pubs/complications_teeth/index.

Office of the Surgeon General. "National Call to Action to Promote Oral Health" (2011), www.surgeongeneral.gov/topics/oralhealth/nationalcalltoaction.

Sharon, Stull, Irene Connolly, and Kellie Murphee. "A Review of the Literature: The Economic Impact of Preventative Dental Hygiene Services." *Journal of Dental Hygiene* (2005), http://goliath.ecnext.com/coms2/gi_0199-4753208/the-economic-impact-of-preventive.

U.S. Department of Health and Human Services. *Oral Health in America: A Report of the Surgeon General.* Rockville, MD: U.S. Department of Health and Human Services, 2000.

U.S. Department of Health and Human Services. *Proposed HHS Recommendation for Fluoride Concentration in Drinking Water for Prevention of Dental Caries.* Washington, DC: U.S. Government Printing Office, January 2011,www.hhs.gov/news/press/2011pres/01/pre_pub_frn_fluoride.html.

U.S. Bureau of Health Professions. "The Professional Practice Environment of Dental Hygienists in the Fifty States and the District of Columbia, 2001." U.S. Government Printing Office, 2004.

World Health Organization. "Social Determinants of Health" (2011), www.who.int/social_determinants/en/.

DEOXYRIBONUCLEIC ACID (DNA)

The benefits for mankind from the discovery of DNA and how it functions have fundamentally changed everything from modern medicine to our legal system. Scientists suggest that information now available through DNA will continue to shape and reshape people's lives in a myriad of ways thanks to improvements in genetic testing, paternity testing, analysis of crime evidence, medical diagnosis, and cloning. Other benefits and uses of DNA include improved testing and more precise dating of archeological discoveries, more specific health tests to determine cell mutations, and the ability to manipulate genes in plants to improve nutrition and drought resistance or other characteristics that will increase food yields. These life-changing discoveries can be traced back to the groundwork done by generations of scientists.

In 1953, U.S. biologist James D. Watson and British chemist Francis Crick discovered a chemical compound, deoxyribonucleic acid, or DNA. Like virtually all scientific breakthroughs, the discovery of DNA did not spring fully formed from Watson's and Crick's brains. It was the result of decades of research and theorizing about the nature of the genetic material.

DNA had been discovered as far back as 1869 by Swiss physician and biologist Johannes Friedrich Miescher, although he knew of no biological role for the compound (which he called nuclein). In fact, scientists knew very little about the structure or function of DNA for nearly seven decades after its discovery. For most of that time, biologists were convinced that unit factors (or genes) must consist of some kind of proteinlike material.

By the early 1950s, most of the clues needed for the deciphering of the DNA structure were in place. The key figures in the research were almost within shouting distance of each other: Watson and Crick at the Cavendish Laboratory at the University of Cambridge and Maurice Wilkins and Rosalind Franklin at King's College, London. While Watson and Crick were manipulating the information they had about DNA from Avery, Chagraff, and other

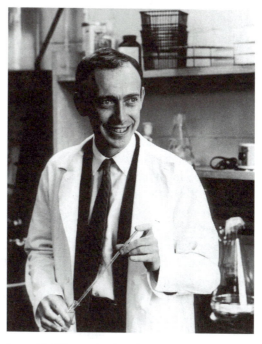

James D. Watson is a U.S. biochemist who shared the Nobel Prize for Physiology or Medicine in 1962 for the (1953) discovery of the molecular structure of deoxyribonucleic acid (DNA). (National Library of Medicine)

researchers, Wilkins and Franklin were taking X-ray photographs of the DNA molecules.

X-ray crystallography is a very powerful, but very difficult, technique for determining the structure of complex molecules by shining X-rays through them. The images obtained by this method are often very difficult to interpret and to translate into three-dimensional models of the molecules. By late 1952, Franklin had obtained extraordinary images of DNA molecules, which appeared to provide the final clue to the compound's structure. She hesitated in announcing her results, however, wanting to further confirm them.

Crick and Watson, who had seen her results, were not so shy. They realized that Franklin's images gave them the last bit of information they needed and, by March 7, 1953, had constructed their model of the DNA molecule. They reported the results of their research in a paper that appeared in the April 25, 1953, issue of the journal *Nature,* titled "A Structure for Deoxyribose Nucleic Acid." They began their paper with the comment: "We wish to suggest a structure for the salt of deoxyribose nucleic acid (D.N.A.). This structure has novel features which are of considerable biological interest" (Watson & Crick, 1953). Watson and Crick (with help from Franklin and others) had unraveled the structure of the DNA molecule. The gene had finally been given a clear and unequivocal chemical and physical structure.

DNA Structure   Watson and Crick discovered that a DNA molecule consists of two very long spaghettilike strands (the "backbone" of the molecule) made of alternating sugar (deoxyribose) and phosphate groups. These two strands are wrapped around each other, a bit like a circular staircase, in a geometric form known as a double helix. Attached to each sugar molecule is one of four nitrogen bases: adenine, cytosine, guanine, or thymine.

The combination of one sugar (deoxyribose) unit and one nitrogen base is called a *nucleoside;* the combination of a sugar, base, and phosphate group is known as a *nucleotide.* To a chemist, then, the long string that makes up a DNA backbone is a *polynucleotide,* many nucleotide units joined to each other. The two strands are then wrapped around each other in such a way that the nitrogen bases are inside the molecule, with complementary bases adjacent to each other.

At this point, a word needs to be said about DNA's perhaps somewhat less well-known cousin, RNA. The two families of compounds are similar in many ways, especially with regard to their importance in the transfer of genetic information from one generation to the next. But structurally, they differ in three important ways. First of all, the sugar in the backbone of an RNA molecule is ribose, not deoxyribose. Second, the four nitrogen bases in RNA are adenine, cytosine, guanine, and uracil, rather than thymine. Third, RNA is a single-stranded molecule and not a double-stranded helix, as in the case of DNA.

Molecular Genetics   The discovery of DNA structure made by Watson and Crick is sometimes cited as being one of the most important discoveries in the history of science. The reason for this accolade is that prior to the discovery, geneticists knew a great deal about the way genetic traits were transmitted from generation to generation. But they knew nothing at all as to how humans might manipulate that process at the most fundamental level—that of cells and molecules. Beyond trial-and-error hybridization experiments, genetic manipulation was essentially a mystery. After Watson and Crick, scientists realized that the genetic material consisted of molecules—molecules of DNA—that could (at least in theory) be synthesized, broken apart, and manipulated in essentially the same way as any other kind of chemical molecule. The opportunities for engineering genes and altering heredity seemed endless.

Before the "at least in theory" could become a practical reality, however, a great many technical problems for working with DNA molecules needed to be solved. Francis Crick was intimately involved in solving the first two of those problems, the mechanism by which genetic information is coded in a DNA molecule, and the process by which that information is used to synthesize proteins in a cell.

In a paper published in 1958, Crick stated two general principles about the function of DNA. The first, which he called the Sequence Hypothesis, says that the specificity of a piece of nucleic acid is expressed solely by the sequence of its bases, and that this sequence is a (simple) code for the amino acid sequence of a particular protein (Crick, 1958, p. 152).

In other words, the genetic information in a DNA molecule consists of some discrete set of nitrogen bases in the molecule. The sequence ATC might translate into one instruction, the sequence TTC into another instruction, the sequence CGC into yet another instruction, and so on. The most likely—but, again, not known—likelihood was that base sequences carry information about the synthesis of amino acids. Amino acids are the basic units from which proteins are made, and the primary function of DNA is to tell a cell how to make proteins.

At this point, Crick (and all other scientists) knew virtually nothing about the code itself, although one piece of information seemed to be obvious: the number of nitrogen bases needed for a specific instruction. Suppose a single nitrogen base codes (carries the information needed) for the synthesis of some specific amino acid—as, for example, adenine codes for the amino acid aspartic acid. But that code can't work because there are only four nitrogen bases and more than 20 amino acids needed for the synthesis of proteins.

Similarly, a two-base code cannot work because the greatest number of amino acids coded for with a two-base system is 16 (4 times 4). But a three-base code would provide enough combinations to code for all known amino acids found in proteins.

Crick called his second hypothesis the Central Dogma. In its simplest form, this hypothesis says that once "information" has passed into protein, it cannot get out again. That is, nucleic acids are able to make other nucleic acids or proteins, but proteins are never able to make nucleic acids.

A number of scientists misunderstood Crick's argument here. They thought that he was saying that the information stored in DNA molecules may be transferred to RNA molecules, which are then used to synthesize proteins. And this information pathway is certainly correct. We now know that it is the primary mechanism by which the information stored in DNA molecules directs the synthesis of proteins. But, as it turns out, other pathways are also possible. For example, RNA molecules are sometimes used to make new DNA molecules. But, as the Central Dogma says, the one prohibited transfer is *from* a protein molecule to any other kind of molecule, protein, or nucleic acid.

The obvious next step in the refinement of DNA technologies was to discover the genetic code, the set of three nitrogen bases (sometimes called a *triad* or a *codon*) that codes for amino acids. That breakthrough occurred in 1966, when U.S. biochemists Marshall Nirenberg and Robert Holley discovered the first element in the code. In an elegantly simple experiment, they prepared a sample of RNA made of only one nitrogen base, uracil. They called the molecule polyuracil RNA because it contained many uracil units joined to each other. When polyuracil RNA was inserted into a cell whose own DNA had been removed, the cell made only one product, the amino acid phenylalanine. The codon UUU, therefore, codes for the amino acid phenylalanine. The first clue to the genetic code had been produced.

The Nirenberg-Holley experiment not only provided the first "letter" in the genetic code—UUU equals phenylalanine—but also suggested a method for breaking the rest of the code. Other researchers were soon constructing synthetic RNA molecules with known base sequences and learning which sequence was responsible for the synthesis of which amino acid. Within a short time, the complete genetic code was known.

Recombinant DNA   By the mid-1960s, scientists had developed a reasonably satisfactory model of the way DNA molecules reproduce themselves and direct the synthesis of proteins in cells. They were beginning to imagine ways in which they could manipulate that process artificially. To do so, they had to develop tools and procedures for working with individual DNA molecules to make the transformations they desired. One of the first steps in that direction arose from the work of the Swiss microbiologist Werner Arber and his colleagues.

Arber was interested in the fact that bacteria appear to have evolved a mechanism for protecting themselves against attack by viruses (called *bacteriophages,* or just *phages*). That mechanism involves the use of enzymes with the ability to make scissorlike cuts in the DNA of the invading phage particles. Arber and his team were able to isolate the specific enzymes used by bacteria for this purpose, enzymes that were given the name *restriction endonucleases* or *restriction enzymes.*

This discovery, for which Arber received a share of the 1978 Nobel Prize for Physiology or Medicine, provided researchers with the first tool they needed in working with DNA molecules, a way of slicing open the molecule. The additional feature needed for that tool, however, was a "recognition" feature that could be used to cut a DNA molecule at any desired and specific point, such as the bond between an adenine nucleotide and a cytosine nucleotide (A – C → A + C) or between a guanine nucleotide and thymine nucleotide (G – T → G + T).

That step was accomplished in 1970, when U.S. molecular biologist Hamilton O. Smith and his colleagues discovered a restriction enzyme that recognizes a specific nitrogen base sequence in a DNA molecule. That enzyme, which they called *endonuclease R* but is now known as *HindII,* "recognizes" the base sequence shown below and cuts it in the center of the sequence, as shown by the arrows.

↓

GT(T/C)(A/G)AC
CA(A/G)(T/C)TG

↑

More than 3,000 restriction enzymes have now been discovered, each with the unique property of recognizing and cutting a DNA molecule within some specific base sequence. Many of these enzymes are commercially available for off-the-shelf use by researchers. With these enzymes, researchers now have a way of cutting apart a DNA molecule at virtually any point within its structure.

A cutting tool, such as restriction enzymes, is essential in manipulating a DNA molecule since it provides a way of opening up the molecule. But another kind of tool is also necessary—one that seals the molecule once a desired change has been made in it. By the mid-1960s, scientists already knew that such tools must exist in nature. That knowledge comes from the fact that DNA molecules have the ability to repair themselves after being damaged.

For example, DNA that has been damaged by exposure to X-rays is often found later to have been repaired by some mechanism. That mechanism, researchers decided, must be some kind of enzyme that knits up the broken pieces of DNA and makes it functional again. The search was on for that enzyme.

In 1967, a molecular geneticist at the National Institutes of Health, Martin Gellert, reported that his research team had found the putative compound, an enzyme known as a ligase (from the Latin *ligare,* to bind). More specifically, since this enzyme repairs damage to DNA molecules by restoring bonds that have been broken, the compound is known as DNA ligase. The discovery of ligases was of significance, because researchers now had the tools both to cut DNA molecules (restriction enzymes) and to put the molecules back together again (DNA ligases).

The first successful use of these tools in the manipulation of a DNA molecule was accomplished in 1972 by a research team headed by American biochemist Paul Berg. Berg worked with two well-studied viruses, the SV40 (for simian virus 40) monkey virus and a bacterial virus known as the (lambda) bacteriophage. The DNA in both viruses consists of closed loops. The first step in this experiment involved cutting open the phage DNA with a restriction enzyme, converting it into a linear molecule. A section of the phage DNA was then removed and treated at both ends with chemical groups that made it sticky (think of a small strip of Velcro at each end of the strip).

Another restriction enzyme was used to cut open the SV40 viral loop, and Velcrolike groups were also added to the ends of the open loop. The sticky strip of phage DNA was then attached to opposite ends of the SV40 open chain, and the SV40 combination was sealed up by treatment with DNA ligase and a variety of other enzymes. The product of this experiment was a single molecule of DNA consisting of base sequences from two different organisms. It was a *recombinant DNA* (rDNA) molecule, the first ever made by humans. The molecule could also be described in other ways, as a chimera, for example, or as a transgenic molecule. The word *chimera* comes from the Greek mythological animal with the body and head of a lion, the tail of a snake, and a goat's head protruding from its spine. The term *transgenic,* similarly, refers to any organism or material resulting from one or more genes from a foreign organism being transplanted into a host organism.

The next step beyond Berg's research was already underway by the time his results were published. At Stanford University, medical researcher Stanley N. Cohen was studying bacteria that are resistant to antibiotics. He knew that bacteria must have this property because of the action of genes stored on their DNA. In the case of bacteria, this DNA exists in the form of circular loops known as *plasmids.* How genes on the plasmid confer antibiotic resistance to bacteria was his research problem.

At virtually the same time, Herbert Boyer at the University of California at San Francisco was working on a line of research similar to that of Berg's, attempting to learn more about the function of restriction enzymes in the common bacterium *Escherichia coli,* usually called simply *E. coli.*

Cohen and Boyer did not know each other and probably had heard little or nothing about each other's work. That situation changed, however, when the two men were both invited to present papers about their work at a joint U.S.–Japan conference on bacterial plasmids held in Honolulu in November 1972. Each was interested to hear about the other's research, and over sandwiches at a local delicatessen, they discussed the possibility of collaborating on a new project. After returning to California, they began a series of experiments that drew on the skills each had developed in working with microorganisms.

Their first experiment was relatively simple in concept, although a technological challenge. They worked with a plasmid that had been invented by Cohen, the pSC101 plasmid (*p* for plasmid; *SC* for "Stanley Cohen"; and *101,* an identifying number). The pSC101 is a very simple plasmid consisting of only two genes. One gene codes for replication of the plasmid, and the second gene codes for resistance to the antibiotic kanamycin. The value of the second gene is that it allows researchers to identify the presence of the gene in an experiment by treating the organisms present with the antibiotic.

Using Boyer's expertise, they cut the plasmid with a restriction enzyme known as *Eco* RI and inserted a new gene into the opened plasmid, a gene that codes for resistance to the antibiotic tetracycline. They then used DNA ligase and other enzymes to seal up the plasmid, which now had three genes: one for replication, one for kanamycin resistance, and one for tetracycline resistance. The altered plasmid was then inserted into a colony of *E. coli* bacteria, and kanamycin and tetracycline were added to the colony. Boyer and Cohen found that some bacteria were killed off by the kanamycin and some by the tetracycline. But some remained healthy, indicating that they had absorbed the altered plasmid into their own genetic material. The experiment demonstrated that it was possible to change the genetic characteristic of an organism (*E. coli* bacteria in this case) by adding a new component (the tetracycline gene in this case) to the host organism.

The next series of Boyer-Cohen experiments was even more impressive. Using the same procedure as described above, they added a gene removed from the

South African toad (*Xenopus laevis*) to the pSC101 plasmid and, again, inserted the plasmid into a colony of *E. coli* bacteria. After a period of time, they found that the toad gene was expressing itself in the *E. coli* colony, and that it continued to do so generation after generation.

Perhaps of equal importance was the consequence of this experiment. Bacteria reproduce quite rapidly; in the case of *E. coli*, reproduction occurs about every 20 minutes. That means that any substance produced by the normal metabolism of the bacteria—the *X. laevis* gene product in this case—could be captured as a product of the bacterium's normal process of reproduction. The bacterium had become a factory for the substance coded for by the toad gene (in this case, nothing other than an RNA molecule).

The Boyer-Cohen experiments have become a classic landmark in the history of DNA technology. Cohen chose to remain at Stanford and continue his research on antibiotic resistance in bacteria. Boyer, however, chose a somewhat different future. In 1976, he and venture capitalist Robert A. Swanson founded Genentech, a company whose purpose was to conduct basic research on recombinant DNA products and to develop those products for commercial use.

In that respect, Genentech was the first company founded to commercialize the products of recombinant DNA research. Before it was a year old, the company had developed its first commercial product, genetically engineered somatostatin, a naturally occurring growth hormone inhibiting hormone that inhibits the production of somatotropin, insulin, gastrin, and other hormones.

Boyer was not the only person to recognize the potential commercial value of his discovery with Cohen. At Stanford University, Neils Reimer, then director of the university's newly established Office of Technology Licensing, tried to convince Cohen to file a patent on the Boyer-Cohen invention, if such it could be called. At first, Cohen was reluctant to seek financial advantage from a scientific discovery. Eventually he relented, however, and three patent applications were filed in 1974, one for the methodology used in the research and two for any products that might result from use of the procedure (one for prokaryotes and one for eukaryotes). The applications were filed in the name of the university.

The U.S. Patent Office agonized for a long time over the question as to whether living organisms and procedures related to them could be patented, but eventually decided to issue the patents, which it did on December 2, 1980; August 28, 1984; and April 26, 1988. The three patents all expired in 1997. By the end of 2001, Stanford and the University of California had realized more than $255 million in profits from licenses to 468 companies. A significant amount of that profit came from 2,442 products that had been developed from the patented procedures. Licensing fees were a modest cost to the companies who had to pay them, considering that the 2,442 products had generated an estimated $35 billion in sales over the life of the patents (Beera, 2009).

David E. Newton

See also Amino Acids; Bacteria; *E. Coli* Infection.

References

Beera, Rajendra K. "The Story of the Cohen-Boyer Patents." *Current Science* 96, no. 6 (March 25, 2009): 760–61.

Begley, Sharon. "Little Lamb, Who Made Thee?" *Newsweek,* March 10, 1997, www.news week.com/id/95479.

"Bioethics and Patent Law: The Case of the Oncomouse." *WIPO Magazine* 3 (June 2006): 16–17, www.wipo.int/wipo_magazine/en/2006/03/article_0006.html.

Choi, Charles Q. "First Extinct-Animal Clone Created." *National Geographic News* (February 10, 2009), http://news.nationalgeographic.com/news/2009/02/090210-bucardo-clone.html.

Crick, F.H.C. "On Protein Synthesis." *Symposia of the Society for Experimental Biology: The Biological Replication of Macromolecules* 12 (1958): 152–53.

Erfo Centrum. "Facts and Figures about Gene Therapy" (2009), www.biomedisch.nl/gentherapie_dynamic/gene_therapy_facts_and_figures.php#Number%20of%20trials%20 1989-2007.

Murphy, Denis J. *People, Plants and Genes: The Story of Crops and Humanity.* New York: Oxford University Press, 2007.

National Human Genome Research Institute. "Cloning" (2009), www.genome.gov/25020028#7.

Smitha, Frank Eugene. "Macrohistory and World Report" (2009), www.fsmitha.com/index.html.

University of British Columbia Faculty of Land and Food Systems. "History of Plant Breeding" (2009), www.landfood.ubc.ca/courses/agro/424/resources/AGRO424_history.pdf.

Watson, J.D., and F.H.C. Crick. "A Structure for Deoxyribose Nucleic Acid." *Nature* 171, no. 4356 (April 25, 1953): 737–38.

DEPRESSION

Most people have periods when they feel sadness, low energy, very little motivation to do anything, and perhaps some degree of despair. These feelings and experiences, which can be normal, overlap with a condition more serious, which should not be ignored: clinical depression. Ordinary depression and clinical depression differ in the number of symptoms, intensity of symptoms, and duration. Clinical depression is a state of emotion, mind, and body that can be serious enough to result in extreme suffering, a lack of motivation or ability to take care of oneself, even suicidal behavior. Clinical depression is a common mental illness that is costly to the individuals who suffer from it as well as to their family and other loved ones and society.

Most commonly, individuals are diagnosed with a depressive disorder in the course of an interview with a qualified mental health professional such as a psychologist or psychiatrist. In the United States and other countries, a mental health professional's diagnostic interview will typically be guided by the *Diagnostic and Statistical Manual of Mental Disorders* (*DSM*), published by the American Psychiatric Association, or the *International Classification of Diseases* (*ICD*), published by the World Health Organization. The *DSM* and *ICD* list all mental disorders and diagnostic indicators (e.g., symptoms) of the disorders. The mental health professional will compare the symptoms that his or her client demonstrates to the lists of symptoms in the *DSM* or *ICD*. The end result of the interview is when the client receives one or more diagnoses.

Clinical depression is a type of mood disorder. Mood disorders in the *DSM* fall into two broad categories: depressive disorders, the type discussed in this article and which have been referred to as clinical depression, and bipolar disorders. Individuals diagnosed with bipolar disorder experience episodes of depression and episodes of mania. A mania involves symptoms that tend to be the opposite of depressive disorders (e.g., elevated mood, high self-esteem, high energy, very little sleep needed, and so forth).

Depressive disorders include major depressive disorder (MDD), dysthymic disorder, and depressive disorder not otherwise specified. To be diagnosed with MDD, an individual must experience at least one major depressive episode. A major depressive episode includes five or more of nine symptoms, each occurring nearly continuously for two weeks or more. The nine symptoms are depressed mood, loss of pleasure or interest, decrease or increase in appetite or significant weight loss or gain, sleep disturbance (insomnia or hypersomnia), psychomotor retardation or agitation, fatigue, feelings of worthlessness or guilt, difficulty concentrating or indecisiveness, and suicidal thoughts or behavior or recurrent thoughts of death. To be diagnosed, at least one of the symptoms must be either depressed mood or loss of pleasure or interest. Additionally, the individual must either feel significant distress or experience significant impairment in social, occupational, or other important functioning.

This sterile description does not convey the extreme suffering that someone afflicted by MDD must experience. The symptoms listed above are emotional, cognitive, motor, and physical and describe a comprehensive experience of both the mind and the body. How a depressed person feels, thinks, moves, sleeps, and eats is determined by his or her depressive state. Clinical depression, including MDD, is common and attacks people from all walks of life. Many famous people from political figures such as Abraham Lincoln and Winston Churchill to celebrities such as Marie Osmond and Brooke Shields have reputedly suffered from clinical depression. A number of individuals have written emotional memoirs about their experiences with depression. One such book, *The Bell Jar*, by award-winning poet Sylvia Plath, eloquently conveys what Plath felt emotionally in the throes of depression. Sadly, Plath committed suicide at age 30 during a depressive episode.

The second type of depressive disorder, dysthymic disorder, involves symptoms that are less severe but typically longer lasting. To be diagnosed, the individual must have experienced a depressed mood for at least two years and must exhibit two or more of the six depressive symptoms (e.g., appetite disturbance, sleep disturbance, low energy). The diagnosis depressive disorder not otherwise specified may be assigned when an individual appears to suffer from a distressing or impairing disorder with depressive features, but does not strictly meet the criteria for MDD, dysthymia, or related disorders (such as the bipolar disorders or particular anxiety disorders). Examples include minor depressive disorder, in which the individual has at least two weeks of depressive symptoms, but with fewer than the five symptoms required for a diagnosis of MDD, or, premenstrual dysphoric disorder, which involves depressive symptoms associated with the premenstrual period of a woman's menstrual cycle.

When an individual is diagnosed with a mood disorder, including MDD and dysthymic disorder, one or more specifiers may be notated to indicate a special feature of the particular individual's depression. The specifiers include: (1) severity level: mild, moderate, or severe; (2) with psychotic features; (3) remission status: in partial remission or in full remission; (4) with catatonic features, which describes a severe psychomotor disturbance; (5) with melancholic features, which involves a lack of pleasure or interest in nearly all activities; (6) with atypical features; and (7) with postpartum onset.

Depression exists in all segments of society. Estimates suggest about 7 percent of adults in the United States experience MDD per year, and an additional 5 percent per year suffer from a milder form of depression. In the United States, lifetime risk that an individual will suffer at least one episode of MDD is about 17 percent. The majority of people who experience one depressive episode experience recurrent episodes. Depressive disorders are at least two times more common in women than in men, although among children, girls and boys are about equally likely to experience depression. Depression occurs at all ages, but the most common age group is people in their 40s. Depression appears to be relatively common in most cultures, with prevalence varying by culture. For instance, prevalence of mood disorders (MDD, dysthymic disorder, and bipolar disorder, combined) per year is estimated to be 9.6 percent in the United States, 6.6 percent in Lebanon, 4.8 percent in Mexico, 3.6 percent in Germany, and 3.1 percent in Japan.

Clinical depression likely has multiple causes. Prominent models of causes are genetic and biological, psychological, and sociocultural. Depression runs in families, which may suggest a genetic predisposition. Results of a large variety of family studies conducted over the past 35 years led to the conclusion that depression risk among first-degree relatives (children, parents, and siblings) of people with depression is two to five times higher than the risk in the general population.

Biological factors associated with depression include brain chemicals called neurotransmitters, hormones, and specific brain structures. Neurotransmitters are involved in transmitting messages between neurons. One or both of two neurotransmitters, norepinephrine and serotonin, may play a significant role in triggering depression; depression is frequently associated with low activity of one or both of these neurotransmitters. Research on depression and neurotransmitters has spanned decades; however, researchers are still unsure about the exact relationship between either of these neurotransmitters and depression. Furthermore, other neurotransmitters may be involved in some cases of depression, and sometimes no neurotransmitter dysfunction is readily identified in a particular case of depression, suggesting a complex relationship between neurotransmitter amount or activity and symptoms of depression.

Hormones are chemicals released by endocrine glands in the body. They determine and regulate many body functions, including growth, body metabolism, and sexual function. A particular hormone, cortisol, involved in stress reactions, tends to be elevated in people suffering from depression. The hormone melatonin, which regulates sleep, may also be involved in some cases of depression.

Several brain areas have also been linked with depression. The prefrontal cortex, located in the front of the brain in the area of the hairline on the forehead, is involved in many functions, including mood, attention, immune function, and complex cognitive processes such as planning and decision making. In many cases of depression, activity in this area is decreased, and in some cases activity is elevated. Researchers are therefore unsure regarding the exact relationship between the prefrontal cortex and depression since the area does appear to dysfunction in depression. Two adjacent areas in the brain located above the ears, the hippocampus and amygdala, may be involved in depression. Both areas are associated with memory functions and emotion. The amygdala is specifically linked with negative emotions, and fear in particular. Studies have shown the production of new neurons is decreased in the hippocampus when an individual is depressed. The production of new neurons has been found to return to normal in the hippocampus when individuals take antidepressant medications. Research on the amygdala and depression has thus far produced inconsistent findings; however, a number of researchers consider the amygdala worthy of continued study.

Research on these three areas—the prefrontal cortex, hippocampus, and amygdala—is ongoing, along with more recently initiated research on additional brain areas, such as Brodmann Area 25 (often called simply Area 25) and the ventricles of the brain. A specific example of a research question for the future is: What part does the decreased production of hippocampal cells play in depression? Does depression lead to decreased production of cells, or the other way around? This question is best addressed through utilizing a longitudinal study design, in which people are studied prior to suffering from depression and are then repeatedly studied over time.

Psychological theories of depression contribute to the understanding of causal factors. These theories include psychodynamic (Freudian), behavioral, and cognitive. Overall, cognitive theories have received the most research support. Perhaps the most influential cognitive theory is the one first proposed by clinical psychologist Aaron Beck in the 1960s. Beck argued that a variety of cognitive factors—including maladaptive attitudes, a negative cognitive triad, and automatic thoughts—lead to depression. Beck stated that, as children, some people develop attitudes that are maladaptive and that make them vulnerable to depression. Examples of such attitudes include, "I have worth only if I achieve highly," "I have worth only if I am perfect," or "I am unlovable." Attitudes such as these can lead to disappointment and feelings of failure and to other forms of more consistent negative thinking, such as the cognitive triad, in which an individual thinks negatively about themselves, the world in general, and their futures. Examples of individual negative thoughts may include that one is ugly, stupid, mean, socially awkward, or klutzy. Negative thoughts about the world could involve thinking that people are naturally bad or that the planet is hopelessly, irrevocably polluted.

Furthermore, an individual who feels that the present is unbearable may also be unable to hope for the future. He or she thinks that negative way life is the way life will always be. These types of underlying belief patterns lead to automatic thoughts in one's ongoing experiences. For instance, depressed individuals may frequently and readily think they are stupid or incompetent, that other people do not like them, or that other people are mean, as a reaction to another person's very small behavior viewed by other individuals as innocuous.

Sociocultural factors can also impact depression. Some sociocultural researchers and theorists emphasize the family and other interpersonal factors as contributing to depression. Depressed people tend to have poorer social skills than nondepressed people, and their social awkwardness may lead to a downward spiral that isolates the individual from others, further increasing depression. For example, many depressed people speak hesitantly and quietly and may appear needy to others, frequently seeking reassurance from others. Other people sense the awkwardness and discomfort of depressed individuals and withdraw from them. This cycle of behavior continues to repeat itself.

Lacking an intimate relationship is associated with depression. In particular, a number of researchers, including Mark Whisman and colleagues, have studied how the quality of marital relationships is associated with depression. The researchers found sadness and marital conflict are moderately correlated, and marital conflict predicts future episodes of MDD. The research findings of Whisman and colleagues were compelling enough that they concluded that preventing marital dissatisfaction may prevent up to 30 percent of cases of MDD among married people.

Gender and culture are other sociocultural factors that impact incidence of depression. Women suffer from depression two times more frequently than men, have more frequent and longer-lasting episodes, and are less responsive to treatment than men. A large number of explanations for the gender difference have been proposed. Explanations include hormonal differences between women and men and the "body dissatisfaction theory," stating the societal pressure women feel to have perfect bodies causes low self-esteem and depression. It is also suggested that differences in life stress, focusing, for example, on the fact that women experience higher rates of poverty, have less satisfying jobs, experience more discrimination than men, and are overburdened with child care and housework may also influence the rate of depression in women. An additional set of explanations are cognitive, such as the rumination theory, which states that women tend to think about and focus on their depressed feelings more than do men, whereas men are more likely to distract themselves from sad feelings. In research, rumination has been shown to perpetuate depression.

Many symptoms of depression are common across cultures, such as feelings of sadness and hopelessness, lack of pleasure, low energy, and inability to concentrate. However, other parts of the clinical picture differ by culture. In Eastern cultures such as China and Nigeria, people more frequently experience physical symptoms including weight loss and sleep disturbance. Western culture is strongly associated with the cognitive symptomatology of depression: people experience negative thought patterns, low self-esteem, and guilt.

Fortunately, in the majority of cases, depression can be successfully treated. Successful treatment provides at least moderate relief from symptoms and can mean a full return to state of mind and level of functioning that existed prior to the depression. A variety of psychological treatments exists; most are forms of psychotherapy. One highly regarded therapy is cognitive therapy, which is based in the cognitive theory of depression associated with Aaron Beck and described above. This type of therapy works on the negative thinking characteristic of depression. It involves having individuals challenge their negative assumptions and automatic thoughts. For instance, in a session of psychotherapy between Beck and a client, the client describes that she is depressed and states that her depression stems from the fact that her husband left her. Beck explores the idea that her depression is caused by her husband's action. Beck challenges her to think carefully about the meaning of the event that she says has so much power. What is the meaning of "David left me?" The client says that one meaning is "David doesn't love me." Beck shows that she cannot logically conclude this, especially since David says that he loves her. Beck points out that David himself may have problems, because he continues to say that he loves her, yet has a pattern of leaving her then coming back. Beck probes, trying to determine if there is a deeper meaning associated with "David left me." The client responds that David's action also means that she is unlovable. Beck points out the logical problem with drawing this conclusion. The fact that David is leaving her does not necessarily suggest that David does not love her, and it certainly does not suggest that she is unlovable; this conclusion is too far removed from the actual event that occurred, abandonment by her husband.

Another effective form of therapy is interpersonal psychotherapy, developed by Gerald Klerman and Myrna Weisman in the 1980s. They argued that four interpersonal issues often cause depression: interpersonal loss, interpersonal role dispute, interpersonal role transition, and interpersonal deficits. First, depression may be associated with a grief reaction following the loss of a loved one through death or abandonment. Therapists guide clients to examine the relationship and uncover difficult emotions, learning to think differently about the relationship and becoming prepared to initiate new ones. Second, interpersonal role disputes may cause and/or maintain depression. This is when the two people involved in a relationship have different ideas about what their roles should be. For instance, one may believe that women and men have specific roles in marriage and another may believe that marriage should be egalitarian. Therapy focuses on teaching clients how to deal with the conflict associated with these divergent assumptions. Third, the client may be experiencing an interpersonal role transition in which a major life change has occurred, such as children leaving the house, divorce, or entering the workforce for the first time. Therapy focuses on developing skills for coping with the new roles. Fourth, some clients may suffer from interpersonal deficits such as social awkwardness, extreme social insecurity, or extreme shyness. Therapy involves helping the individual to recognize the effect that his or her behavior may have on others and teaching social skills.

Two forms of biological treatment are equally effective to cognitive therapy and interpersonal therapy: antidepressant medications and electroconvulsive therapy (ECT). Three broad classes of antidepressant medications are available: monoamine oxidase (MAO) inhibitors, tricyclics, and second-generation antidepressants. In general, the second-generation antidepressants offer the best combination of effectiveness and low side effects. This group was first developed in the 1980s and includes fluoxetine (Prozac), sertraline (Zoloft), escitalopram (Lexapro), and venlafaxine (Effexor). These medications operate on the neurotransmitter serotonin, increasing the activity of serotonin in the brain. Some operate on another neurotransmitter or more than one neurotransmitter. For instance, venlafaxine affects both serotonin and norepinephrine. The second-generation antidepressants are often the first medications that a physician may try with a client; since they are not effective in all cases, tricyclics and MAO inhibitors are also available. Tricyclics are about equally effective to second-generation antidepressants, but they pose a greater risk of overdose and more troublesome side effects. MAO inhibitors are also considered less effective than the other two categories, although they can be the best choice for some individuals. MAO inhibitors create serious reactions when they are ingested along with the chemical tyramine, present in foods including some cheeses, wines, and bananas. Dietary restrictions are necessary when an individual is taking MAO inhibitors.

The other effective biological treatment for depression is electroconvulsive therapy. In ECT, two electrodes are placed on the head of the patient, introducing an electrical charge of 64 to 140 volts. The electricity causes a brain seizure lasting from about one-half minute to a few minutes. The majority of patients experience improvement in their depression after 6 to 12 treatments, which are administered over about two to four weeks. ECT is most effective for severe depressions and depressions that include some psychotic features, such as delusions (for instance, when someone believes they are the devil). While researchers remain uncertain why ECT is effective, some psychologists and psychiatrists believe that ECT should not be used at all. The procedure can appear frightening; it has been described by critics as barbaric. Additionally, memory loss can be a side effect, and some believe that neurological damage is a risk from ECT. For these reasons, ECT tends to be a procedure of last resort.

In recent years, several new biological treatments for depression have shown promising preliminary results. These include vagus nerve stimulation, transcranial magnetic stimulation, and deep brain stimulation. Currently, and likely into the near future, much of the primary research on new treatments for depression involve biological treatments rather than physical choices such as ECT.

Gretchen M. Reevy

See also Bipolar Disorder; Psychosomatic Health Care; Stress.

References

American Psychiatric Association. *Diagnostic and Statistical Manual of Mental Disorders,* 4th ed., text rev. Washington, DC: American Psychiatric Association, 2000.

Beck, Aaron T., and Brad A. Alford. *Depression: Causes and Treatment.* Philadelphia: University of Pennsylvania Press, 2009.

Comer, Ronald J. *Abnormal Psychology.* New York: Worth, 2010.

Imel, Zac E., Melanie B. Malterer, Kevin M. McKay, and Bruce E. Wampold. "A Meta-analysis of Psychotherapy and Medication in Unipolar Depression and Dysthymia." *Journal of Affective Disorders* 110, no. 3 (2008): 197–206.

Plath, Sylvia. *The Bell Jar.* New York: Harper Collins, 2006. First published 1963.

Preston, John D., John H. O'Neal, and Mary C. Taluga. *Handbook of Clinical Psychopharmacology for Therapists,* 6th ed. Oakland, CA: New Harbinger, 2010.

Taube-Schiff, Marlene, and Mark A. Lau. "Major Depressive Disorder." In *Handbook of Psychological Assessment, Case Conceptualization, and Treatment, Vol. 1: Adults,* edited by Michel Hersen and Johan Rosqvist, 319–51. Hoboken, NJ: John Wiley, 2008.

Whisman, Mark A., and Martha L. Bruce. "Marital Dissatisfaction and Incidence of Major Depressive Episode in a Community Sample." *Journal of Abnormal Psychology* 108, no. 4 (1999): 674–78.

DIABETES

Diabetes is a disease in which the body can no longer produce or properly use insulin, a hormone required to convert sugars and starches from the food we eat into the energy we need. It is one of the most common chronic illnesses today, affecting an estimated 17 million people in the United States and an estimated 120 million people worldwide. It is affecting an increasing number of people. The World Health Organization predicts that the total number of people with diabetes worldwide will rise to 300 million by 2025.

There are two major types of diabetes: In Type 1, sometimes called juvenile diabetes or insulin-dependent diabetes, the pancreas no longer produces insulin. Between 5 and 10 percent of people diagnosed with diabetes have Type 1 diabetes. That's between 500,000 and 1 million people in the United States. It usually strikes children or young adults, though it can develop at any age. It occurs when the body's immune system mistakenly attacks the insulin-producing cells in the pancreas. People with Type 1 diabetes must take daily insulin injections to stay alive. While the cause of Type 1 diabetes is unknown, it is likely that heredity plays a role. However, in susceptible individuals, a virus can trigger the disease.

In Type 2 diabetes, the body does produce insulin, but either makes too little or has become resistant to it. More than 90 percent of people with diabetes have Type 2, and it most often strikes older people and those with a history of obesity and inactivity, though increasingly it is appearing in younger people—even children—who are overweight and inactive. People with Type 2 diabetes can often control their blood sugar levels through weight loss, exercise, and better nutrition, but many also need oral medications and/or insulin.

A third type of diabetes, gestational diabetes, is a temporary condition that occurs during pregnancy, when the body fails to produce the extra insulin needed

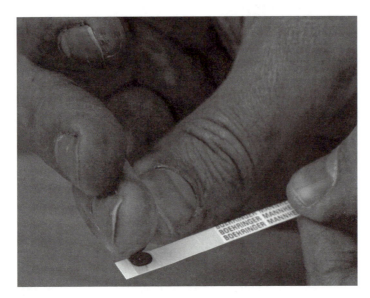

Man pricks his finger to check the glucose level in his blood. Tight glucose control, including frequent blood glucose monitoring, significantly reduces organ damage caused by diabetes. (National Institutes of Health)

during some pregnancies. Gestational diabetes requires that the pregnant woman monitor her food and blood sugar levels carefully. It usually goes away after the pregnancy, but women who have had it are at an increased risk of later developing Type 2 diabetes.

Heredity plays a role in development of Type 1 diabetes. Siblings of people with Type 1 as well as children of parents with Type 1 are at a higher risk of developing the disease. Type 1 most often strikes in puberty, according to researchers, though it can occur at any age. Type 2 diabetes has a hereditary factor as well—people with a family history of Type 2 are more likely to develop the disease themselves. And some racial and ethnic groups have higher rates of diabetes. African Americans and Latinos are nearly twice as likely to develop Type 2 diabetes as the general population.

The warning signs for Type 1 diabetes include frequent urination, excessive thirst, unusual hunger, extreme fatigue, and unexplained weight loss. Victims of Type 2 diabetes can experience the same symptoms, as well as blurred vision, tingling or numbness in the hands or feet, and cuts, bruises, and infections that are slow to heal. Often, though, people with Type 2 diabetes will have no symptoms at all, and the disease won't be discovered until they have developed complications.

Diabetes is the seventh leading cause of death in the United States and the sixth leading cause of death by disease. Each year, nearly 200,000 people die as a result of diabetes and its long-term complications, which include blindness, kidney disease, heart disease, stroke, nerve disease, and amputations. It is often described as a silent killer because in its Type 2 form, it can go undetected for years. It is only when serious and sometimes life-threatening complications develop that many people learn they have the disease. Complications of diabetes—which often take years to develop—stem in many instances from the damage that high blood sugar levels do to the tiny blood vessels in the body. In instances of kidney failure, for example, damage has been done to the blood vessels inside the kidney that act as filters to remove wastes, chemicals, and excess water from the blood. Poorly controlled diabetes can cause blindness by damaging the tiny blood vessels in the retina.

The most serious short-term complication of Type 1 diabetes is called ketoacidosis. When the body doesn't have enough insulin, it begins to burn fat for energy. Burning fat produces ketones, an acid that can poison the body, leading to coma and even death. Ketoacidosis usually develops slowly—early warning signs include thirst, a dry mouth, frequent urination, and high levels of ketones in the urine. Later, the person may feel nausea, have a fruity odor on the breath, or have difficulty breathing. Ketoacidosis is a serious condition that requires immediate medical attention.

People with diabetes must take a lot of responsibility to make sure their treatment plan works. People with diabetes must balance a variety of factors every day—deciding what to eat and when, or determining how much medication to take and when to take it. Physical activity or illness can also mean adjusting the treatment regimen. The best way to learn that responsibility is to seek advice from a team of health care professionals.

A primary care physician is a good place to start, but treating diabetes almost always involves specialists in other areas as well. A diabetes care team usually involves an eye doctor, a dietitian, and a certified diabetes educator. If complications arise, a patient might be sent to other specialists.

For people with Type 1 diabetes, insulin is the only option. But there are a wide variety of approaches to insulin therapy. There are more than twenty kinds of insulin available—some act very quickly or peak at different times, and some last all day long. There are also different ways to deliver insulin—syringes, insulin pens, and insulin pumps.

Most people with Type 1 begin by taking two injections of two types of insulin per day. Later they move to taking multiple injections, usually three or four per day, depending on what they're eating or their level of activity. A person with Type 1 diabetes often calculates the amount of carbohydrates she will consume and then injects herself with a number of units of insulin. This formula depends on the individual's reaction to insulin as well as expected activity level.

Injecting insulin before every meal or snack is the most targeted approach to diabetes treatment and allows the greatest flexibility, but some diabetics find it cumbersome. Another approach is to inject a specific amount of insulin in the morning and then eat only those foods that will be covered by that amount of insulin. The second approach is more regimented and doesn't allow for spontaneous snacking.

Another recent innovation in insulin delivery is the insulin pump, a device that looks like a beeper and provides a steady, incremental dose of fast-acting insulin through a tiny tube inserted in the person's abdomen. Insulin pumps are the most expensive approach to diabetes care, but the device is the closest thing to the normal delivery of insulin that a person with diabetes can achieve. Pumps can be programmed to deliver different amounts of insulin at different times of the day or night, giving the person the ability to fine-tune their treatment regimen.

If you have an insulin-dependent diabetic friend, or if you are insulin-dependent yourself, make sure you discuss this openly. There's the possibility that insulin-dependent diabetics may need help at some point. They may experience an episode of hypoglycemia (low blood sugar) and need help getting a snack or sugared drink. Hypoglycemia occurs when the person has either taken more insulin than needed for the carbohydrates consumed or is particularly active. The other risk is developing hyperglycemia, or high blood sugar. That happens when the person hasn't taken enough insulin or has eaten more carbohydrates than the insulin can cover. A fast-acting insulin can help counteract these spikes. It's much less intimidating to help a diabetic prepare an insulin injection or provide a sweet snack if you've discussed the symptoms and what to do in advance.

Millions of Americans were introduced to the difficulties of living with Type 1 diabetes thanks to rock music star Bret Michaels, who was diagnosed with Type 1 diabetes when he was a child. Michaels appeared and was the final winner on NBC's "Celebrity Apprentice" with Donald Trump during the 2010 season. Michaels spoke out about his challenges managing the disease while living the rock star lifestyle, and he named the American Diabetes Association (ADA) as his charity of choice during the program. Michaels supports ADA Diabetes Camps and his winnings on the show, which totaled almost $400,000, were donated to the ADA.

People with Type 2 diabetes have a different set of treatment options. Sometimes, Type 2 diabetes can be controlled through diet and exercise alone. In many cases, though, the body needs help. In people with Type 2, the body doesn't make enough insulin and doesn't use the insulin it does make very well.

Oral medications can help the body reduce blood sugar levels. There are three classes of drugs for Type 2. The first kind stimulates the body to produce more insulin. The second makes the body more sensitive to the insulin it does have. The third blocks the breakdown of starches and certain sugars, which slows the rise of blood sugar levels. Sometimes people with Type 2 will take a combination of oral medications or will take pills in combination with insulin. For every person with Type 2, medication combined with improved nutrition and regular exercise is the best treatment.

A key part of self-treatment of diabetes is frequent blood sugar testing. Pharmacies sell a variety of small blood glucose monitors and test strips that diabetics can (and should) carry with them. The diabetic places a drop of blood on the test strip and within a minute or so has a reading of the blood sugar level. The general goal is to achieve blood sugar levels as close to normal as possible. People without diabetes generally maintain blood sugar levels between 70 and

120 milligrams per deciliter before eating and less than 180 milligrams per deciliter after eating.

People with diabetes can also gauge how well they're controlling their blood sugar by taking a glycated hemoglobin test every three months. The test, done through a doctor's office, measures the presence of excess glucose in the blood over a three- or four-month period and gives a better picture of the effectiveness of the person's diabetes care than a single test on a glucose monitor.

Research has shown that the best way to avoid complications is to keep blood sugar levels as close to normal as possible. A 10-year study that was completed in 1993 showed the benefits of tight control. The Diabetes Control and Complications Trial (DCCT) followed 1,441 people with Type 1 diabetes for several years. Half of the participants followed a standard diabetes treatment, while the other half followed an intensive-control regimen of multiple injections and frequent blood sugar testing.

Those who followed the intensive-control regimen had significantly fewer complications. Only half as many developed signs of kidney disease, nerve disease was reduced by two-thirds, and only one-quarter as many developed diabetic eye disease. Achieving tight control means taking several injections of insulin every day or using an insulin pump to mimic the release of insulin that occurs in people without diabetes. It also means doing several blood tests a day to gauge how much insulin is needed.

Though the DCCT only followed people with Type 1, researchers believe tight control can have the same effect on people with Type 2. Since most people with Type 2 diabetes do not take insulin, they must take a different approach to tight control. Losing weight is one of the best ways to bring down glucose levels. Regular exercise helps, too, not only to bring down weight but in helping to reduce glucose levels. A recent study of 1,263 men with Type 2 diabetes showed that, over 12 years, the men who did not exercise and stay active were more than twice as likely to die as those who exercised.

Tight control has obvious benefits, but it's not necessarily the right choice for everyone. The DCCT found that people who followed tight control had three times the number of low blood glucose episodes as those using conventional treatment. Plus, people using the tight control approach gained more weight than those on conventional treatment—an average of 10 pounds, according to the DCCT.

Those who should avoid tight control include people who already have complications; young children (whose developing brains need glucose); and the elderly, who can suffer strokes or heart attacks from episodes of hypoglycemia.

As the number of people with diabetes increases in the United States, so do concerns that older adults with diabetes may be at greater risk for mental decline and dementia. Research released in the January 2010 issue of the *British Journal of Psychiatry* provided evidence of just such a scenario. The four-year study followed participants over the age of 65 who had mild cognitive impairment (memory loss greater than normal for an individual's age but does not meet the criteria for dementia), and researchers found that those participants with diabetes had nearly three times the risk of developing dementia or Alzheimer's disease as those without diabetes. Scientists are continuing to study the possible link between diabetes in older adults and this higher risk for dementia.

Marjolijn Bijlefeld and Sharon Zoumbaris

See also Alzheimer's Disease; Exercise; Immune System/Lymphatic System.

References

American Diabetes Association. *American Diabetes Association Complete Guide to Diabetes.* Alexandria, VA: American Diabetes Association, 2011.

American Diabetes Association, www.diabetes.org.

Beaser, Richard S., and Amy Peterson Campbell. *The Joslin Guide to Diabetes: A Program for Managing Your Treatment.* New York: Simon & Schuster, 2005.

Bunker, Katie. "Star Turns: Bret Michaels Rocks 'Celebrity Apprentice,' Raising $390,000 and Counting for the American Diabetes Association." *Diabetes Forecast* 63, no. 7 (July 2010): 61–62.

"Diabetes: A Major Threat to the Brain: Diabetes Can Cause Major Changes in the Brain Over Time and May Increase the Risk of Vascular Dementia and Alzheimer's Disease." *Mind, Mood and Memory* 6, no. 7 (July 2010): 1–2.

"Eli Lilly and Co." *Indianapolis Business Journal* (May 9, 2011): 13A.

Greene, Bob. *The Best Life Guide to Managing Diabetes and Pre-diabetes.* New York: Simon & Schuster, 2009.

Hirsch, James S. *Cheating Destiny: Living with Diabetes, America's Biggest Epidemic.* Boston: Houghton Mifflin, 2006.

Hurley, Dan. *Diabetes Rising: How a Rare Disease Became a Modern Pandemic and What to Do about It.* New York: Kaplan, 2010.

Hurley, Dan. "Steps Forward, and Backward, in Treating Diabetes." *New York Times* (July 20, 2010): D5.

Kaufman, Francinie Ratner. *Diabesity: The Obesity-Diabetes Epidemic That Threatens America and What We Must Do to Stop It.* New York: Bantam Books, 2005.

DIETARY GUIDELINES FOR AMERICANS

The Dietary Guidelines for Americans are the basic foundation of the U.S. government's' MyPlate system, released in 2011. MyPlate replaces the U.S. Department of Agriculture's MyPyramid, introduced in 2005 to spice up the original Food Guide Pyramid unveiled in 1992. According to nutritionists, the pyramid had become too complicated for average Americans to understand.

The report of the 2010 Dietary Guidelines for Americans is distinctly different from any previous report in a few significant ways. First, it addresses an American public that continues to grow more overweight and obese. Also, the Dietary Guidelines Advisory Committee (DGAC) for the first time has available a state-of-the-art web-based electronic system and methodology called the Nutrition Evidence Library to provide answers to its scientific questions concerning data analyses, food pattern modeling analyses, and other issues.

The guidelines, originally released in 1977 as Dietary Goals for the American People, were at first merely concerned with complementary nutrient-based and food-based recommendations. At that time, they focused on energy balance and recommended that Americans consume only as much energy in the form of calories as they expended. The latest set of recommendations observes that the most significant negative health trend among U.S. children in the past 40 years has been a dramatic increase in obesity. According to the report, the prevalence of overweight and obesity has doubled among children ages 2 to 11 years since the 1970s and tripled among adolescents aged 12 to 19 years old (DGAC, 2010).

To combat this growing health problem, the 2010 guidelines suggest a diet that includes a healthy balance of nutritious foods with an emphasis on eating fresh fruits and vegetables. They call for a stronger focus on calorie control combined with increased physical activity and a reduction of salt by 40 percent, lowering the maximum daily intake from 2,300 milligrams (mg) to 1,500 mg. Surprisingly to some Americans, the report does not recommend dietary supplements; instead it suggests that a daily multivitamin or mineral supplement does not offer health benefits to anyone eating a healthy, varied diet (Sawyer, 2010).

The guidelines are reviewed every five years based on the latest research, labeling, and nutrition information and are considered the core of the government's general food and nutrition policy. Following their initial release in 1977 by the U.S. Senate Select Committee on Nutrition and Human Needs led by Senator George McGovern, they were placed under the direction of the U.S. Department of Agriculture (USDA) and the U.S. Department of Health and Human Services (HHS), which at that time was called the Department of Health, Education and Welfare.

In early 1980, the two departments collaborated and released another brochure titled *Nutrition and Your Health: Dietary Guidelines for Americans,* which described seven principles for a healthy diet and suggested ways to make healthy daily food choices. However, even though the recommendations were presented as basic nutritional goals, they were met with some controversy from a variety of industry and scientific groups. The debate led Congress to create an advisory committee that would provide impartial and expert advice to be used in developing future editions. The first advisory committee was composed of scientific experts from outside the federal government who developed the 1985 report titled *Nutrition and Your Health: Dietary Guidelines for Americans.*

A second scientific advisory committee reviewed the guidelines in 1989 and revised the guidelines based in part on the 1988 *Surgeon General's Report on Nutrition and Health* and the 1989 National Research Council's report *Diet and Health: Implications for Reducing Chronic Disease Risk.*

The report in 1990 promoted healthy eating through variety and moderation rather than restrictions. For the first time, it provided recommendations for specific amounts of dietary fat and saturated fat. The seven principals in this report included: eat a variety of foods; balance the foods eaten with physical activity to maintain or improve weight; choose a diet with plenty of grain products, vegetables, and fruits; choose a diet low in fat, saturated fat, and cholesterol; choose a diet moderate in sugars; choose a diet moderate in salt and sodium; and drink alcoholic beverages in moderation.

With the passage of the 1990 National Nutrition Monitoring and Related Research Act, the 1995 guidelines became the first report mandated by law. The act directed the secretaries of the USDA and HHS to jointly issue a report every five years. The 2000 guidelines presented A-B-C (aim, build, choose) steps. A was designed to aim for fitness by being physically active each day. B was to build a healthy base through food choices from the Food Pyramid and a variety of fruits, vegetables, and whole grains. The C was to choose sensibly from foods that were low in fat and cholesterol and limited in sugars and salt. The most notable changes between the 1995 and 2000 guidelines included greater emphasis on limiting sugar and salt and on lowering fat and cholesterol.

Since the release of the 2005 Dietary Guidelines, food safety concerns have escalated in the United States following recalls of foods contaminated with bacteria or adulterated with nonfood substances. The committee recommended four basic food safety principles—clean, separate, cook, and chill—and encouraged Americans to practice safety as they prepared healthy food and to practice good nutrition.

Unfortunately, despite drastic changes in the 2010 Advisory Committee's recommendations that also included increased physical activity, Americans are still facing a rising rate of obesity and related diseases, including heart disease, diabetes, and cancer. In its latest report, the committee advised Americans to consume nutrient-dense foods in the proper proportions and noted that, in the United States, adults consume less than 20 percent of the recommended intake for whole grains, less than 60 percent for vegetables, less than 50 percent of the recommended intake for fruits, and less than 60 percent for milk and milk products.

In its final statement, the report also called on the food industry to work with all segments of society—from parents to policymakers and everyone else in between—to take responsibility in creating gradual and steady change to help current and future generations achieve the goal of eating a more nutritious diet and living more healthy and productive lives. Success toward that goal will be measured by any changes that occur when the 2015 DGAC convenes.

The 13 independent experts that make up the 2010 DGAC are affiliated with universities throughout the country and are nationally recognized in the fields of nutrition and health. During the review of the guidelines, the committee held six public meetings during two years, and the transcripts of all public comments and meeting minutes are posted online. The use of webinar technology for showing the public meetings increased attendance by almost half.

Sharon Zoumbaris

See also Cholesterol; Exercise; Fats; MyPlate.

References

Sawyer, Antoaneta. "A Review of the New 2010 Dietary Guidelines for Americans." Examiner.com (June 18, 2010), www.examiner.com/diets-in-milwaukee.

United States Department of Agriculture. "Report of the DGAC on the Dietary Guidelines for Americans, 2010," www.cnpp.usda.gov/dietaryguidelines.htm.

United States Department of Agriculture and U.S. Department of Health and Human Services. *Report of the Dietary Guidelines Advisory Committee on the Dietary Guidelines for Americans, 2000.* Washington, DC: USDA, Agricultural Research Service, 2000.

U.S. Congress. National Nutrition Monitoring and Related Research Act of 1990, Public Law 445, 101st Congress, 2nd Session, Section 301, 7 USC 5341, October 22, 1990.

USDA Center for Nutrition Policy and Promotion. "USDA's Nutrition Evidence Library," www.cnpp.usda.gov/NEL.htm.

U.S. Senate Select Committee on Nutrition and Human Needs. *Dietary Goals for the United States,* 2nd ed. Washington, DC: U.S. Government Printing Office, 1997.

DIETARY REFERENCE INTAKES (DRI)

One thing every person has in common is the need for food. When it comes to what we eat, we often choose our foods based on anything or everything but what our bodies need. And a diet deficient in nutrients over time will result in health problems.

Enter Dietary Reference Intakes (DRI), a set of nutrient-based reference values that estimate what we need to eat to be healthy. The DRIs were determined by the Institute of Medicine, a private, nonprofit organization paid to provide health policy advice to the U.S. government.

These values are based on the scientific evaluation of four categories: estimated average requirements (EAR); recommended dietary allowance (RDA); adequate intake (AI); and tolerable upper intake level (UL). That alphabet soup also takes into account age and gender.

The EAR is the average amount needed to meet the requirements of a particular age group or gender and is a useful tool when assessing the nutrition of a particular group rather than an individual. The RDAs are the nutrient requirements established for healthy individuals, and those are based on the EAR. The AI is a number or value set as a goal for individual intake of nutrients when an RDA cannot be determined. Finally, the UL is the highest daily intake of any nutrient that has been shown to pose no risk of ill health for an individual.

Of course, these recommendations did not develop overnight. The RDA was introduced in the 1940s as the government responded to the growth of scientific knowledge about the roles nutrients played in human health. It was after World War II when food rationing in the United States and Europe was ending that the government began releasing food guides to improve health and nutrition. A committee set up by the U.S. National Academy of Sciences was put to work to develop standard daily allowances for each type of nutrient. The committee, named the Food and Nutrition Board, released its recommendations in 1941.

The United States Department of Agriculture went on to release the Basic Seven food guide in 1943; later this became the foundation for the 1968 RDAs, which were revised every 5 to 10 years. In 2006, the RDAs were renamed Reference Daily Intakes or RDIs in order to broaden the existing guidelines, and they were added to food labels. The concept behind the DRIs is that they represent a shift in emphasis from preventing deficiency to decreasing the risk of chronic disease through nutrition. For example, current DRI levels are expected to reduce the risk of osteoporosis, diet-related cancers, and cardiovascular disease. Since 1998, the Institute of Medicine has issued eight volumes of DRIs. However, the older RDIs remain on nutrition labels rather than the newer DRIs.

DRIs are used most frequently in the composition of menus for schools, hospitals, nursing homes, and prisons because they encompass the entire spectrum of nutrients—calcium, related vitamins and minerals, macronutrients, carbohydrates, dietary fats, fiber, protein, amino acids, electrolytes and fluids, and other food components—that play a beneficial role in human health.

Sharon Zoumbaris

See also Institute of Medicine (IOM); National School Lunch Program (NSLP); U.S. Department of Agriculture (USDA).

References

Institute of Medicine. "Dietary Reference Intakes for Calcium and Vitamin D" (November 2010), www.iom.edu/vitamind.

Nestle, Marion. *Food Politics*. Berkeley: University of California Press, 2002.

United States Department of Agriculture. "Dietary Guidelines," http://fnic.nal.usda.gov.

United States Department of Agriculture. "Dietary Reference Intakes (DRI)," http://fnic.nal.usda.gov.

United States Department of Agriculture. "RDA Chart," www.nal.usda.gov/fnic/dga/rda.pdf.

DIETARY SUPPLEMENTS

The U.S. government defines dietary supplements as products that contain a dietary ingredient such as vitamins, minerals, amino acids, botanicals, or other substances that can supplement the diet. They are usually swallowed and come in many forms, including capsules, tablets, powders, and even energy bars and liquids. They can be purchased in stores, pharmacies, convenience stories, specialty shops, over the Internet, through direct sales representatives, and from catalogs.

Government Legislation The Dietary Supplement Health and Education Act of 1994 is the main law that defines what products are classified as dietary supplements and what types of claims their manufacturers can make about any possible health benefits. Federal law requires they be labeled as supplements

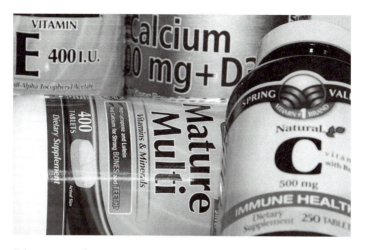

Dietary supplements come in many forms including capsules, tablets, powders, energy bars, and liquids. (Jennifer Pitiquen/Dreamstime.com)

(a subset of foods, not drugs), with the term *dietary supplement* or a variation of their ingredient such as *herbal supplement* or *calcium supplement* clearly on the label. They can make claims or statements about the effect on the structure or function of the body. They cannot, however, claim to cure, treat, prevent, or diagnose specific diseases without U.S. Food and Drug Administration (FDA) authorization. For example, on a calcium supplement, the label can state that regular exercise and a healthy diet with enough calcium can help women maintain good bone health, but it cannot say that this supplement will prevent or cure osteoporosis.

Since dietary supplements are regulated by the FDA and do not have to be reviewed for their safety before they are sold, their labeling is required to be truthful and not misleading. Quality control is left to the manufacturer, supplier, or others in the production process. To improve quality, the FDA issued good manufacturing practices for dietary supplements in 2007 with the expectation that manufacturers would guarantee the identity, purity, strength, and composition of their products to protect the public from contamination, improper packaging, or labeling.

Unfortunately, that is not always the case. A congressional investigation of dietary herbal supplements reported finding trace amounts of lead, mercury, and other heavy metals in nearly all products tested in the spring of 2010 (Harris, 2010). However, the levels of the heavy metal contaminants did not exceed established limits. That same report found that 16 of the 40 supplements tested contained pesticide residues that may have exceeded legal limits. There were also several misleading health claims according to the report, prepared by the Government Accountability Office.

What does this mean for Americans who are swallowing dietary supplements in increasing numbers? Supplements have gained mainstream popularity, with more than half of adults taking them, according to a report in 2011 by the

National Center for Health Statistics at the Centers for Disease Control. However, more important than the numbers of people taking these supplements are the possibilities that supplements have ingredients that may interact with medications and cause unwanted interactions or side effects or may contain harmful substances.

Popular Supplements With some 29,000 dietary supplement products on the market, it is important for consumers to be educated about their safety and effectiveness. The most popular supplement categories are multivitamins, meal replacements, sports nutrition supplements, calcium, B vitamins, vitamin C, glucosamine and chondroitin, vitamin D, and fish oil.

Multivitamins were first introduced to consumers in the 1950s to offset the effects of an explosion of overprocessed foods. Americans from all walks of life had become more interested in low cost and convenience than in nutrition. In the process, they had filled their kitchens with items like Wonder Bread, a white, fluffy loaf that promised to "build strong bodies 12 ways." The enrichment was necessary because all the bread's original nutrients were processed out of it. Still, no research exists that demonstrates multivitamins are necessary, and the government's 2010 dietary guidelines do not recommend any vitamin supplement for a healthy population consuming a variety of foods.

Meal replacements are marketed to dieters who want to lose weight by substituting diet shakes, bars, or prepackaged meals for their regular foods. However, one important drawback to meal replacements is that they are processed foods; although they contain added vitamins and minerals, they lack fiber, antioxidants, and the other health benefits associated with eating fresh foods, especially fruits and vegetables.

Sports nutrition supplements include a vast array of powders, drinks, gels, bars, and pills, and they contain vitamins, amino acids, minerals, herbs, and other botanicals. These products were developed for serious athletes but are routinely purchased and used by everyone from recreational athletes to couch potatoes. Sport drinks are especially popular. Unfortunately, studies have shown that they are more acidic than orange juice and may contribute to the erosion of tooth enamel. They often contain high amounts of sodium and caffeine, which is a factor in lower calcium levels, because calcium is excreted through urine and both salt and caffeine greatly increase urine output.

In fact, our national intake of caffeine and sodium is sky-high. The latest report from the Institute of Medicine (IOM) released in April 2010 strongly recommends that Americans lower the amount of sodium in their diets. The IOM estimates the average American eats about 4,000 milligrams (mg) of sodium per day (IOM, 2010). The institute recommends only 1,500 mg of sodium a day, and 1,200 mg for anyone over 70. Americans also consume about 45 million pounds of caffeine each year in the form of coffee, soft drinks, food, and drugs.

Calcium is the next most popular dietary supplement in the United States and is often lacking in the average U.S. diet. Given the high number of Americans who eat and drink excessive amounts of sodium and caffeine, a lack of calcium may be due in part to the diuretic effects of many daily food and beverage choices.

The B vitamins include B1 or thiamine, B2 or riboflavin, B3 or niacin, B5 or pantothenic acid, B6 or pyridoxine, B7 or biotin, B9 or folic acid, and B12. Most people do not need vitamin B supplements, and overuse can create problems. Vitamin B3, also known as niacin, is used to lower cholesterol, but it can also cause liver damage and prevent the absorption of medications if too much is taken. It should only be used under a doctor's supervision. Vitamin B6 has been promoted in the treatment of everything from depression to premenstrual syndrome, but even doses less than 500 milligrams per day may cause nerve damage and numbness in the arms and legs.

Vitamin B9, also known as folic acid, has been added to all enriched food products—such as breads, cereals, flours, pasta, and other grains—since 1996. That was the year the FDA required bakers to add enough folic acid to enriched white flour to raise the average intake by an estimated 70 to 120 micrograms a day. Since 1996, instances of neural tube birth defects such as spina bifida and anencephaly have dropped in the United States. However, researchers now worry that an overabundance of folic acid may raise the risk of colon cancer or accelerate other forms of cancer, such as leukemia. Vitamin B12 deficiencies are rare, but adults over age 50 do have a reduced ability to absorb it. Unfortunately, folic acid can make a B12 deficiency worse and can cause anemia. Doctors recommend not taking folic acid and B12 together to prevent this situation.

Americans can thank Linus Pauling, a two-time Nobel Prize winner, for our love affair with vitamin C. At age 65, when most people consider retirement, Pauling began his research on the therapeutic effects of vitamin C. He published his opinions in 1970 in a book that claimed that large amounts of vitamin C will cure the common cold and some forms of cancer. There is still no definitive scientific proof that megadoses of vitamin C have any benefits, and many scientists argue that excess intake of the vitamin is a waste of money and may actually be harmful. Still, when a cold strikes, many consumers take vitamin C.

The combination of glucosamine and chondroitin is sold as a one-two punch for people suffering from arthritis and joint pain. But these supplements, taken alone or in combination, were not found to provide significant relief from osteoarthritis pain in a study published in the *New England Journal of Medicine* (Ernst, Vassiliou, Pelletier, Clegg, & Reda, 2006) as well as in later studies in 2007 and 2008. Still, word of mouth keeps these supplements on the best-sellers list.

Vitamin D is an essential vitamin manufactured in the skin during exposure to the sun. It is fat soluble and responsible for regulating the absorption and use of calcium and phosphorous in a healthy person. This vitamin also helps build normal bones, cartilage, and teeth. It can be manufactured in the body with as little as a half-hour of sunlight. Unfortunately, vitamin D is highly toxic, and excessive consumption can cause nausea, loss of appetite, and kidney damage. Prolonged use of megadoses may result in kidney failure and death.

Omega-3 fatty acids are a booming supplement, sold for the prevention of heart disease. The American Heart Association (AHA) recommends eating fatty fish twice a week, whether from natural sources or supplements, However, there is no definitive scientific evidence that omega-3 oil supplements have any benefit in healthy individuals. Researchers are concerned that excessive fish oil consumption, whether from natural sources or supplements, may increase the risk of stroke and weaken the immune system.

Earlier Problems Although supplement makers are supposed to formulate their products according to defined chemical criteria and make sure the products contain just what the labels describe, neither the government nor the industry sets any meaningful standards for their actual contents. Worse than ineffective supplements are those that do real harm. The story of ephedra is a prime example of what can go wrong.

Products with ephedra were finally banned in the United States after almost 10 years of being linked to growing numbers of heart attacks, strokes, seizures, and deaths. The ephedra plant, known as *ma huang* in Chinese, had been used for centuries in China to treat coughs, colds, fever, sweating, congestion, shortness of breath, and water retention. The herb was processed into a drug called ephedrine that appeared in the United States in weight-loss formulas. The FDA banned the combination of ephedrine and caffeine in 1983 based on growing concerns about the safety of the drug mixture. Problems continued because even though the two ingredients together were illegal, ephedra, the natural herb, was still legal in the United States.

Unfortunately for consumers, ephedra was classified as an herb and not a drug, so its use in diet pills continued, along with its potentially deadly consequences. Finally, in 2003, it appeared that ephedra might have played a role in the death of Baltimore Orioles pitcher Steve Bechler. The ensuing public outrage helped the FDA push through a ban on ephedra in March 2004.

Congress did respond to concerns about how difficult it was for the FDA to ban ephedra sales even after thousands of people suffered serious health problems. They passed the Dietary Supplement and Nonprescription Drug Consumer Protection Act in December 2006. The act mandated that manufacturers of dietary supplements and nonprescription drugs notify the FDA about serious adverse problems related to their products, especially deaths, life-threatening events, hospitalizations, significant disabilities, birth defects, or the need for medical intervention based on their products. Manufacturers were also required to add a contact telephone number or address to their product labels for consumers.

Another tragic case that involved a dietary supplement began in 1994 when a growing number of patients from a Belgian weight-loss clinic developed severe kidney disease. By the time the herb aristolochia was identified as the culprit, there were 105 documented cases of rapid kidney failure. Some 30 of the women died, and at least half of the rest had to have kidney transplants. The herb and its derivative, aristolochic acid, were quickly banned in seven European countries, as well as in Egypt, Japan, Canada, and Venezuela.

In the United States, the FDA acted within the scope of its powers, and in May 2000 wrote a letter to manufacturers and distributors urging them to stop selling supplements containing aristolochic acid. By the time the FDA wrote a second letter, again asking companies to stop selling the dangerous herb, at least two new cases of kidney failure linked to aristolochia were reported in the United States.

How can it be that this ancient Chinese herb was never found to be toxic before? Apparently one of its most insidious features is that damage or illness occurs years after the herb is taken. The delayed symptoms kept people from understanding its toxicity until the Belgian doctors linked the pieces together. An editorial published in the June 2004 issue of the journal *Nephrology* described the hundreds of cases that have since been linked to aristolochic acid poisoning in China. The director of the renal division of Peking University First Hospital in Beijing added more bad news: aristolochic acid is extremely carcinogenic, so patients who survived the initial crisis could face cancer later in their lives.

A 2006 study in *Clinical Toxicology* examined raw herbs purchased from Chinese wholesalers and found that four of the six contained aristolochic acid; of seven manufactured products examined, two contained it as well (Cheung, Xue, Leung, Chan, & Li, 2006). This raised serious concerns about the safety of Chinese herbal remedies. Researchers suggested lax regulatory controls, widespread misidentification, and incorrect herbs substituted by suppliers as key reasons for the problem (Cheung et al., 2006). Aristolochic acid was still available online according to a 2008 article in *Kidney International*. The article reported that despite FDA warnings about the safety of botanical remedies containing aristolochic acid, these herbs were still being sold via the Internet (Debelle, Vanherweghem, & Nortier, 2008).

Before using a dietary supplement, consumers should check with their health care professionals and ask themselves several important questions, including whether the supplement interacts with any prescription or over-the-counter medicines they are taking; if there are any side effects; what the correct dose for that individual product is; if there are any foods, drugs or other supplements that should be avoided while taking the product; and where to get more information about the product or dietary supplements in general. Additional resources about dietary supplements include web-based resources such as PubMed (www.ncbi.nlm.nih.gov/pubmed/) through the National Institutes of Health, which is the federal focal point for medical research in the United States, and on the FDA website (www.fda.gov). Consumers should also consult their health care provider if they have any questions.

Sharon Zoumbaris

See also Ephedra/Ephedrine; Pauling, Linus; Vitamins.

References

Barrett, Stephen E. "Quackwatch," www.quackwatch.com/.

Brody, Jane E. "Potential for Harm in Dietary Supplements." *New York Times* (April 8, 2008): F7.

Cheung, Thomas P., Charlie Xue, Kelvin Leung, Kelvin Chan, and Chun G. Li. "Aristolochic Acids Detected in Some Raw Chinese Medicinal Herbs and Manufactured Herbal Products." *Clinical Toxicology* 44, no. 4 (June 2006): 371.

Debelle, Frederic D., Jean-Louis Vanherweghem, and Joelle L. Nortier. "Aristolochic Acid Nephropathy: A Worldwide Problem." *Kidney International* 74 (July 2, 2008): 158–169.

Ernst, E., Vassiliou, V. S., J. P. Pelletier, D. O. Clegg, and D. J. Reda. "Glucosamine and Chondroitin Sulfate for Knee Osteoarthritis." *New England Journal of Medicine* 354, no. 20 (May 18, 2006): 2184–85.

Harris, Gardner. "Study Finds Supplements Contain Contaminants." *New York Times* (May 25, 2010), www.nytimes.com.

Institute of Medicine of the National Academies. "Strategies to Reduce Sodium Intake in the United States" (April 20, 2010), www.iom.edu/Reports/2010/Strategies-to-Reduce-Sodium-Intake-in-the-United-States.aspx.

Jacobson, Michael F. "Supplement Scams." *Nutrition Action Healthletter* 34, no. 7 (September 2007): 2.

Johnson, Michael. "Senate Hearing Criticizes Lack of Supplement Regulation by FDA, DEA." *Drug Store News* 31, no. 13 (October 26, 2009): 29.

National Center for Health Statistics. "Dietary Supplement Use among U.S. Adults Has Increased Since NHANES III (1988–1994)." NCHS Data Brief, no. 61 (April 2011), www.cdc.gov/nchs/data/databriefs/db61.pdf.

Singer, Natasha. "Ingredients of Shady Origins, Posing as Supplements." *New York Times* (August 28, 2011), www.nytimes.com/2011/08/28/business/supplement-drugs-may-contain-dangerous-ingredients.html?_r=2&ref=business.

Solorio, Season. "More Consumers Consider Themselves Regular Supplement Users, Annual Survey Results Show." Council for Responsible Nutrition, October 4, 2007, www.crnusa.org/prpdfs/CRN_PR_100407_ConsumerConfidence.pdf.

"Toxic Herb Sold via Internet." *Better Nutrition* 66, no. 1 (January 2004): 22.

DIETING

Dieting practices include various regimens and products that aim to reduce the amount of fat in the human body, specifically those that involve modifying one's intake of various types of food and calories. Since antiquity, physicians have recommended various kinds of diets for maintaining ideal body weight, but not until the 20th century did dieting become widespread and popular for all classes. Some of the most high-tech practices related to dieting and weight loss currently include medical surgeries and pharmaceutical supplements.

Origins of Modern Dieting Thomas Venner's 1620 work *Via Recta* first used the term *obesity* and described it as a hazard of the genteel classes. He argued that a return to a balanced diet and an exercise regimen could cure individuals of their acquired "fleshiness." In the 18th and 19th centuries, *corpulence* was the preferred term in writings on health, regarding it as a self-inflicted condition that resulted from overindulgence. Once a marker of wealth and status, by the late 19th and early 20th centuries, the fat body became considered a symbol of excess and pathology. Dieting regimens placed the onus upon individuals to cure themselves.

One of the early mass diets was generated by the 1863 publication of William Banting's pamphlet *A Letter on Corpulence Addressed to the Public,* which sold thousands. In it, Banting describes obesity as the most distressing of all the "parasites that affect humanity" and argues that obesity and a proper diet are widely misunderstood. Banting detailed how he "cured" himself of his own excesses after trying, in vain, to reduce his weight through various forms of exercise, trying sea air and Turkish bathing, eating only light food, and consuming gallons of "psychic and liver potassae." The only tactic that worked, he argued, was to reduce his consumption of starch and sugar. After Banting, the active participation in weight-loss regimes became a populist pastime. It was not until the beginning of the 20th century, however, that weight-loss strategies became widely available and practiced.

Currently in the West, the diet industry is enjoying a time of massive popularity given the current public health warnings about obesity and its various comorbidities (heart disease, diabetes, cancer, and many others). Weight-loss services, gyms, and prepared diet food companies are advertising in every available media format.

Rise of Fad Diets   Following the popularity of William Banting's diet regimen in the mid-19th century, a slew of radical diets promising quick weight loss appeared in the early 20th century. These new fad diets drew millions of adherents in Western societies in the wake of the shift in bodily aesthetics from corpulence to slimness in the late 19th century.

In 1917, Lulu Hunt Peters published *Diet and Health, With Key to the Calories,* which advocated a diet plan that limited one's intake to 1,200 calories per day. The influence of Peters's thesis has endured for nearly a century, with nutritionists continuing to prescribe diet plans between 1,200 and 1,500 calories per day for weight loss in obese patients. Calorie counting also continues to be the cornerstone of many popular diet regimens.

In the 1920s, cigarette companies began to address the increasing public concern with slenderness by promoting cigarettes as a means of suppressing the appetite and maintaining a good figure. The 1930s saw the emergence of the first marketed diet pills. These drugs contained dinitrophenol, a central ingredient in insecticides, dyes, and explosives. However, research conducted by doctors at the time also found that the chemical had the ability to raise one's metabolism, thus enabling one to burn calories more easily. By the mid-1930s, thousands of U.S. dieters had tried dinitrophenol. However, following numerous cases of blindness and some deaths, the drug was banned.

In addition to diet aids such as tobacco and pills, food combinations became the focus of diet fads into the 1930s. The Hay diet, developed by William Hay, encouraged dieters to separate foods at mealtimes, suggesting that's one's body could not cope with numerous combinations of foods simultaneously. The Hay diet encourages followers to eat meat, dairy, bread, potatoes, and fruit at separate meals, in combination with the administering of enemas several times weekly.

Food fads and diet aids and supplements came together in the 1960s with a diet plan devised by Herman Taller. Taller rejected the importance of counting calories and instead insisted that a high-protein diet could be enjoyed without consequence, provided dieters supplemented their food intake with a pill (invented by Taller) that contained polyunsaturated vegetable oil. Taller published his diet plan in the book *Calories Don't Count,* which sold more than 2 million copies.

In the 1970s, food fads continued, with the grapefruit diet (also known as the Hollywood diet) enjoying widespread appeal among women seeking rapid weight loss. The diet promised a loss of 10 pounds in two weeks and involved variants from eating half a grapefruit prior to each meal (with no more than a mere 800 calories consumed daily) to simply drinking grapefruit juice and eating the fruit for 18 days. The diet was condemned as dangerous and hazardous to the health of dieters, and yet it continued to be popular, and it is still promoted as an effective crash diet.

Beginning in the 1970s, anticarbohydrate fad diets promised to be the new and ultimate weight-loss solution. The best known and most enduring of these diets was the Atkins diet (known formally as the Atkins Nutritional Approach), developed by Robert Atkins (1930–2003) in 1972. Atkins devised the diet to address his own weight problem; it is based on a commitment to a high-protein, low-carbohydrate daily food intake. Thousands of patients sought treatment from Atkins, and in the early years of the 21st century, the Atkins diet continued to be one of the most popular fad diets, with celebrity adherents endorsing its effectiveness and ensuring its ongoing influence.

Numerous other fad diets emerged in the latter part of the 20th century, many concerned with finding a fine balance or ratio for food intake. One such popular diet is the Zone diet, devised by Barry Sears (1947–), which is concerned primarily with achieving optimal hormone balance, particularly insulin levels. Sears suggests that a particular intake ratio of protein to carbohydrate affects a harmony in one's hormone levels, thus triggering weight loss.

One of the more recent fad diets developed in Miami, Florida, by Arthur Agatson is the South Beach diet. This plan designates "good carbs" and "good fats" and positions these as the cornerstones of the diet plan for weight loss and cardiac health. Agatson draws on evidence that suggests that refined ("bad") carbohydrates are absorbed by the body too rapidly, affecting insulin's ability to metabolize fats and sugars. Similarly, he insists on the link between "bad fats" and cardiovascular disease.

In the last few decades, diet fads have been propelled by the endorsements of celebrities who have allegedly had weight-loss successes with particular food regimens. In light of this, the term *fad diet* has come to be replaced more commonly with "*celebrity diet*—a variety of which are routinely offered in women's magazines.

Weight-Loss Companies   Jenny Craig, an American woman, cofounded her highly successful weight-loss company of the same name in 1983 following weight gain after pregnancy. Craig pioneered a prepackaged food diet program that became one of the most well known weight-loss solutions in the West. The Jenny Craig plan consists of more than 500 weight-loss centers as well as an extensive line of packaged foods. The core of the Jenny Craig diet program (and of many other similar organizations) is the diet plan: usually a menu grid of seven days, prescribing foods to be eaten at breakfast, lunch, and dinner (with snacks) that is limited to between 1,200 and 1,500 calories daily, depending on one's starting weight.

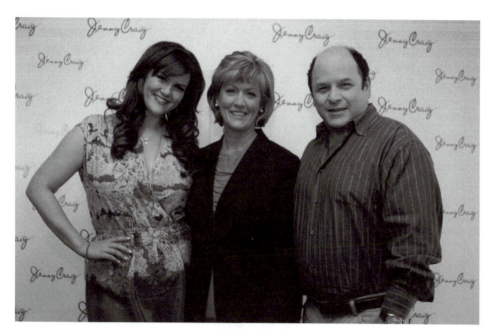

Actress Sara Rue, on left, Jenny Craig CEO Patti Larchet, and actor Jason Alexander pose for a photo at Jenny Craig's New Year's weight-loss resolution "check-in" at the SLS Hotel Beverly Hills in California on February 3, 2010. Alexander signed on as a Jenny Craig spokesman in 2010. (AP/Wide World Photos)

Many weight-loss companies provide services, including weekly consultations or meetings in order for the client to be weighed in and to provide social support for weight loss. Between weekly meetings, many plans insist that one record one's daily eating and activity patterns as well as any difficulties or food challenges one may face. This is often known as a food diary, in which one must detail precisely what is eaten at each meal, at each snack time, the size of portions, the times at which one eats, and so on.

What marks the diet strategy of Jenny Craig and similar weight-loss organizations, such as Weight Watchers, is total vigilance. Weight-loss organizations generally advocate highly regulated food intake. Ironically, food does not become a secondary concern for the fat body, but instead eating is brought to the fore and is scrutinized more intensely than ever before. Weighing out portions of meat, learning what constitutes a fat or bread exchange, and careful negotiation of dining out with friends makes eating a matter of constant surveillance.

Gender and Dieting   Although both men and women are overweight, overwhelmingly, the target audience for modern advertising about diets and food intake regulation is women. Some feminists have argued that dieting amounts to a form of disciplining women's bodies to conform to the pressures of normative beauty ideals that are highly gendered. Others have linked the Western obsession with dieting to eating disorders.

Feminist theorist Susan Bordo looks at the phenomenon of dieting and the endlessly fraught relationship women have with food in her best-selling book *Unbearable Weight*. She argues that society insists this relationship must be stringently managed; that the image of a woman surrendering herself to delicious food with abandon is taboo. Bordo argues that there is a moral panic about excessive desire in contemporary Western societies. To allow desires to run unchecked connotes a modern understanding of addiction. All women are supposed to have a desire for food, beset by a number of anxieties about her intake, and, as Bordo highlights, many advertising campaigns generate food anxieties.

Analyzing advertisers' manipulation of the problem of weight watching for the contemporary woman, Bordo argues that diet food advertising targets women's anxieties by proposing guilt-free solutions to their desire for food and hunger for satisfaction. Bordo explores the current trope of control used in food advertisements, which suggests that women are constantly battling their desire for food. Words such as *mastery* and *control* feature prominently now in advertisements targeting women.

Dieting, Control, and Loss of Pleasure Dale Atrens has argued that food has replaced sex as the leading source of guilt in our society. His work *The Power of Pleasure* is a rebuttal of the ascetic restraint and self-denial of the dieting culture. Atrens argues that in following constant and massive trends such as low-fat, low-salt, high-protein, and low-carbohydrate diets, we are endangering our health rather than improving it. Atrens exposes a "new Puritanism" in dieting culture that suggests that ill health results from unbridled passions and is therefore a symptom of moral weakness. In this logic, fat people are victims of their own "sins." Atrens notes that the eating practices of our everyday lives have taken on an almost religious significance. One's status as a "believer" or an "infidel" is to be found in the condition of one's body.

Many alternative modes of eating have been posited in order to redress the problems with dieting, particularly where they affect women's sense of self and lived experiences. One such model is proposed by psychotherapist Susie Orbach in her landmark text *Fat Is a Feminist Issue*. Orbach's central theory is that fat women eat compulsively to stay fat, in order to create a sexual buffer between themselves and a repressive patriarchal society. The conception that fat surrounds a female body as a kind of armor to protect against one's sexuality, or the exploitation of it, is central.

Orbach posits that women are taught from a very young age that women's bodies are coveted as sexual commodities, that they must be aesthetically pleasing in order to fulfill feminine roles (Orbach, 1984, p. 20). The role of women is a sexualized one, and female participation in society is regulated by the attractiveness of women's bodies and what they can offer. Fat emerges as a barrier to a fulfillment of traditional female sexual roles that are upheld by a continuing maintenance of the body (Orbach, 1984, p. 43). In response to diet practices and a weight-loss culture, Orbach urges women to be more accepting of their bodies. Rather than promoting diets as a response to excess weight, Orbach suggests the need to reconnect to one's body and appetite, to eat only when hungry, and to reject the notion of dieting.

Critics of Orbach have argued that her thesis automatically links fatness to compulsive overeating. Some women argue that their weight is caused by genetic or physiological issues or that it resulted from pregnancy and childbearing.

A Global Epidemic of Obesity   Despite the long history of diet regimens and the immense expansion of the weight-loss industry in Western countries (and its opponents such as Orbach), the World Health Organization has declared that the world (but with particular emphasis on the West) is in the grip of an obesity epidemic. Studies have confirmed that the number of people now considered clinically (and often morbidly) obese has risen steadily and accounts for the dramatic increases in rates of heart disease, diabetes, and other obesity-related illnesses. Given this, obesity has begun to be reconceptualized within medical discourses as a disease rather than as an effect of the absence of individual moral fortitude and self-control.

However, the moral aspersions cast on people deemed as fat persist in the popular imagination. Morality and medicine are thus irrevocably intertwined in discourses about obesity, and a panic has emerged about the disease of obesity and how best to treat it, given the relative failure of a range of dieting practices. In response to the moral panic engendered in and through medical discourses and Western public health directives, drastic (and mainly irreversible) surgical techniques and interventions into the obese body have been developed and have grown in popularity as last-resort options for those deemed obese. These procedures are known as bariatric or weight-loss surgeries, and while they vary in specific surgical techniques, all share a common premise: to alter the shape, size, or function of a patient's stomach to force a regulation and reduction of one's food intake.

Bariatric Surgery   In the past decade, surgery has become a significant weight-loss practice for people who have been determined to be obese, especially for those deemed morbidly obese (or have a body mass index [BMI] of 40 or higher). Various bariatric procedures involve creating malabsorption (interfering with the body's ability to absorb nutrients that are ingested) or restriction (severely limiting the amount of food a person eats to the point of feeling full). Gastric bypass involves dividing the patient's stomach into two sections, consisting of a smaller upper pouch and a larger lower section. A section of the patient's intestine is rerouted to the smaller upper pouch, thereby bypassing the larger stomach section (and the volume of food it can potentially hold). While this is clearly major surgery, what is appealing about bariatric surgeries is the fact that they are most often undertaken via laparoscopy, or "keyhole surgery." This means that, rather than one long incision, a series of very small incisions are made, and tools are inserted (one of these a camera) to conduct the procedure and minimize invasiveness and patient recovery times.

Bariatric surgery has a number of variant procedures, including laparoscopic gastric band, which is reversible. The gastric band (of which there are a number of types) is a silicone structure that encircles the stomach, creating a small upper pouch and larger lower pouch. The band has on its inner surface an adjustable balloon that can be filled with saline to increase a patient's restriction or deflated to allow greater food intake (for example, during pregnancy). Gastric banding has become increasingly popular, given that it has fewer risks than radical bypass surgery, and a patient's food intake can be adjusted after surgery simply via local anesthetic.

The result of bariatric surgery is to radically limit the amount of food a patient can ingest, thereby reducing the calories absorbed by the body, or to decrease the amount of nutrients absorbed by food that is ingested, or both. The result is rapid and dramatic weight loss. It should be noted that patients are routinely screened for eligibility for this procedure prior to undergoing surgery, but the baseline BMI varies according to whether a patient is clinically diagnosed as being morbidly obese or whether a patient is obese with associated comorbidities (having a BMI between 35 and 40).

The increased popularity of bariatric surgeries over the last decade demonstrates the fact that these procedures have come to be regarded as another option for those wishing to lose weight. Weight loss is popularly understood as a task that is defined by deprivation, hardship, and work: rigidly monitoring one's food intake and exercise is required in any diet, and is often not a pleasurable or enjoyable experience. Because of this dominant way of imagining the project of weight loss, bariatric surgical interventions are simultaneously appealing to those who have undertaken numerous diets previously and are regarded by others as radical procedures deployed by those who have failed in previous attempts to lose weight. Weight-loss surgeries have been conceptualized by many as a quick-fix option and a way out of living in a fat body in a culture that abhors excess flesh. These processes are linked to cultural understandings about morality.

Samantha Murray

See also Atkins, Robert C.; Bariatric Surgery; Calories; Fats; Weight Watchers.

References

Atrens, Dale. *The Power of Pleasure.* Sydney, Australia: Duffy and Snellgrove, 2000.

Bordo, Susan. *Unbearable Weight: Feminism, Western Culture, and the Body.* Berkeley: University of California Press, 1993.

Chernin, Kim. *The Obsession: Reflections on the Tyranny of Slenderness.* New York: Harper Perennial, 1994.

Orbach, Susie. *Fat Is a Feminist Issue.* London: Arrow Books, 1978.

DIETING, ONLINE RESOURCES

The Internet has expanded rapidly since its early days and now provides entertainment, news, financial links, and endless social networking opportunities for a wide international audience. Among the fastest growing online services is Internet dieting.

Dieting is never easy, and many Americans are turning to the privacy of Internet dieting since it does not require meetings or weigh-ins. Instead, support comes from diet forums where people share anxieties and dilemmas with others from the comfort and anonymity of their home at all hours of the day or night.

Thousands of diet websites exist, and most do not make any money or profit according to Marketdata Enterprises, a market research firm, founded in 1979, that has tracked the U.S. weight loss market since 1989. Marketdata found in its 2010 analysis that with many revenue-generating dieting sites the trend is moving toward free, advertiser-supported sites with free tools for tracking food and activities (PRWeb Newswire, 2011). The fee-based diet programs continue to grow and they offer the same online tools as their free counterparts along with e-mail counseling from nutritionists or dietitians. Both free and fee-based sites also provide meal planning, menu ideas, and recipes. The difference is that fee-based sites offer the opportunity to buy the diet program or diet products added to the cost of their services.

Among Marketdata's major findings, the online dieting market was worth some $910 million in 2010 with the share of dieters that use websites growing from just over 17 percent in 2005 to some 24 percent in 2010 (PRWeb Newswire, 2011). At the same time, statistics showed the number of dieters using a diet center dropped by that same amount—about 7 percent from 2005 to 2010.

Reasons dieters give for switching to online dieting include the 24/7 access, the privacy, and anonymity. Many dieters are very self-conscious about their appearance and fear being judged by others, so by participating online they do not have to see a coach or other group members face to face. Another plus are the chat rooms, diet forums, and other websites, which can provide a much wider support system than just the members of a local weight-loss group. When online, dieters can find others who share their diet frustrations as well as others who are willing to share their weight-loss successes beyond their own geographic community, state, or country. All this support can provide valuable motivation.

Cost is another plus for those involved with Internet dieting; even websites that charge subscription or registration fees are much less expensive than meeting with a nutritionist or personal trainer or joining a weight-loss program, especially one that requires prepackaged meals. In fact, established weight-loss programs have taken note of the growth in Internet dieting and now offer a much more visible online presence. According to Marketdata, Weight Watchers has increased its number of website users to 1 million paid subscribers as of late 2010, making its website the fastest growing division of the company and bringing in over $196 million in revenue for 2009 (PRWeb Newswire, 2011).

However, there are negatives as well as positives to online dieting. The biggest concern among health professionals is with the sites offering misinformation and bad advice. Another key concern among health care professionals is that while some websites claim close contact or relationships with doctors and nutritionists, they may actually use peer information, and their message boards may be completely unmonitored from a health or nutrition standpoint. Another key issue is the lack of accountability for the individual dieter. It becomes much easier for those looking for any excuse to avoid dieting to simply not log on. There is no one to question their lack of motivation, which would be more likely to happen if the dieter was missing an appointment with a nutritionist or weighing in with a diet group. Internet dieting websites also work better for users with computer skills to make the most of the tools or programs. For those who are not computer savvy, their lack of skill could lead to higher costs or frustration as product marketing on some websites could camouflage hidden fees.

Internet dieting sites differ in their approach even as they offer the same tools and information. Popular websites include eDiets.com, WeightWatchers.com, Fit Day.com, PersonalDiets.com, MyNetDiary.com, SparkPeople.com, and South-beachdiet.com just to name a few. Do they work? While the American Dietetic Association offers no specific opinion on their success rate, they do recommend dieters stay away from quick-fix or fad diets. Instead, to be effective, online weight-loss programs should include key components such as diet recommendations, recipes and menus, a tracking system or food diary tool, exercise recommendations, a social aspect to offer contact with other members such as chat rooms or bulletin boards, and the opportunity for individual feedback or nutrition counseling.

Dieters are advised to be watchful for scam sites, which often promise a quick fix and make weight-loss claims that sound too good to be true. These sites may also push products that are advertised on their site. Dieters should pay close attention to costs associated with these sites and be especially wary of hidden fees. If something sounds too good to be true, it probably is too good to be true. In addition, it may actually turn out to contain something like spam, a type of electronic messaging system that sends bulk messages indiscriminately in large volumes, or it may hide viruses that can damage individual computers.

Among individual dieting Internet sites, eDiets.com is an early industry leader, in operation since 1998 with home meal delivery since 2006. eDiets continues to offer a growing assortment of services and provides diets for weight loss, seasonal eating, a glycemic diet, Mediterranean diet, plus an eating plan based on Bill Phillips's book, *Eating for Life*. Under the heading of healthy living plans, the website offers a wheat-free meal strategy, a heart-smart or low-sodium plan, a hypoglycemic/low-sugar eating program, a vegetarian eating plan, and several other choices for specific dietary needs.

It also offers meal delivery for seven days or five days of food. Other services include a personalized fitness plan, live phone support from certified and registered dietitians, and 24/7 online member support. A variety of costs are associated with membership, including subscriptions to the online weight-loss program and subscriptions to the meal delivery program. The company, based in Fort Lauderdale, Florida, also generates revenue through the sale of advertising and products from its online store and earns licensing revenues for the use of its materials by other nutrition websites.

Weight Watchers online, another industry giant, has a stylish website with online tools that track eating progress. It provides customized meal plans, a list of power foods, restaurant guides, and healthier versions of favorite recipes. It also offers instant "Problem Solvers" for everyday challenges and workouts for all fitness levels with video demonstrations. It offers special sign-up promotions along with a standard monthly plan at just under $50 for the first month and $17.95 for each additional month.

SparkPeople, a free Internet dieting website, boasts 5 million website visits per month. It offers tools such as a calorie counter and meal plans, a fitness program, a motivation system of earned awards and trophies, and feedback reports about individual weight loss progress. The site features recipes and a variety of blogs about subjects such as SparkSavings, which has tools and tips for managing personal finances, BabyFit.com, and SparkTeens, a modified version of the main website geared for 13- to 17-year-olds.

Still, Internet dieting is not for everyone, and those interested in joining an online program should consider some important points before paying subscription rates or fees. Is online dieting is a good lifestyle fit? Is there a free option that does the same thing? What kind of specific support will be offered to members? Who developed the program? Do services include a registered dietitian or any qualified health professionals? Also, is the site medically, nutritionally, and psychologically supervised? Individuals should ask themselves whether they are self-motivated enough for an online program; is the website easy to navigate, and are the tools easy to understand and use. Dieters should also consider if they can afford the price, if the program includes accountability, and, finally, if there is a cancellation policy or a guarantee of weight loss.

Sharon Zoumbaris

See also Calories; Dieting; Exercise; Weight Watchers.

References

DeAvila, Joseph. "The Social-Networking Diet." *TecTrends* (October 10, 2007).

Downie, Chris. *The Spark: The 28-Day Breakthrough Plan for Losing Weight, Getting Fit and Transforming Your Life.* Carlsbad, CA: Hay House, 2009.

eDiets.com. "eDiets Online Diet Plans," http://healthnews.ediets.com/start.

Lofshult, Diane. "How Effective Is Cyberdieting?" *IDEA Fitness Journal* 1, no. 2 (July–August 2004): 130.

Platkin, Charles Stuart. *The Diet Detective's Count Down: 7,500 of Your Favorite Food Counts with Their Exercise Equivalents for Walking, Running, Biking, Swimming, Yoga and Dance.* New York: Fireside/Simon & Schuster, 2007.

PRWeb Newswire. "Online Dieting Represents a $910 Million Market" (January 12, 2011), www.prweb.com/releases/2011/01/prweb4961684.htm.

"Quick Fixes Aren't the Answer for Healthful Weight Control: Learn to Spot Fads and Steer Clear Then Seek Proven, Long-Term Solutions." *American Dietetic Association* (January 17, 2007), www.eatright.org.

SparkPeople.com. "Lose Weight, Get Fit and Feel Great with a New Approach to Weight Loss," www.sparkpeople.com.

Stroup, Katherine. "Desktop Dieting: Is the Internet the Answer to Losing Those Extra Pounds?" *Newsweek* (May 20, 2002): 70.

DIETS, FAD

What will Americans do to lose weight? Just about anything, it seems. Over the past century, a variety of quick and easy fixes have flooded the market. Many of these products or devices are costly; some are not safe; and some are simply outrageous. Consider a bristle brush to scrub fat away or magic weight-loss earrings.

Dietitians and physicians will say that there is only one fundamental combination to help most people lose weight: eat less and exercise more. Through its Dietary Guidelines for Americans, the government recommends an assortment of foods: vegetables, fruits, grains, fat-free or low-fat milk products, fish, lean meat, poultry, and beans.

While weight loss may not seem like a topic of debate, there are distinct and seemingly opposing voices. Indeed, the voices of those who advocate a low-carbohydrate diet have gained volume recently. In essence, they say that the emphasis on low-fat diets over the past few decades has not resulted in weight loss for Americans. In fact, just the opposite—more American adults and children are overweight and obese today than just a decade ago. They blame carbohydrates, which cause insulin levels to spike, which in turn make people feel hungrier again sooner. They say that diets rich in high-fat foods and low in carbohydrates will help people lose weight.

Yet that doesn't mean that Americans should immediately forgo the salad and order more fries. The headlines may be more sensational than the truth. Much of mainstream medicine still stands by its emphasis on a balanced diet limiting high-fat and high-cholesterol foods.

What is happening with the current debate mirrors what happens so often with weight-loss topics: Americans are looking for a quick fix. People want to eat a food or type of food that will make the pounds disappear. Or they want to avoid a food or certain foods that will cause them to put on weight.

There's no doubt that people have lost some weight following specific diet plans. But is it the best way, or even the only way to lose weight? For most people, moderation may do the trick. Cut down on sweets, cut down on fats, cut down on carbohydrates. Increase your level of daily physical activity. The result is fewer calories consumed and more calories burned. In the long run, this combination results in long-lasting weight maintenance, not just a quick-fix weight loss.

In all cases, before starting a diet to aggressively lose weight, see a doctor. Too sudden or rapid a weight loss can have severe consequences. And realize, too, that losing weight is just one part of healthy living. Maintaining a good weight and a diet that provides you with enough energy to feel good and be active is a lifelong goal.

Early History of Fad Diets In dieting, as in life, everybody wants a quick answer, a quick meal, and quick success. The elusive promise of quick weight loss is the driving force behind the popularity of best-selling books, powders, liquids, pills, and programs. Each year these new fad diets appear on the scene—everything from high-protein, low-carbohydrate plans to fasting and liquid meals. And Americans—teens included—desperate to lose weight, embrace them enthusiastically. At any given time, 15 percent to 35 percent of Americans are actively dieting. And they have good reason to be concerned about losing weight since the latest findings from the Centers for Disease Control and Prevention's (CDC) National Health and Nutrition Examination Survey showed more than 72 million American adults were considered obese in 2008. Additionally, some 17 percent of children and adolescents aged 2 to 19 were also obese (Ogden, 2010).

These sobering statistics go a long way toward explaining why the lure of quick, easy weight-loss schemes is so hard to resist. Unfortunately, fad diets aren't healthy and don't work for the long haul. Consider this: some 80 percent of all dieters will regain their lost weight in one to five years (Wing, 2005), Americans spend more than $40 billion on dieting and diet-related products each year (Marketdata, 2007).

Not only are diet theories and products nothing new, they date back centuries to a time when people had no scientific understanding of digestion and food assimilation. And while today's consumers make their decisions based on improved research and understanding of how the body works, they still fall victim to fad diets that focus on one true aspect of nutrition, which is then exaggerated to an extreme. For women in particular, the lure of fast, effortless weight loss is strongly tied to the demands of fashion and beauty.

Thinness as a beauty ideal surfaced in the early 1800s with the emerging Victorian woman. This thin, genteel, docile creature replaced the idealized voluptuous women painted in the 16th and 17th centuries by artists like Rembrandt and Rubens. And as thinness became the defining feature of beauty in the United States, an 18-inch waist became the holy grail of physical perfection. Unfortunately, this measurement was so out of line with normal body dimensions that to achieve it most women resorted to a practice called tightlacing, a procedure immortalized in Margaret Mitchell's *Gone With the Wind*. This extreme corset tightening eventually caused headaches, fainting spells, and uterine and spinal disorders.

In the 1830s, as literacy increased, technology advanced, and the publishing industry expanded, American women became the target of medical advice books as well as beauty manuals, all of which encouraged thinness. Still, there were critics like writer Harriet Beecher Stowe who vigorously lamented the increasing problems associated with dieting and the national preoccupation with thinness.

Lois Banner, in *American Beauty*, quoted Beecher Stowe's opinion of the misuse of dieting by American women. "We in America have got so far out of the way of a womanhood that has any vigor of outline or opulence of physical proportions, that, when we see a woman made as a woman ought to be, she strikes us as a monster. Our willowy girls are afraid of nothing so much as growing stout; and if a young lady begins to round into proportions like the women in Titian's or Gorgione's picture, she is distressed above measure, and begins to make secret inquiries into reducing diet, and to cling desperately to the strongest corset."

A decade earlier, English poet Lord Byron influenced beauty and diet practices and standards in the United States as well as in Europe. According to scholars, Byron was known for his tendency to gain weight. By 1822 the poet had starved himself into what biographers call an unnatural thinness. In fact, Banner, in *American Beauty,* traces the popularity of drinking vinegar to lose weight to Byron, whose favorite weight-loss regimen was to subsist for some days on vinegar and water. But Byron's most lasting contribution to the popularity of fad diets came from his statement that the sight of a woman eating was disgusting. Biographer Leslie A. Marchand attributed this quote to the poet in *Byron: A Portrait.* "A woman," Byron wrote, "should never be seen eating or drinking, unless it be lobster salad and champagne, the only truly feminine and becoming viands." Following this remark, fashion historians say women in Europe and the United States took up systematic fasting. Indeed, thanks to Byron and other cultural factors, dieting was commonplace by 1900.

Others who influenced society's early love affair with diets included Englishman William Banting, credited with writing the first diet book. Born in 1797, by age 40 the 5-foot-5-inch Banting was extremely obese. He consulted doctor after doctor, but nothing helped, and his growing girth was ruining his life. By age 60, he was unable to stoop and tie his shoes, and he walked backward down the stairs to lessen the stress on his joints. Finally, in 1863 at age 66, he consulted William Harvey, a surgeon known for his starch-free and sugar-free diet treatment for diabetes.

Banting immediately lost weight by eating only lean meats and dry toast and eventually went from a high of 202 pounds to a comfortable 156 pounds. Eager to share his success with the world, Banting wrote his diet book, a testimonial titled *A Letter on Corpulence.* Following its publication, *banting* or *to bant,* meaning to diet, became a household word in England and in the United States. At his death in 1878, more than 58,000 copies of his diet book had been sold, and a total of 12 editions had been published between 1863 and 1902.

Meanwhile, in the United States in 1837, talk of diet and health nearly incited a riot in Boston. Sylvester Graham, an evangelical New England preacher and speaker faced an angry mob one evening as he attempted to lecture on food and hygiene reform. Graham was a controversial figure whose spartan views on diet and drinking had strongly divided the Boston crowd. Critics of Grahamism included the writer Ralph Waldo Emerson, who mocked Graham as "the prophet of bran bread and pumpkins." While Graham was also called the father of all modern diet crazes, he is most widely remembered as the namesake of the graham cracker.

His career as a lecturer grew out of his earlier study of human physiology, diet, and nutrition, a choice largely influenced by his 1830 appointment as general agent for the Pennsylvania Temperance Society. During this time, Graham developed the "Graham system," as he liked to call it, based on the French vitalist school of medicine. He believed nutrition had moral as well as physical qualities, and any desire for food or drink, except for stark hunger and thirst, was depraved. Gluttony was a debilitating expression of an unhealthy urge, and Graham was determined to launch an all-out war on debauchery and gluttony.

Graham was one of the first U.S. health reformers to reach a mass audience via lectures. He traveled a circuit through Massachusetts, Rhode Island, Maine, New York, New Jersey, and Pennsylvania. In his talks he recommended a strictly vegetarian diet but did allow for a small daily ration of roasted beef or boiled mutton for those who wanted some meat. He did not believe in cooking vegetables—or in warm food in general, since he considered heat a stimulant. And he was particularly adamant about the evils of commercially baked white bread, made from highly refined flour. Graham argued that any good wife and mother must feed her family homemade, coarse bread, served stale after 24 hours.

Long after Graham's death in 1851, his followers, called Grahamites, whose ranks included John Harvey Kellogg of cornflake fame, would continue to advocate vegetarianism, temperance, and bran bread. Many of the most ardent Grahamites were women who were attracted to his recommendations on diet, health care, and dress reform, which criticized disfiguring corsets and advocated loose, comfortable clothing. And while knowledge about nutrition would not be discovered until the early 20th century, Graham was also ahead of his time in understanding the importance of fiber in the diet. Even though the modern version of graham crackers are a far cry from the coarse, whole-wheat bread Graham championed in his time, he was clearly an early voice in preaching that you are what you eat.

Sylvester Graham died in 1851, but his influence on the U.S. diet was only beginning. Per capita meat consumption began to decline as Americans shed their fears of fresh fruit and vegetables and began to eat more balanced meals. Graham had moved public opinion away from gluttony and poor digestion toward slenderness and eating to produce good health. Although Graham died in the 19th century, his way of thinking significantly influenced another man who founded a 20th-century version of Grahamism. Like Graham, Bernard Adolphus McFadden, born in 1868 near Mill Spring, Missouri, believed there was a specific way to eat and live that would produce ultimate health and longevity. He was a man who practiced what he preached, and historians believe his philosophy, known as physical culture, is largely at the root of today's health and fitness consciousness in the United States.

The core belief of McFadden's philosophy was that people got sick because of poor diet, lack of proper exercise, stale air, lack of sunshine, tobacco, alcohol, and drugs. Like Graham, McFadden believed meat should play a minor part in the diet. He preferred fruits, vegetables, and whole grains, and, like Graham, he also thought white bread was the worst food a person could eat. He advocated fasting on a regular basis and believed it was a cure for all ailments.

Another important component of his physical culture regime was regular exercise, such as walking, and he encouraged women not to wear corsets or any kind of restrictive clothing. In 1892 Bernard McFadden changed his first name to Bernarr and his last name to Macfadden. His third wife, Mary, wrote in her book titled *Dumbbells and Carrot Strips* that Macfadden believed the changes would glamorize his name while at the same time making him sound more robust.

Macfadden's ultimate philosophy of health was shaped by his early years as a sickly child. By the time he was 11, both his parents were dead—his father of alcoholism and his mother of tuberculosis. He finally overcame his poor health when relatives in Illinois took him in. Working on their farm turned him into a strong, healthy teenager. At 5-feet-6-inches tall, he was not a big man but he had incredible stamina and energy and developed his 145 pounds into a powerful upper body and a strong chest.

In 1899 Macfadden launched *Physical Culture* magazine with its motto, "Weakness is a Crime: Don't Be a Criminal." It was an immediate success, and by the 1930s, his publishing empire included *True Story, True Romances, Photoplay,* and the sensational tabloids *Midnight* and the *New York Graphic,* a publication where young Walter Winchell got his start as a writer. At the same time, Macfadden also began to organize and promote bodybuilding competitions for men and women. Macfadden was so convinced he was right about health and nutrition that he campaigned to be the country's first secretary of health in the cabinet of President Franklin D. Roosevelt. When that failed, he campaigned for the Republican nomination for president in 1936, promoting himself through his publications and funding campaign expenses with money from his business. The results were disastrous: stockholders ousted him from his publishing company, he failed to win the nomination, and he lost a great deal of money.

Macfadden's eventual undoing came from his need to carry his ideas to an extreme. In 1955 he developed a urinary tract blockage. Since he believed fasting was a cure for all ailments, he attempted to treat his final illness by fasting but instead became severely emaciated. By the time he reached a hospital, doctors could do nothing to save him. He died October 12, 1955.

At the same time that U.S. men and women were trimming their waistlines through programs like Macfadden's physical culture, medical doctors were telling patients that obesity was bad for their health. This advice added authority to the new insurance industry ideal height-and-weight charts. Many insurance companies had been charging larger premiums for heavy clients since the 1830s, but as more middle-class families bought policies and as medical examinations became mandatory, Americans now looked to these ideal tables as an important indicator of their overall health. Self-styled obesity experts quickly followed, and those entrepreneurs helped shape the lucrative diet business with a hastily created array of prescription and patent medicines guaranteed to dissolve and expel unwanted fat.

These early digestive cures included Berledets, made of boric acid, cornstarch, milk, and sugar, and Human Ease, a combination of sodium bicarbonate and lard. Sassafras tea was a chief ingredient in Densmore's Corpulency Cure, while mineral water made up the bulk of Lucile Kimball's powder, along with a little soap and Epsom salt. Arsenic, used for years to stimulate the flow of digestive juices, was turned into an obesity tablet by mixing it with strychnine, caffeine, and phytolacca. Hillel Schwartz describes in *Never Satisfied* how Phytoline, made from phytolacca or pokeberry, a well-known emetic and purgative, was created and marketed as a fat-dissolving preparation.

In 1936, another manufactured drug, dinitrophenol, was sold as a weight-loss medicine. Dinitrophenol, a derivative of benzene, was commonly used in the synthesis of different color dyes. At low dosages it would speed up metabolism. Unfortunately, dieters quickly experienced serious side effects: rashes, loss of the sense of taste, and blindness from cataracts. Some who exceeded the recommended dosages of dinitrophenol died from hyperpyremia, a condition where the body literally burns itself up, according to Carl Malmberg in *Diet and Die*. Finally, the government in 1938 banned dinitrophenol. The American Medical Association's *Nostrums and Quackery* series, first published in 1912, detailed these and some of the other most blatant examples of the various fake obesity cures.

Early diet books were also growing in popularity, such as Lulu Hunt Peter's *Diet and Health* and Vance Thompson's *Eat and Grow Thin,* which reached its 112th printing in 1931. The early 1930s also saw the introduction of another new weight-loss product, the diet drink. One of the best-known reducing drinks was Dr. Stoll's Diet Aid, sold through beauty parlors in the 1930s. A combination of milk chocolate, starch, and an extract of roasted whole wheat and bran, users mixed it by the teaspoon into a cup of water as a diet substitute for breakfast and lunch.

Twenty years later in 1959, doctors at the Rockefeller Institute, studying metabolic changes, mixed together evaporated milk, corn oil, dextrose, and water and created another low-calorie diet drink whose balance of protein, fat, and carbohydrate closely resembled breast milk. Metrecal, a product of the Mead Johnson Company, famous for its Pablum baby food, reawakened the public's interest in diet drinks. Today Nestlé, another distributor of infant formulas, markets Metrecal under the brand name Carnation Slender.

Even at the height of the Depression, the diet industry was flourishing, soon to grow by leaps and bounds with the introduction of amphetamines in the late 1930s. First used clinically in the mid-1930s to treat narcolepsy, a rare disorder resulting in an uncontrollable tendency to sleep, amphetamines skyrocketed in use when doctors began prescribing them for appetite suppression and the treatment of depression. At the time, pharmacologists were actually looking for a synthetic substitute for the expensive ephedrine, which had been used to treat asthma.

Under the trade names Benzedrine, Methedrine, and Dexedrine, amphetamines, with their clear effect on appetite and weight loss became the new darling of the diet industry. Amphetamines stimulate the central nervous system by increasing heart rates and blood pressure while reducing fatigue. However, people who use amphetamines on a regular basis build up a tolerance to them until dieters need higher doses to achieve the same effects. Soon widespread use by dieters in the 1930s created related problems of drug dependency and addiction. As early as 1943, the American Medical Association publicly opposed the use of amphetamines for the treatment of obesity because of problems of dependence, but doctors continued to recommend them for dieters. Five years later, doctors began prescribing Dexedrine as the drug of choice for weight loss and justified it by adding a prescription for barbiturates to calm the amphetamine jitters.

With dieting now a growing national pastime, diet foods became fashionable. For example, in New York, Minneapolis, and five other cities, Stouffer's restaurants offered special low-calorie lunches, and the Pennsylvania Railroad featured a 470-calorie "Streamliner" on its dining car menus. Some 80 percent of U.S. supermarkets added dietetic departments filled with low-calorie foods whose sales totaled $25 million according to an August 10, 1953, article in *Time*. Post-war Americans began joining dieting groups. Take Off Pounds Sensibly (TOPS) was the first of the group programs and boasted a membership of 30,000 by the late 1950s. Overeaters Anonymous was started in 1960, Weight Watchers in 1961, and the Diet Workshop in 1965.

Calories Don't Count was the catchy title of a diet book written in 1960 by Herman Taller, a Rumanian-born physician who practiced obstetrics in Brooklyn. He told people they could eat as many protein and fatty foods as they wanted, but he recommended that dieters severely cut back on carbohydrates. His diet also prescribed six capsules a day of safflower oil. While book sales jumped to more than a million copies in less than a year, in 1962 Taller was fined $7,000 for violating the federal Food, Drug and Cosmetic Act and was sharply criticized by the U.S. Food and Drug Administration (FDA).

FDA Commissioner George Larrick, quoted in the July 13, 1962, issue of *Time*, said, "This best-selling book was deliberately created and used to promote these worthless safflower oil capsules for the treatment of obesity, cardiovascular diseases and other serious conditions. One of its main purposes was to promote the sale of a commercial product in which Dr. Taller had a financial interest." Larrick went on to say that there is no easy, simple substitute for weight loss, but added that in the end calories do count.

And so today's consumers find themselves inundated with every kind of diet product and program from Dr. Atkins to the Zone. To lose unwanted pounds, desperate dieters continue to look for magic pills and easy programs from Slim Fast to Nutri/System or Jenny Craig, from herbal capsules, skin patches, or pills to liposuction. Yet, in most cases, the pounds come back once the fad diet ends. And as Americans move into a new century, the dieting public seems ready to embrace a whole new crop of schemes and fads no matter how far-fetched. Yet the real solution has always been available. Simply eat more fruits, vegetables, and whole-grain food; eat fewer junk and fast foods; and, most important, exercise. Experts recommend at least 30 minutes of vigorous activity five days a week. If you can't find 30 minutes, try two 15-minute intervals, or even three 10-minute intervals.

Marjolijn Bijlefeld and Sharon Zoumbaris

See also Dietary Guidelines for Americans; Eating Disorders; Fast food; Graham, Sylvester; Kellogg, John Harvey; Weight Watchers.

References

Adams, Samuel Hopkins. *The Great American Fraud*. Denver: Nostalgic American Research Foundation, 1978.
Banner, Lois W. *American Beauty*. New York: Alfred A. Knopf, 1983.
"Benzedrine and Dieting." *Newsweek*, September 8, 1947, 48–49.
"Calories Do Count." *Time*, July 13, 1962: 56–57.

Cambridge World History of Food. New York: Cambridge University Press, 2000.

Malmberg, Carl. *Diet and Die.* New York: Hillman-Curl, 1935.

Marketdata Enterprises. "U.S. Weight Loss and Diet Control Market" (2007), www.marketdataenterprises.com.

Ogden, C.L., M.M. Lamb, M.D. Carroll, and K.M. Flegal. "Obesity and Socioeconomic Status in Adults: United States 1988–1994 and 2005–2008." NCHS Data Brief, no. 50. Hyattsville, MD: National Center for Health Statistics, 2010.

Ogden, C.L., M.M. Lamb, M.D. Carroll, and K.M. Flegal. "Obesity and Socioeconomic Status in Children: United States 1988–1994 and 2005–2008." NCHS Data Brief, no. 51. Hyattsville, MD: National Center for Health Statistics, 2010.

Pillsbury, Richard. *No Foreign Food: The American Diet in Time and Place.* Boulder, CO: Westview Press, 1998.

Roberts, Paul. "The New Food Anxiety." *Psychology Today,* March–April 1998, 30–40.

Schwartz, Hillel. *Never Satisfied: A Cultural History of Diets, Fantasies and Fat.* New York: Macmillan, 1986.

Wing, Rena R., and Suzanne Phelan. "Long-term Weight Loss Maintenance." *American Journal of Clinical Nutrition* 82, no. 1 (July 2005): 2225–55.

DOCTORS IN THE MEDIA

Doctors have always held a position of authority in U.S. society, so the combination of celebrity and physician has created a situation where patients now trust their health to men and women they've never met. In the early days of celebrity physicians, Dr. Benjamin Spock wrote best-selling books giving advice to parents who wanted help raising their children in the 1960s. In the 1970s and 1980s, Dr. Ruth Westheimer talked about sex over the radio with millions of Americans during her popular call-in show, *Sexually Speaking.*

Like Dr. Ruth, other top celebrity doctors have earned their celebrity status through radio, television, books, and now the Internet. They include Dr. Deepak Chopra, Dr. Phil, Dr. Oz, Dr. Drew, Dr. Sanjay Gupta, Dr. Andrew Weil, and Dr. Kevin Pho. Two of the men on this list were launched by talk show host Oprah Winfrey. Both Dr. Phil and Dr. Oz started as frequent guests on Winfrey's daytime show.

Mehmet Oz, a cardiothoracic surgeon, first appeared on Winfrey's program in 2004, and in 2009 her production company, Harpo Productions, launched his television show, *The Dr. Oz Show.* He has also published over 10 books and numerous articles and was named to *Time* magazine's 2008 list of the 100 Most Influential People. Dr. Phil McGraw met Winfrey during a 1996 lawsuit. McGraw's company, Courtroom Sciences, works with trial lawyers to conduct mock trials, behavioral analysis, and mediation. After McGraw's company helped Winfrey win the case, he appeared as an expert on her show. He launched his own nationally syndicated talk show in 2002 and has published several books, four of which made the *New York Times* best-seller list.

Dr. Deepak Chopra is a speaker, writer, and follower of Ayurveda and alternative medicine. He was the founding president of the American Association of Ayurvedic Medicine, served on the National Institutes of Health Ad Hoc Panel on

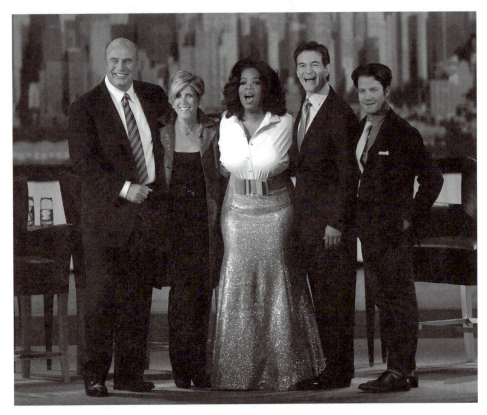

Oprah Winfrey is pictured with celebrity doctors Dr. Phil McGraw and Dr. Mehmet Oz. Also pictured are Suze Orman and Nate Berkus. (AP/Wide World Photos)

Alternative Medicine, and founded the Chopra Center for Well Being in California. Chopra has written over 50 books.

Dr. Sanjay Gupta has made a name for himself as a medical correspondent on the broadcast network CNN, where he has won numerous awards for his reporting on a range of medical and scientific topics. He is also a neurosurgeon and has written two books and was named one of the Ten Most Influential Celebrities by *Forbes* magazine in 2011.

Dr. Drew Pinsky launched his celebrity career following a successful radio show, *Loveline*. Pinsky is board certified in internal and addiction medicine and runs a private practice along with his television show, *Celebrity Rehab with Dr. Drew*. His show features other celebrities who are struggling with treatment for drugs and sex. He has written a book and coauthored an academic study on celebrities and narcissism, which was published in the *Journal of Research in Personality*.

Dr. Andrew Weil, who graduated from Harvard Medical School in the 1960s, is best known for his approach to integrative medicine and his extensive publishing on integrative medicine and health. In 1994 he founded the Arizona Center for Integrative Medicine, which trains health professions in the techniques of integrative medicine, a type of medicine that seeks to create a partnership between the patient and doctor and combines conventional Western medicine with alternative or complementary treatments such as acupuncture, biofeedback, and yoga.

Kevin Pho may be the future of celebrity doctors. He is a primary care physician who is board certified in internal medicine and a member of *USA Today*'s Board of Contributors. He frequently tweets and blogs about health care, drawing hundreds of visitors per day ("Blogging It," 2004). While most celebrity doctors still practice medicine, medical experts say it's important for Americans to develop a relationship with a primary health physician, someone they can reach when real health problems arise.

Sharon Zoumbaris

See also Online Health Resources; Primary Care Physicians.

References

Albiniak, Paige. "Oz Feeling Great and Powerful: Sources Say Fox, NBC Want Established Oprah Spinoff." *Broadcast and Cable* 140, no. 24 (June 14, 2010): 28.

"America's Doctor, Dr. Mehmet Oz and Jeff Arnold Launch Sharecare.com, an Online Health and Wellness Platform Providing Consumers with Expert Information to Live Healthier Lives." *Cardiovascular Week* (October 18, 2010): 45.

"Blogging It; Docs Take to Web to Offer Their Opinions, Reach Public." *Modern Healthcare* 34, no. 37 (September 13, 2004): 42.

Chopra, Deepak. *Quantum Healing: Exploring the Frontiers of Mind/Body Medicine.* New York: Bantam, 1990.

"KevinMD.com Joins the HCPLive.com Network." *Cancer Weekly* (March 24, 2009): 838.

Schardt, David. "Supplementing Their Income: How Celebrities Turn Trust into Cash." *Nutrition Action Healthletter* 33, no. 1 (January–February 2006): 1 (5).

DREAM THERAPY

Dreams can be understood as inner experiences occurring during sleep in which a narrative is created from images. These experiences sometimes are kept private and sometimes are shared. Dreams also are associated with physiological indicators that occur during sleep, such as rapid eye movements and brainwave patterns similar to those found in the waking state. Some people claim not to have dreams at all, but the physiological indicators suggest that all of us dream (although some of us may not remember our dreams). Others only dimly recollect their dreams, except for an occasional one that stands out as exceptionally vivid. And the values of dreams are controversial, as some people appreciate and even diligently try to explore their dreams, while others discount them as meaningless.

Value of Dreams Dreams can be used in psychotherapy by engaging with dream content and process within a healing context. This can include dream interpretation and other ways of working with dreams. It can be performed individually (e.g., using self-analysis via keeping a dream journal), by a client working with an individual therapist, or by sharing dreams in a group setting. Throughout history and across cultures, dreams have been used in therapeutic ways. In ancient Assyria, Babylonia, and Egypt, dreams were viewed as divine messages offering advice on important topics, including healing. In ancient Greece and Rome, people would sleep in special temples in hopes of having a dream visitation by a deity with the power to diagnose and heal sickness. Ancient Greek philosophers were among the first to try to rationally understand dreams, such as Aristotle's rejection of the popular belief of his time that dreams come from deities, instead claiming they reflect states of embodiment, such as health issues.

Contemporary Western culture increasingly ascribes to rationality, emphasizing observable facts, and consequently many Westerners pay little attention to dreams, believing they have no practical value. Someone considered impractical is often disparagingly called a "dreamer." But within the modern Western world, there still are people who value dreams, including some Western mental health professionals who use dream therapy for healing.

Psychotherapy is a broad collection of methods used to address psychological difficulties in life. These may include distress while adjusting to relationships or work, as well as dealing with specific psychological problems, such as anxiety and depression. Most psychotherapy involves a verbal dialogue between a client (or patient) and a mental health practitioner. Some psychotherapies occasionally address dreams, but there are a few specific therapeutic approaches focusing primarily or even exclusively on dreams; both fit the term *dream therapy*. However, there are also many mental health professionals who never work with or ever ask clients about their dreams.

Therapeutic Use of Dreams   Sigmund Freud (1899/2008) introduced dream therapy to the modern West as the founder of psychoanalysis, one of the earliest forms of psychotherapy. Many of his insights were gleaned from previous traditions of dream work, such as those stemming from the biblical story of Joseph's interpreting the Egyptian pharaoh's dreams. However, Freud brought these into the modern Western rational context. Freud believed dreams both reflected wish fulfillment on the part of the dreamer as well as revealing valuable hidden (i.e., unconscious) information based on unresolved childhood conflicts, which he suggested could be uncovered through a type of nonjudgmental awareness (i.e., free association).

Freudian dream work focused on interpreting dream content brought forward through free association based on its supposed meaning related to the dreamer's early life conflicts. Through unraveling dream symbolism, Freud encouraged bringing unconscious material into awareness through dreams, allowing for clients to increase their ability to live more rationally without being overly controlled by their unconscious forces. Many psychotherapists working within the psychoanalytic tradition later modified and extended Freud's initial contributions to dream therapy, such as Carl Jung (1948/1974), whose approach emphasized interpreting the healthy, as well as the problematic, aspects of dreams. He thought that dreams represent a creative striving for wholeness and not just psychopathology.

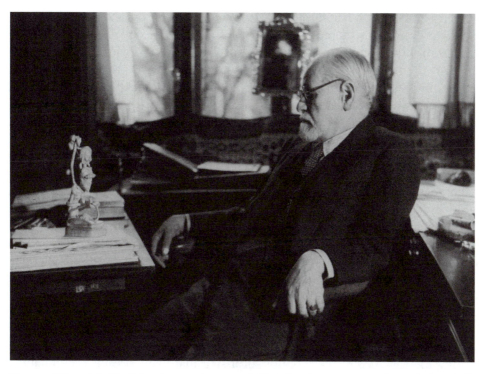

Sigmund Freud devised the therapy for mental disorders known as psychoanalysis, which involves uncovering repressed psychological traumas so that the patient can confront and overcome them. Though the specifics of many of his theories no longer command the wide acceptance they once did, the general framework for psychotherapy that he created has exercised an enormous influence on the theory and practice of psychology. (Library of Congress)

Consequently Jungian dream interpretations are usually much broader than Freudian, often amplifying dream images to examine their cultural and even spiritual implications. F.C. "Fritz" Perls (1969), working within the gestalt therapy tradition, expanded this approach further by discussing dreams as a type of inner theater in which dreamers are the playwrights, players, producers, prompters, public, and even the critics of their own dreams, which often represent disowned aspects of the dreamer. His approach to psychotherapy emphasized reenacting various aspects of the dream, asking clients to take each part of the dream as a role to be explored for its potential meaning. Pesant and Zadra (2004) provide a good review of these and many other traditions of psychotherapy that incorporate dream therapy, such as cognitive approaches in which dreams are used to identify errors in thinking and maladaptive beliefs. There are also many specific dream therapies, such as the Dream Interview Method (Delaney, 1993) in which the therapist (i.e., interviewer) assumes a naïve perspective and asks for a detailed subjective description of all aspects of the dream, and then explores how the dream could be used to achieve meaningful life changes. And some, like

Eudell-Simmons and Hilsenroth (2007), have proposed ways to integrate various approaches to dream therapy.

Dream Interpretation   One main concern regarding dream therapy focuses on how to interpret symbolism in dreams. Many systems propose that a specific symbol has a true meaning (e.g., assuming that a snake always represents a phallus), whereas others look more flexibly in a constructivist way (e.g., that a dream's meaning is co-constructed by clients interacting with therapists) for creating meanings useful to the client. We urge the rejection of simplistic works on dream interpretation that proclaim any symbol be treated with one meaning. A symbol is an image that has a deeper meaning, and dream symbols may have more than one meaning.

In addition to working with dreams in a general way, sometimes an unpleasant dream itself can indicate the need for psychotherapy, especially if it is a recurrent nightmare. Such dreams may or may not be related to a psychological problem, like trauma or stress, but could also be triggered by other factors, such as an undiagnosed physical illness or even medication side effects. However, posttraumatic nightmares or other problematic dreams may not disappear without professional help. It is important to consider multiple vantages before concluding that unpleasant dreams indicate a need for dream therapy. One of the functions of dreams is the downloading and working through of emotions experienced during the day. As a result, it is not surprising that many dreams are unhappy, confusing, or even terrifying.

Another intriguing area of growing interest involves lucid dreaming (i.e., a state where a person is aware of being in a dream while he or she is dreaming). It has been speculated that this unusual phenomenon might shed light on some psychoses, where people may be having waking dreams but do not know they are dreaming. In this regard, hallucinations common in psychoses might be similar to lucid dreaming. Also, from a growth perspective, lucid dreams offer an avenue for people to begin to work therapeutically with their own dreams in vivo (i.e., while they are dreaming), which is a practice found in some cultures. This is just one of many exciting frontiers of dream therapy (see Krippner & Ellis, 2009).

Although few contemporary psychotherapists use dream therapy, it is an area that remains of great interest to some. Pesant and Zadra (2004) and Hill and Rochlen (2009) reviewed the research literature on the effectiveness of various studies on dream therapy. Although the older research does not provide a clear picture of whether dream therapy may be effective, Clara Hill's cognitive-experiential method demonstrated its utility in several studies, such as providing increased client satisfaction, especially for those who were highly motivated to work with their dreams. One reason for the success of Hill's method may be its incorporation of insights gained in dream therapy into a client's daily behavior. The research data as a whole suggest that dream therapy can increase clients' self-insights about central issues in their lives and facilitate their productive involvement in therapy, as well enriching clinicians' understanding of their clients. Although dream therapy remains controversial, as psychologists who have worked extensively with many clients while focusing on dreams, we think exploring dreams within therapeutic contexts can be both meaningful and useful.

Harris Friedman and Stanley Krippner*

See also Depression; Stress.

References

Delaney, G. "The Changing Roles of Dream Interpreters in the Understanding of Dreams." *International Journal of Psychosomatics* 40, no. 1 (1993): 6–8.

Eudell-Simmons, E., and M. Hilsenroth. "The Use of Dreams in Psychotherapy: An Integrative Model." *Journal of Psychotherapy Integration* 17, no. 4 (2007): 330–56.

Freud, S. *The Interpretation of Dreams.* Translated by J. Crick. New York: Oxford University Press, 2008. (Original work published 1899)

Hill, C.E., and A.B. Rochlen. "Working with Dreams: A Cognitive-Experiential Model." In *Perchance to Dream: The Frontiers of Dream Psychology,* edited by S. Krippner and D. Ellis, 71–77. New York: Nova Science, 2009.

Jung, C.G. "General Aspects of Dream Psychology." In *Dreams,* by C.G. Jung, 23–66. Translated by R. Hull. Princeton, NJ: Princeton University Press, 1974. (Original work published 1948)

Krippner, S., and D. Ellis, eds. *Perchance to Dream: The Frontiers of Dream Psychology.* New York: Nova Science, 2009.

Perls, F.C. *Ego, Hunger and Aggression: The Beginning of Gestalt Therapy.* New York: Random House, 1969.

Pesant, N., and A. Zadra. "Working with Dreams in Therapy: What Do We Know and What Should We Do?" *Clinical Psychology Review* 24, no. 5 (2004): 489–512.

DRUGS, RECREATIONAL

Recreational drugs are drugs which are often used for recreational purposes. In other terms, these drugs are described as *club drugs* or *designer drugs*, often used when teens and young adults gather at bars, nightclubs, concerts, and parties. These substances include cocaine, methamphetamine, MDMA (Ecstasy), ketamine, and gamma hydroxybutyrate (GHB). Other recreational drugs are marijuana and opiates, but these drugs have particular effects and concerns of their own and are discussed in the entries on medical marijuana and smoking.

Recreational drugs have a variety of general effects on both the brain and the body. Cocaine is a strong stimulant of the central nervous system, greatly increasing levels of dopamine (the internal, chemical brain transmitter associated with pleasure) in the brain's reward center. Methamphetamine was developed from its parent drug, amphetamine, except that at comparable doses,

*Preparation of the Dream Therapy entry was supported by the Saybrook University Chair for the Study of Consciousness.

methamphetamine gets into the brain at much higher levels, making it a much more efficient way to affect the central nervous system and increase production of dopamine. MDMA or Ecstasy is similar to methamphetamine, with a hallucinogenic addition.

Ketamine is a short-term anesthetic, called a disassociative, which means that it impedes the brain's sensory connection to the physical body. And GHB is a legitimate, prescribed central nervous system depressant used for narcolepsy (a sleep disorder). GHB and a similar drug, Rohypnol, sedate users and have been used to commit sexual assaults (also known as date rape, drug rape, or drug-assisted assault). The use of these last drugs causes unsuspecting victims to be incapacitated, thus preventing resistance to sexual assault.

Broadly described, the control status of recreational drugs varies from drug to drug. A substance's control status is described according to the Controlled Substances Act of 1970, which serves as the foundation for the U.S. government's legal battle against drugs of abuse. While the recreational drugs mentioned here generally involve a pleasurable, euphoric effect, there are differences in the illegality of each individual drug.

Cocaine is a Schedule II drug, meaning this drug has a high potential for abuse, with severe governmental restrictions. It was historically used as a painkiller for dentistry and for surgical operations on eyes and throats. Now, however, cocaine is viewed primarily as a powerfully addictive stimulant. Methamphetamine (as well as its parent drug, amphetamine) is also a Schedule II stimulant. This means that both cocaine and methamphetamine are very likely to be abused and are legally available only through prescriptions. Ketamine is a Schedule III drug (a drug with less potential of abuse than Schedules I and II), an anesthetic causing distortion of sight and sound as well as feelings of detachment. It does require a prescription for purchase. The depressant GHB is a Schedule II drug with restrictions so severe that it requires a patient registry for legal prescriptions. The synthetic, psychoactive MDMA (Ecstasy) is a Schedule I drug, meaning it has a high potential for abuse with no known medical use for treatment in the United States.

There are several ways cocaine can be administered: snorting, injecting, and smoking. Snorting (intranasal) is the process of inhaling cocaine powder through the nostrils, where it is absorbed into the bloodstream through the nasal tissues. Injection involves intravenous use, where the drug accesses the bloodstream directly and the intensity of cocaine's effects is heightened. The final mode of ingesting cocaine is by smoking, where the cocaine vapor or smoke is inhaled into the lungs. This can be achieved through the use of either freebase or crack cocaine, both of which are solid varieties of cocaine. The effect of smoke inhalation is virtually as fast as injection and includes increased energy, reduced fatigue, mental alertness, and a euphoric state of well-being.

Other recreational drugs have several routes of administration. MDMA is almost always taken orally, in tablets. Ketamine is usually injected, although it can be snorted like cocaine. Methamphetamine is taken orally, intranasally, by needle injection, or by smoking. GHB is usually taken orally, either in liquid or powder form (in capsules or tablets).

Recreational drugs are known by a broad number of street names or slang terms. Cocaine is known as coke, C, snow, crack, candy, rock, freebase, and toot. Amphetamines are known as pep pills, bennies, uppers, and speed. Methamphetamine is known as meth, ice, crank, tweak, crystal meth, biker's coffee, stove top, trash, and go fast. GHB may be called goop, grievous bodily harm, liquid ecstasy, and liquid X. Ketamine is known as cat valium, K, special K, kit kat, vitamin K. And MDMA, in addition to Ecstasy, is called E, XTC, hug drug, lover's speed, peace, and STP.

The short-term effects of these drugs varies, usually with what begins as a beneficial or pleasurable feeling in almost all cases. However, there are distinct differences, especially in the long-term, depending on the type of drug and how it acts on the brain and the rest of the body.

For cocaine, common initial reactions are euphoria, talkativeness, increased blood pressure, and heart rate. Users can be energetic and mentally alert. Since cocaine produces such pleasurable effects and is so addictive, considerable study has been done on this drug and these effects. Cocaine acts on levels of the brain chemical (neurotransmitter) dopamine and blocks dopamine from being removed from the brain, thereby causing an excess of dopamine (or "rush") to accumulate in the brain. Thus, euphoria is a common effect. This high can decrease the immediate need for food and sleep. However, the initial rush wears off quickly, in anywhere from just 5 minutes to up to 30 minutes. This almost always leaves

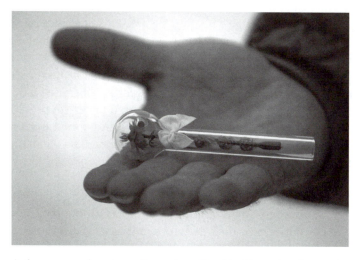

A drug counselor at an alternative school holds a pipe for smoking crystal methamphetamine, which some kids call a "bubble," in Lake Elmo, Minnesota, on February 24, 2005. Methamphetamines are one of many popular recreational drugs. (AP/Wide World Photos)

users with feelings of discomfort, depression, and an increasing desire to experience the drug or feel the high again and again.

Amphetamine's effects are fairly strong, and similar to methamphetamine, but not as efficient and potent. Therefore, just the latter will be discussed here. Methamphetamine's short-term effects are an intense rush or euphoric sensation upon immediate use. The high can be effective and can last up to half a day by some reports. Repeated uses over a period of many hours can lead to a "run," or an extended period of intoxication. High levels of dopamine are believed to accumulate in the brain during this time as the rush continues.

MDMA, or Ecstasy, produces feelings of increased energy, emotional warmth, even openness to complete strangers. These short-term effects come from the brain chemical or neurotransmitter serotonin. MDMA binds to the serotonin transporter in the brain, and increases and prolongs the signals. It also causes an excessive release of serotonin. Users' tactile sensations increase, causing the feeling of touch to become more pleasurable. MDMA can also produce short-term feelings of confusion, depression, intense jaw clenching, and inability to concentrate.

Ketamine's effects vary depending on how much is taken, and in what way. Low-dose intoxication can cause impaired attention and memory. In the short-term, at higher doses, the results can vary from feelings of weightlessness to out-of-body feelings to near-death experiences. Some people find the loss of control over their bodies disconcerting. This drug has also been used as a date rape drug.

Another substance used for recreational purposes is amyl nitrite, an inhalant. While it has medicinal purposes, when used recreationally it expands blood vessels, which results in lowering of blood pressure. This is also considered a party drug and is common on the nightclub scene. Amyl nitrite is made available in ampules, also known as "poppers." These are held to the nostrils for quick inhalation, and are especially sought after to enhance sexual arousal or stimulation. This general type of drug called nitrites are chemicals that cause vasodilation, and so have some legitimate health use and are still used in certain procedures today. However, some variations of these nitrites have been banned from prescription use since the 1990s. Even though they have been banned, they remain popular in their illegal or nonprescribed form among a certain segment of teens and young adults.

The short-term results of GHB can vary, even from use to use with the same person. After an initial feeling of euphoria and relaxation, other more unpleasant effects can occur. These include nausea, dizziness, drowsiness, and visual disturbances. Since GHB is a Schedule II drug and has little medical use by itself, it is often illegally manufactured. This can lead to a wide variance in purity and strength of the drug and can account for the inconsistence of effects felt by users.

The long-term effects of these recreational drugs vary widely. All of them are considered extremely liable to abuse, if not addiction, if taken with any sort of regularity. The American Psychiatric Association's *Diagnostic and Statistical Manual of Mental Disorders* defines substance abuse using the following criteria. The abuse has one or more maladaptive patterns of use, resulting in clinically significant impairment or distress. This includes (1) recurrent failure to fulfill major role obligations; (2) recurrent use in physically hazardous situations; (3) recurrent substance-related legal problems; and (4) continued use despite persistent or recurrent social or interpersonal problems due to use.

Long-term cocaine use is likely to increase and lead to abuse. It is a powerfully, highly addictive drug. With repeated exposure of the brain to cocaine, the brain begins to adapt. The internal pleasure receptors or the reward pathway of the brain, where dopamine occurs, become less and less sensitive. Thus, tolerance can develop. Repeated users report that they seek the pleasure of their initial high but fail to find it. So they are driven to repeat the experience over and over, sometimes with greater and greater amounts of the drug, chasing that initial high. Users can also take the drug in binges, using repeatedly and at increasingly higher doses. This can lead to feelings of increased irritability, restlessness, panic attacks, intense desire for isolation, and paranoia.

Cocaine also has a number of long-term effects on the physical body. It increases body temperature, heart rate. and blood pressure. Since cocaine often decreases appetite, habitual users can become malnourished. If users snort over an extended time, they can lose the sense of smell, have nosebleeds, difficulty in swallowing, and a chronic runny nose. Injecting cocaine over a period of time and at higher and higher levels can increase the possibility of contracting HIV/AIDS and other blood-borne diseases. Users can also develop severe allergic reactions.

If cocaine use increases over an extended period of time, the usage can cause the abuser to have an erratic heartbeat as well as a loss of concentration and coordination. Extended abuse can even lead to psychosis, which involves losing touch with reality and having auditory and visual hallucinations. Even after withdrawal symptoms have disappeared and after extended periods of abstinence, sudden cravings for cocaine may surface many months, even years, after last reported use.

Long-term use of methamphetamine can lead to violent behavior, anxiety, confusion, and insomnia. Abusers can become psychotic, as well. Paranoia sometimes leads to homicidal as well as suicidal thoughts. In addition, research has shown that prolonged exposure to even low levels of meth can lead to significant damage done to the dopamine-producing cells in the brain, as well as to nerve cells that contain serotonin.

MDMA or Ecstasy can have many of the same physical effects as cocaine, but since a large number of the drug users in the documented studies reported using other substances at the same time, there are a variety of opinions on the exact long-term effects of MDMA. Those long-term effects include confusion, depression, sleep difficulties, and intense anxiety. Any of these problems can occur at any time after taking the drug, from as quickly as immediately after ingestion to weeks or even months after taking the drug. There is some documentation that MDMA includes similar effects of a stimulant, which are increases in heart rate and blood pressure, but these findings are still not conclusive.

Ketamine has not been widely studied on its own. However, ketamine has been noted as often being used with MDMA. What little is known about ketamine is that there are reports of LSD-type flashbacks and a deterioration of short-term memory as well as potentially fatal respiratory problems. GHB is another drug often used in combination with other drugs, often in the club or party atmosphere, earning it the designation of a recreational drug. This type of use does not aid research on GHB alone. Other than physical and psychological dependence and occasional insomnia, anxiety, and trembling, which may or may not occur anywhere from 3 to 12 days after stopping the drugs, researchers have not been able to conclusively discover much about the drug's long-term effects.

Recreational drugs have a variety of trafficking trends. Different drugs are more popular with individual subpopulations. For example, MDMA was initially favored by white teens and young adults for recreational purposes (at raves and nightclubs). However, use of this drug has recently spread over the general population, affecting a wider range of ethnicities. GHB and ketamine and the lesser known benzodiazepine Rohypnol are often taken in combination with other drugs. The yearly *Monitoring the Future* survey shows the use of these drugs to be consistently low among high school age youth over approximately the past 10 years.

One particular subpopulation where these drugs are used is in environments—often clubs, but not always—where men have sex with men. Some report using these recreational drugs as part of a multidrug experience that may also include marijuana, sildenafil citrate (Viagra), and other legal and illegal substances.

Cocaine remains sadly popular in both urban and rural areas, with the notable exception of crack cocaine use. Crack use has decreased slightly in the adolescent and young adult age groups in both urban and rural areas, according to the 2008 National Survey on Drug Use and Health.

The use of recreational drugs is easily detected by blood or urine analysis, with the exception of GHB, which is not usually included in a toxicity screen. However, other drugs are not as quickly diagnosed by a visual examination, for example in an emergency room visit. This is often because certain drugs taken at the same time cause other, more serious clinical situations.

In the case of recreational drugs taken one after the other, a "cocktail" effect can occur. In certain clubs, there are reports of the existence of an area or room where people who are unwell can be assessed, and discreet inquiry made as to the kinds of drugs they may have ingested. However, there is very little published data concerning the possible existence of these areas or rooms.

The different scheduling (see the Controlled Substances Act of 1970 for further information) of these various controlled substances causes a number of legal consequences for possessing and selling these drugs. These vary from misdemeanors to felonies with mandatory jail time. The use of drug courts (intensive, community-based judicial and case management programs) has been shown to be effective in dealing with many drug cases. Much of the drug and criminal justice research done in this area has shown that adaptive interventions, such as drug court supervision, enhance recovery success rates.

Inpatient drug and alcohol detoxification units have gained some familiarity with the more exotic illegal substances. Many urban hospital emergency departments have dealt with them as well. This kind of critical care treatment is needed primarily for medical stabilization. The better option would be to provide an abuser who wanted to stop drug use with knowledgeable medical and clinical care beyond their initial treatment.

Cognitive-behavioral intervention, coupled with changing the abuser's thinking, expectations, and behavior about their drug use is considered an effective treatment. Support groups (such as Narcotics Anonymous, Cocaine Anonymous, and Alcoholics Anonymous) have also been effective in the long term for many drug users. These groups also provide excellent sources of camaraderie and support for the abusing person who is willing to stop his or her drug use.

Elizabeth Jones

See also Addiction; Medical Marijuana; Smoking.

References

American Psychiatric Association. *Diagnostic and Statistical Manual of Mental Disorders,* 4th ed. text rev. Washington, DC; American Psychiatric Association, 2000.

Hanson, G.R., P.J. Venturelli, and A.E. Fleckenstein. "Appendix B: Drugs of Use and Abuse." In *Drugs and Society,* 9th ed., 570–75. Burlington, MA: Jones and Bartlett, 2006.

National Institute on Drug Abuse. "Club Drugs (GHB, Ketamine, and Rohypnol)." *NIDA InfoFacts* (July 2010), National Institutes of Health, U.S. Department of Health and Human Services, http://drugabuse.gov/infofacts/infofactsindex.html.

National Institute on Drug Abuse. "Cocaine." *NIDA InfoFacts* (March 2010), National Institute on Drug Abuse, National Institutes of Health, U.S. Department of Health and Human Services.

National Institute on Drug Abuse. "MDMA (Ecstacy)." *NIDA InfoFacts* (December 2010), National Institute on Drug Abuse, National Institutes of Health, U.S. Department of Health and Human Services.

National Institute on Drug Abuse. "Methamphetamine." *NIDA InfoFacts* (March 2010), National Institute on Drug Abuse, National Institutes of Health, U.S. Department of Health and Human Services.

National Institute on Drug Abuse. "High-Risk Drug Offenders Do Better with Close Judicial Supervision." *NIDA Notes* 22, no. 2 (December 2008), www.drugabuse.gov/NIDA_notes/NNVol22N2/HighRisk.html.

National Institute on Drug Abuse. "Research Report Series—Cocaine Abuse and Addiction" (2006), National Institutes of Health, U.S. Department of Health and Human Services, www.nida.nih.gov/researchreports/cocaine/references.html.

National Institute on Drug Abuse. "Research Report Series—Methamphetamine Abuse and Addiction" (2006), National Institutes of Health, U.S. Department of Health and Human Services, http://drugabuse.gov/reesearchreports/methamp/methamph.html.

NZ (New Zealand) Drug Foundation. "Cocaine: What It Is," www.drugfoundation.org.nz/cocaine/what-it-is.

NZ (New Zealand) Drug Foundation. "Ecstasy: What It Is," www.drugfoundation.org.nz/ecstasy/what-it-is.

NZ (New Zealand) Drug Foundation. "GHB: What It Is," www.drugfoundation.org.nz/ghb/what-it-is.

NZ (New Zealand) Drug Foundation. "Ketamine: What It Is," www.drugfoundation.org.nz/ketamine/what-it-is.

U.S. Department of Justice, Drug Enforcement Administration. *Drug Fact Sheet—GHB. Get Smart about Drugs, A Resource for Parents from the DEA,*), www.justice.gov/dea/pubs/abuse/drug_data_sheets/ghb_DrugDataSheet.pdf.

U.S. Department of Justice, Drug Enforcement Administration. *Drug Fact Sheet—Methamphetamine. Get Smart about Drugs, A Resource for Parents from the DEA,* www.justice.gov/dea/pubs/abuse/drug_data_sheets/methamphetamine_DrugDataSheet.pdf1.

Van Dusen, V., and A.R. Spies. "An Overview and Update of the Controlled Substances Act of 1970," *Pharmacy Times* (February 1, 2007), www.pharmacytimes.com/print.php?url=2007-02-6309.

West, E., P. Cameron, G. O'Reilly, O.H. Drummer, and A. Bystrzycki. "Accuracy of Current Clinical Diagnosis in Recreational Drug-Related Attendance to the Emergency Department." *Emergency Medicine Australasia* 20 (2008): 333–38.

Wood, D.M., M. Nicolaou, and P.I. Dargan. "Epidemiology of Recreational Drug Toxicity in a Nightclub Environment." *Substance Use and Misuse* 44 (2009): 1495–502.

E

EATING DISORDERS

Eating disorders encompass a range of disturbances related to food consumption. The American Psychiatric Association, in the fourth edition of its *Diagnostic and Statistical Manual of Mental Disorders* (*DSM*), states that the two most serious eating disorders are anorexia nervosa and bulimia nervosa. In the former, the patient refuses to maintain normal weight; in the latter, he or she binges on food and controls weight gain with fasting, excessive exercise, or purging by self-induced vomiting, the use of laxatives and diuretics, or taking enemas. Both types of eating disorders are extremely serious, and anorexia, particularly, can quickly become life-threatening.

According to the National Institute of Mental Health (NIMH), over the course of a lifetime, up to 6 percent of the adult population in the United States will develop anorexia nervosa, up to 1 percent will have bulimia nervosa, and another 2.8 percent will suffer from binge eating disorder. According to figures released by the National Association of Anorexia Nervosa and Associated Eating Disorders, an estimated 6 percent of those with anorexia die each year as a result of their illness, making it one of the top psychiatric illnesses that lead to death.

Characteristics Anorexia is characterized by a resistance to maintaining a healthy body weight, an intense fear of gaining weight, and other extreme behaviors that result in severe weight loss. People with anorexia see themselves as overweight even when they are dangerously thin. Bulimia generally is characterized by recurrent episodes of binge eating, followed by self-induced purging behaviors. People with bulimia often have normal weight, but, like those with anorexia, they are intensely dissatisfied with the appearance of their bodies. Eating disorders involve multiple biological, behavioral, and social factors that are not well understood.

A study funded by NIMH reported in August 2006 that Internet-based intervention programs may help some college-age, high-risk women avoid developing an eating disorder. Although it cannot be assumed that all people at risk would benefit from such online approaches to prevention, the programs may serve as valuable screening tools to help susceptible individuals seek treatment before the disease has progressed (NIMH, 2006).

A third manifestation of eating disorders is known as a bingeing and purging disorder. Unlike bulimics, the individuals eat normally, but still feel compelled to purge even though they maintain near-normal weight. Comprising a fourth type of eating disorder are food addictions (overeating addictions), which can often lead to obesity; a compulsive desire to gorge on sweets is a common example. Although obesity is considered by some to be an eating disorder because it involves an unhealthy relationship with food, it is not specifically characterized as such in the *DSM;* however, the manual discusses obesity within the context of a mental health disorder if there are psychological factors contributing to its cause.

The complexity of eating disorders makes many difficult to treat. Like other compulsive behaviors, proper diagnosis is critical, and the earlier a diagnosis is made, the better; but this is often complicated by the fact that shame and a distorted sense of body image—known as body dysmorphic disorder—deter patients from asking for help. This delays treatment until after the illness has become life-threatening, making therapeutic interventions more difficult. Treatment for an eating disorder can be costly, and insurance policies do not cover many of the costs of care. A Senate bill proposed in 2010 by Senator Daylin Leach would require insurance companies to provide coverage for residential care in the treatment of eating disorders. That bill is an example of the growing support for insurance coverage for those with eating disorders being proposed by legislators such as Leach as well as physicians and mental health professionals.

Long associated with a low self-esteem, eating disorders stem from a complex mix of biological, environmental, and genetic causes. Although males are not exempt, the condition disproportionately affects females. At some time in their lives, anywhere from 5 to 10 percent of girls and women suffer from eating disorders that usually appear during adolescence or early adulthood. The disease is frequently accompanied by anxiety or depression, and, in many cases, it is likely that each disorder reinforces or exacerbates the symptoms of the others.

Prevalence among Males Although eating disorders primarily affect girls and women, boys and men are also vulnerable. One in four preadolescent cases of anorexia occurs in boys, and binge-eating disorder affects females and males about equally. Like females who have eating disorders, males with the illness have a warped sense of body image and often have muscle dysmorphia, a type of disorder that is characterized by an extreme concern with becoming more muscular. Some boys with the disorder want to lose weight, while others want to gain weight or bulk up.

Boys who think they are too small are at a greater risk for using steroids or other dangerous drugs to increase muscle mass. Boys with eating disorders exhibit the same types of emotional, physical, and behavioral signs and symptoms as girls, but, for a variety of reasons—including that the disease is often considered a female disorder—boys are less likely to be diagnosed (NIMH, 2011).

Eating disorders do not necessarily meet all the same diagnostic criteria. While bulimia is frequently regarded as an impulse control disorder, some aspects of anorexia nervosa meet the *DSM* definitions for major depressive disorder, social phobia, and obsessive-compulsive disorder. Nevertheless, researchers are intrigued that in people with eating disorders and in those addicted either to substances or to compulsive behaviors, key neurological activity in specific regions of the brain is so similar. This may help explain why eating disorders are often accompanied by a history of substance abuse. The progressive nature of eating disorders mirrors that of substance abuse; like drug addiction or an addiction to pathological gambling, the behavior continues in spite of negative consequences, and the individual experiences intense craving to repeat the behavior despite periods of abstinence.

These findings have tempered the prevailing wisdom of prior decades, which held that eating disorders arose out of psychological and family influences, particularly a history of abuse, repression of emotional expression, parental neglect or hostility, and a somewhat obsessive need to control one's environment. Nevertheless, despite the undeniable influence of biological factors, a cultural emphasis on thinness increases the possibility that a psychologically vulnerable adolescent girl or young woman will develop an eating disorder. One study reported in 2008 that girls who ate meals at the table with their families five or more times per week were significantly less likely to develop eating disorders than their peers. Although the same result was not shown for boys, the study authors suggest that teenage girls might be much more heavily influenced by quality time spent with families, especially in terms of developing a healthy relationship with food and in associating good eating habits with positive family interaction.

Treatment varies depending on the characteristics of the individual eating disorder and is best developed around a combined approach of cognitive-behavioral therapy and medications to address contributory neurochemical imbalances; pharmaceutical approaches are particularly helpful if used early in treatment before the patient has learned new coping strategies in therapy. In some instances, family therapy is advisable to address relationship issues and interpersonal dysfunction, especially in situations in which adolescent patients are still living at home. In severe cases, hospitalization may be necessary, both to institute nutritional therapy and because eating disorders of long standing can result in serious damage to the liver and pancreas and cause heart arrhythmias and mental impairments. Death from starvation is possible.

Prevalence of Eating Disorders Previously, eating disorders were most often seen in adolescents or young adults, but reports early in 2008 indicated that they are being diagnosed in people in their 30s and 40s as well. Women and girls are more likely to develop an eating disorder than men and boys. Males seem to account for an estimated 5 to 25 percent of patients with anorexia or bulimia, although many reports suggest they suffer the same number of binge-eating disorders as women. Eating disorders frequently co-exist with other psychiatric illnesses such as depression, substance abuse, or anxiety disorders. People with eating disorders also can suffer from numerous organic problems, such as heart disease or kidney failure, which could be fatal. Results from a large-scale national survey suggest that binge-eating disorder is more prevalent than both anorexia nervosa and bulimia nervosa (NIMH, 2007, 2011).

FAQs about Eating Disorders   The National Institute of Mental Health has published a list of frequently asked questions about eating disorders from which the following questions are adapted:

1. What are eating disorders?
   Eating disorders are often long-term illnesses that may require long-term treatment. They frequently occur with other mental disorders such as depression, substance abuse, and anxiety disorders. The earlier these disorders are diagnosed and treated, the better the chances are for full recovery.
2. Who has eating disorders?
   Research shows that more than 90 percent of those who have eating disorders are women between the ages of 12 and 25. However, increasing numbers of older women and men have them, and hundreds of thousands of boys are affected as well.
3. What are the symptoms of eating disorders?

   - Anorexia nervosa: People who have anorexia develop unusual eating habits such as avoiding food and meals, picking out a few foods and eating them in small amounts, weighing their food, and counting the calories of everything they eat. They may exercise excessively. A refusal to maintain normal weight is a key feature of anorexia.
   - Bulimia nervosa: People who have bulimia eat an excessive amount of food in a single episode and almost immediately make themselves vomit or use laxatives or diuretics (water pills) to get rid of the food in their bodies. This behavior often is referred to as the binge-purge cycle. Like people with anorexia, people with bulimia have an intense fear of gaining any excess weight but generally maintain near-normal weight levels.
   - Binge-eating disorder: People with this recently recognized disorder have frequent episodes of compulsive overeating, but unlike those with bulimia, they do not purge their bodies of food. During these food binges, they often eat alone and very quickly, regardless of whether they feel hungry or full. They often feel shame or guilt over their actions. Unlike anorexia and bulimia, binge-eating disorder occurs almost as often in men as in women.

4. What medical problems can arise as a result of eating disorders?

   - Anorexia nervosa: Anorexia can slow the heart rate and lower blood pressure, increasing the chance of heart failure. Those who use drugs to stimulate vomiting, bowel movements, or urination are also at high risk for heart failure. Starvation can also result in heart failure and damage the brain. Anorexia may also cause hair and nails to grow brittle. Skin may dry out, become yellow, and develop a covering of soft hair called lanugo. Mild anemia, swollen joints, reduced muscle mass, and light-headedness also commonly occur. Severe cases of anorexia can lead to brittle bones that break easily as a result of calcium loss.

- Bulimia nervosa: The acid in vomit can wear down the outer layer of the teeth, inflame and damage the esophagus, and enlarge the glands near the cheeks. Damage to the stomach can also occur from frequent vomiting. Irregular heartbeats, heart failure, and death may result from chemical imbalances and the loss of important minerals such as potassium. Peptic ulcers, inflammation of the pancreas, and long-term constipation are also consequences of bulimia.

- Binge-eating disorder: Binge-eating disorder can cause high blood pressure and high cholesterol levels. Other effects of binge-eating disorder include fatigue, joint pain, Type 2 diabetes, gallbladder disease, and heart disease.

5. What is required for a formal diagnosis of an eating disorder?

- Anorexia nervosa: Weighs at least 15 percent below what is considered normal for others of the same height and age; misses at least three consecutive menstrual cycles (if a female of childbearing age); has an intense fear of gaining weight; refuses to maintain the minimal normal body weight; and believes he or she is overweight though in reality is dangerously thin.

- Bulimia nervosa: At least two binge-purge cycles per week, on average, for at least three months; lacks control over eating behavior; and seems obsessed with body shape and weight.

- Binge-eating disorder: At least two binge-eating episodes per week, on average, for six months; lacks control over eating behavior.

6. How are eating disorders treated?

- Anorexia nervosa: The first goal for the treatment of anorexia is to restore a healthy weight. This may require hospitalization. Once a person's physical condition is stable, treatment usually involves individual psychotherapy and family therapy during which parents help their child learn to eat again and maintain healthy eating habits on his or her own. Behavioral therapy also has been effective for helping a person return to healthy eating habits. Supportive group therapy may follow, and self-help groups within communities may provide ongoing support.

- Bulimia nervosa: Unless malnutrition is severe, any substance abuse problems that may be present at the time the eating disorder is diagnosed are usually treated first. The next goal of treatment is to reduce or eliminate the person's binge-eating and purging behavior. Behavioral therapy has proven effective in achieving this goal. Psychotherapy can help prevent the eating disorder from recurring and address issues that led to the disorder. Studies have also found that antidepressants may help. As with anorexia, family therapy is also recommended.

- Binge-eating disorder: The goals and strategies for treating binge-eating disorder are similar to those for bulimia.

Kathryn H. Hollen

See also Addiction; Anorexia Nervosa; Bulimia Nervosa; Obesity; Obsessive-Compulsive Disorder (OCD).

References

American Psychiatric Association. *Diagnostic and Statistical Manual of Mental Disorders,* 4th ed., text rev. Washington, DC: American Psychiatric Association, 2000.

Davis, Caroline. "Addiction and the Eating Disorders." *Psychiatric Times* (February 2001), www.psychiatrictimes.com/p010259.html.

Erickson, Carlton K. *The Science of Addiction: From Neurobiology to Treatment.* New York: Norton, 2007.

Grant, Jon E., and S.W. Kim. *Stop Me Because I Can't Stop Myself: Taking Control of Impulsive Behavior.* New York: McGraw-Hill, 2003.

Hyman, S.E., and R.C. Malenka. "Addiction and the Brain: The Neurobiology of Compulsion and Its Persistence." *Nature Reviews Neuroscience* 2, no. 10 (2001), 695–703.

Kalivas, P.W., and Nora Volkow. "The Neural Basis of Addiction: A Pathology of Motivation and Choice." *American Journal of Psychiatry* 162, no. 8 (August 2005): 1403–13.

National Institute of Mental Health. "College Women at Risk for Eating Disorder May Benefit from Online Intervention" (August 7, 2006), www.nimh.nih.gov/science-news/2006/college-women-at-risk-for-eating-disorder-may-benefit-from-online-intervention.shtml.

National Institute of Mental Health. www.apps.nimh.nih.gov/health/publications/eating-disorders/how-are-men-and-boys-affected.shtml.

National Institute of Mental Health. "Study Tracks Prevalence of Eating Disorders" (February 9, 2007), www.nimh.nih.gov/science-news/2007/study-tracks-prevalence-of-eating-disorders.shtml.

National Institute of Mental Health. "What Are Eating Disorders?" (July 21, 2011), Bethesda, MD: National Institute of Mental Health, 2011, www.nimh.nih.gov/health/publications/eating-disorders/what-are-eating-disorders.shtml.

National Institute on Drug Abuse. *The Science of Addiction: Drugs, Brains, and Behavior.* NIH Publication No. 07-5605, Bethesda, MD: National Institute of Health, February 2007.

Nestler, Eric J., and Robert Malenka. "The Addicted Brain." *Scientific American* (September 2007), www.sciam.com/article.cfm?chanID=sa006&colID=1&articleID=0001E632-978A-1019-978A83414B7F0101.

Neumark-Sztainer, Dianne, Marla Eisenberg, Jayne Fulkerson, Mary Story, and Nicole Larson. "Family Meals and Disordered Eating in Adolescents." *Archives of Pediatrics and Adolescent Medicine* 162, no. 1 (2008): 17–22.

Ozelli, Kristin Leutwyler. "This Is Your Brain on Food." *Scientific American* 297, no. 3 (September 2007): 84–85.

Potenza, Marc N. "Should Addictive Disorders Include Non-Substance-Related Conditions?" *Addiction* 101, no. s1 (2006): 142–51.

Sacker, Ira, and Sheila Buff. *Regaining Your Self: Breaking Free from the Eating Disorder Identity: A Bold New Approach.* New York: Hyperion, 2007.

Substance Abuse and Mental Health Services Administration. "Eating Disorders." Rockville, MD, 2011, http://mentalhealth.samhsa.gov/publications/allpubs/ken98-0047/default.asp.

E. COLI INFECTION

E. coli infection is caused by a strain of *Escherichia coli* bacteria. Although most strains of *E. coli* are not dangerous and normally live in the lower intestines of humans and animals, this particular strain—described by the alphanumeric combination O15:H7—produces chemicals that can cause serious illness in humans. *E. coli* infections primarily result from eating undercooked ground beef, although the bacteria can also spread through other methods. About 73,000 cases of infection occur in the United States on an annual basis. Of these cases, less than 0.1 percent ends in death.

E. coli is not just a problem for Americans, as evidenced by the May 2011 outbreak in Germany that eventually killed 50 people and left over 4,300 people ill in some 15 European countries. Health officials in Europe finally signaled the end to that outbreak in July 2011. Initially the source of contamination was unclear, and many Europeans were frightened of eating fresh vegetables after experts recommended they avoid salads. The source was eventually identified as Egyptian fenugreek seeds, although Spanish cucumbers were blamed early in the investigation. Many of the fenugreek seeds were used to produce sprouts.

The European Commission announced in July 2011 a compensation package for fruit and vegetable producers from member states if those individuals suffered heavy revenue losses over the summer. The European Union also banned additional imports of the seeds from Egypt for several additional months. The outbreak illustrated the reach of global markets since the seeds were imported by only one distributor in Germany but were eventually sold to 54 different companies in Germany and some 16 companies in almost a dozen other European countries ("Seeds Linked to E. coli Outbreak," 2011).

French officials confirmed later in the summer that the *E. coli* strain that sickened people in Germany was genetically similar to the one that caused illness in the Bordeaux region of France in June.

For years undercooked ground beef was considered the main source of *E. coli* infection. Other sources of infection now include raw milk, unpasteurized juice, eggs, vegetables and fruits, or drinking or swimming in water contaminated by waste. Although meat is often contaminated during slaughter and processing, consumers can prevent *E. coli* infection by thoroughly cooking ground beef. Individuals can also prevent the spread of *E. coli* in the kitchen by washing their hands and properly handling uncooked foods. They can also wash fruits and vegetables before they slice them, and consumers should be very careful not to use the same utensils or cutting boards for raw meat and fresh fruits or vegetables.

The main symptoms of *E. coli* infection include stomach cramps and bloody diarrhea, although some cases of infection present no symptoms at all. While symptoms of infection usually disappear in 5 to 10 days without treatment, young children and the elderly are more susceptible to complications from the infection, which include a serious condition called hemolytic uremic syndrome. This condition, which occurs in 2 to 7 percent of people infected with *E. coli,* destroys red blood cells and leads to kidney failure. Some individuals with hemolytic uremic syndrome may suffer a lifetime of complications and require continual kidney dialysis.

In 1993, four children died and hundreds of others became sick from *E. coli* after eating undercooked hamburgers served at the Jack in the Box fast-food chain. Consequently, Jack in the Box developed food handling regulations of the highest standard, which other fast food franchises have adopted to ensure the safety of their food. Federal agencies currently face the challenge of developing preventive measures at farms and slaughterhouses to reduce the contamination of meat. In addition, officials continue to promote the use of irradiation, which increases the safety of meat by killing harmful organisms.

Michele Morrone

See also Food-borne Illness; Irradiation; Vegetables.

Further Reading

Bell, Chris, and Alec Kyriakides. *E. Coli: A Practical Approach to the Organism and Its Control in Foods.* Oxford: Blackwell Scientific, 1999.

Cliver, Dean O., and Hans P. Riemann. *Foodborne Diseases,* 2nd ed. Burlington, MA: Academic Press, 2002.

Nuthall, Keith. "EU: E. coli Compensation Fund Increased." *Just-food.com* (July 29, 2011), www.just-food.com/news/e-coli-compensation-fund-increased_id116123.aspx.

"Seeds Linked to E. coli Outbreak Still Being Sold." *Consumer Health News* (July 5, 2011), www.healthday.com.

EDIBLE SCHOOLYARD PROJECT

The Edible Schoolyard is a nutrition and garden project that originated in Berkeley, California. The program has several affiliates across the country in states from California to New York and North Carolina. Started by chef Alice Waters, the idea was to create an organic garden that could then be integrated into a school's curriculum and lunch program. This would provide students an opportunity to grow, prepare, serve, and eat their own food, an experience that Waters believes will encourage children's awareness of and appreciation for fresh food and ultimately for the environment.

The program began in 1995 at Martin Luther King Jr. Middle School in Berkeley, California, after Waters and the school administration met to discuss that school's lunch problems. Budget cuts had closed the cafeteria, and students were eating fast food from Styrofoam containers, sitting on the school blacktop.

With donations from the community and from fundraising, the school was able create a one-acre garden. The first crop was a simple cover crop, but today the acre contains vegetables, fruits, herbs, and flowers.

At first students participated in the garden once a month, but now each student at King Middle School attends up to 30 sessions in the kitchen and garden classrooms depending on their grade level. The King school is now a model for other Edible Schoolyard programs, with math classes measuring garden beds, science classes studying soil erosion and drainage, and history classes studying the use of corn among world cultures.

The idea of the Edible Schoolyard project is more than the introduction of fruits and vegetables into the school lunch menu. According the program website, each project incorporates lessons about botany and history of foods, of showing rather than telling students about the health consequences of their eating habits and engaging them in an interactive

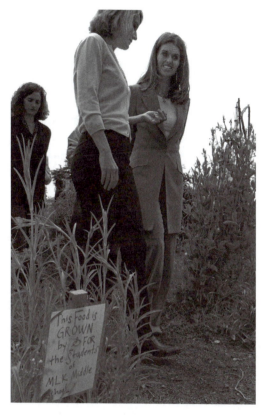

California first lady Maria Shriver, right, is given a tour of the Edible Schoolyard project by Katrina Heron, center, director of the Chez Panisse Foundation, at a middle school in Berkeley, California, on April 20, 2004. (AP/Wide World Photos)

education that brings with it a new understanding of food, health, and the environment. Supporters of the program compare the need for nutrition education in schools to the addition of physical education classes into public schools by President John Kennedy, who felt that U.S. schoolchildren needed to be more physically active and fit.

While few argue against introducing children to the pleasure of growing, harvesting, and eating fresh vegetables, critics of the program feel its integration into the entire school curriculum keeps students from having the time for core subjects such as math and reading.

The Chez Panisse Foundation was developed in 1995 to assist in creating funding for Edible Schoolyard programs and has assisted in establishing affiliate programs in Greensboro, North Carolina; Los Angeles; New Orleans; Brooklyn, New York; and San Francisco. The foundation also provides technical assistance to the affiliates while they work to introduce local, state, and national policy recommendations. For example, the foundation provided a three-year grant to the Berkeley Unified School District to overhaul its public school lunch program. The Berkeley school district serves every student a free breakfast and began cooking its meals from scratch using local fruits and vegetables rather than the frozen or canned commodity food from the federal government.

In 2010 actor Jake Gyllenhaal joined the Chez Panisse Foundation as the newly appointed ambassador for the Edible Schoolyard program. Gyllenhaal will work to raise awareness for the program and to encourage other school districts to adopt the Edible Education model for their students. Gyllenhaal visited the Edible Schoolyard site in Brooklyn in fall 2010 and planted the first tree with students at school PS 216.

Sharon Zoumbaris

See also National School Lunch Program (NSLP); Waters, Alice.

References

"The Edible Schoolyard." *Chez Panisse Foundation,* http://chezpanissefoundation.org.
"Fighting the Flab: Nutrition in Schools." *The Economist* (June 5, 2010): 38.
Waters, Alice. "Eating for Credit." *New York Times* (February 24, 2006): A23.

ENVIRONMENTAL HEALTH

"There was once a town in the heart of America where all life seemed to live in harmony with its surroundings," reads the first line in *Silent Spring* (Carson, 1962). The book, written by nature author and biologist Rachel Carson in the early 1960s, focused a spotlight on environmental poisoning and its link to emerging health issues. That beginning sentence refers to an anonymous U.S. town where the effects of the pesticide DDT "silenced all life, from fruit, fish, and birds to human children" (Carson, 1962). Carson's work was a catalyst in raising public awareness of how the environment influences and changes human health and wellness.

Now half a century later, incidences of cancer, asthma, autism, and allergies continue to rise and in many cases are blamed on exposure to the growing list of toxins in our daily lives. Consider the medical waste in municipal water, or baby bottles that leach chemicals into the milk, bleach in cotton bedding and electromagnetic frequencies from a host of electronic devices. Are they improving our lives or making us sick?

In microbiology, a toxin is a poisonous substance produced by living organisms or cells. A biotoxin, such as a snake's predatory venom or a bee's defensive stinger, relates to a toxin's biological source. According to the Society of Toxicology, toxicity is the biological effect of a substance; in this context, the words *toxicity* and *hazard* are used interchangeably. Toxicology is the study of the adverse effects of chemical, physical, or biological agents on people, animals, and the environment.

Environmental toxins vary by nature, type, and impact with each inherently presenting a threat to the health of the environment and humankind. The list of hazardous environmental toxins seems endless. Sources range from plastics, chemicals, gases, drugs, industrial and human waste, food, electromagnetic fields, radioactive materials, noise, climate warming, pollution, and emissions to bacteria, viruses, germs, and infectious agents.

In addressing the impact of environmental toxins, different organizations and groups describe environmental health in different terms. One of the most widely accepted definitions comes from the World Health Organization (WHO). According to the WHO, environmental health is made up of external human variables—from physical and chemical to biological—and their related aspects, which impact a person's life. In this definition, the WHO includes targeted disease prevention, the creation of health-supportive environments, and the evaluation and control of environmental factors that can potentially affect health.

The link between personal lifestyle choices such as smoking, overeating, and too much alcohol and adverse health effects is well established. Health care providers can confidently advise individuals on how these bad habits are putting them at risk for serious ailments. However, identifying an individual's risk of exposure to environmental hazards is more challenging. People come in contact every day with various forms of physical energy, natural or manmade chemical substances, and living matter, leaving a wide range of mediums such as air and water as potential hazards. Human health is a complicated issue that can be altered by many things, including choice, perception, and genetics.

Chemicals and other environmental sources may be triggers that cue genes to act in an unhealthy manner. Environmental toxins in combination with a genetic predisposition is but one of many theories in the search to unravel the mysteries behind certain neurological diseases, autoimmune disorders, endocrine problems, and pediatric cancers.

A team of Washington State University (WSU) scientists discovered that exposure to an environmental toxin during embryonic development can cause an animal, along with most of its descendents, to develop adult-onset illnesses such as cancer and kidney disease. Investigators exposed pregnant rats to a fungicide commonly used in grape vineyards during the period that the sex of the animals' offspring was being determined. At that development stage, the genes of the male embryo's sex cells (future sperm) are highly vulnerable to reprogramming (Washington State University, 2007).

The WSU research highlights the potential long-term health hazards of environmental toxins on health. It represents an epigenetics study of gene expression. Epigenetics involves changes to genes that don't affect the underlying DNA sequence (each person's genetic roadmap) but do affect how genes eventually express themselves. These changes can be transmitted from one generation to the next. Environmental epigenetics concentrates on how toxins, lifestyle choices (e.g., diet, smoking), and other factors activate the chemical switches that regulate gene expression.

Environmentally based health hazards are a particular challenge in at-risk populations such as the disabled, the poor, children, the unemployed, the underserved, and those already in a diminished health state. Poor environmental quality takes its heaviest toll on such individuals. Environmental health policy

Environmental Toxins

Five everyday chemicals have been linked to serious ailments, including behavioral issues, cancer, and sexual problems. They are BPA, polybrominated diphenyl ethers or PBDEs, phthalates, PFOA, and formaldehyde.

BPA—Bisphenol A—is a type of lightweight, clear, almost unbreakable, heat-resistant plastic used in nearly every industry in the manufacture of plastic water bottles, baby bottles, reusable food containers, jar lids, dental sealants, and electrical and electronic equipment. The Environmental Protection Agency has placed BPA on a concern list.

PBDEs—Polybrominated diphenyl ethers—are chemicals used to make flame retardant materials. They accumulate in human fatty tissue and in the environment. Evidence shows that PBDEs cause liver toxicity, thyroid toxicity, and neurodevelopmental toxicity. They are found in furniture foam, plastic TV cabinets, consumer electronics, coatings for draperies and upholstery, as well as in plastics for personal computers and small appliances.

Phthalates are found in packaging materials used in the production of foods and beverages. Associated problems include reproductive difficulties and an increased risk of cancer and liver disease. Phthalates are most commonly ingested through drinking water discharge from rubber and chemical factories.

PFOA—perfluoroocatonic acid—is a synthetic chemical not currently regulated under federal environmental laws that is used in the manufacture of nonstick cookware and all-weather clothing. Studies indicate that PFOA can cause developmental health effects in laboratory animals. PFOA is used by companies such as DuPont, which has agreed to eliminate PFOA emissions and products by 2015.

Formaldehyde is widely used in many consumer products, including permanent press clothing, draperies, and in pressed wood building materials. It has been shown to cause cancer in animals; asthma attacks in people; eye, nose, and throat irritation; and skin rash. In 2010 the EPA posted a formaldehyde review with comments for the public on its website.

must address, control, and ease the societal and environmental factors that can increase exposure to toxins and disease for these disparate groups.

On the other hand, nuclear accidents such as those that occurred at power plants in Three Mile Island, Pennsylvania, in the United States; Chernobyl in the Ukraine; and Fukushima in Japan present a health hazard for entire populations. Population health threats are difficult to relate to the individual scale; what may cause asthma, cancer, or infertility in one person may not in another. Epidemiologists—scientists who follow disease footprints within populations—develop long-term data by measuring the incidence of disease occurrence and associating it with different characteristics of populations and environments. At best, health care providers can use this information to caution individuals about population-based health problems.

Public-sector agencies deal with larger considerations and view environmental health in the context of preventing or controlling disease, injury, and disability related to the interactions between people and their environment. Maintaining and sustaining a healthy environment is vital to increasing quality of life and years of healthy life. A 2006 WHO report on the estimate of the environmental burden of disease noted that worldwide approximately 25 percent of all deaths and the total disease burden can be attributed to divergent, far-reaching environmental factors (Pruss-Ustun & Corvalan, 2006). These factors include exposure to hazardous substances in the air, water, soil, and food; natural and technological disasters; physical hazards; nutritional deficiencies; and the human-made or "built" environment.

In an effort to improve the environment, the U.S. Department of Health and Human Services Healthy People 2020 initiative pinpoints six theme-based environmental health objectives. Each of the following themes centers on an area of environmental health with a need for improvement:

1. Outdoor air quality: Cancer, premature death, and long-term damage to respiratory and cardiovascular systems are associated with bad air quality. Unhealthy air emissions have been reduced, yet a 2010 U.S. Environmental Protection Agency report states that in 2008 nearly 127 million people lived in U.S. counties that exceeded national air quality standards.
2. Surface and ground water: Surface and ground water quality relates to drinking water and recreational water. Mild to severe illness can develop from infectious agents or chemical contamination.
3. Toxic Substances and hazardous wastes: Ongoing research is being developed for a better understanding of how exposure to toxic substances and hazardous wastes affects human health.
4. Homes and communities: People spend the majority of their time at home, work, or school and may be exposed to indoor air pollution, inadequate heating and ventilation, structural problems, electrical and fire hazards, and lead-based paint.
5. Infrastructure and surveillance: A collaborative approach using personnel, surveillance systems, and education to investigate and respond to disease, monitoring for hazards, and educating the public is necessary to prevent exposure to environmental hazards.
6. Global environmental health: A reduction in the incidence of disease can be achieved by improving water quality and sanitation and increasing access to adequate water and sanitation facilities.

Public health remains a number-one priority in developed countries, including the United States. To improve the health of its citizens, the U.S. Public Health

Service Commissioned Corps began more than 200 years ago. Public health experts and medical practitioners can set forth guidelines for good health practices, legislators can establish laws and regulations to reinforce community health standards, and epidemiologists can set up large population health studies; still, individual behavior may have the most impact on disease prevention and how healthy the environment is.

A person's home may contain an abundance of potential environmental toxins. Chemicals, additives, preservatives, and synthetic materials are everywhere. Many have known health hazards for humans or have demonstrated adverse effects in animal models and can be found in common household products. A special 2010 Earth Day edition of *Time* magazine on the environment lists the federal government's top 10 household toxins (Park, 2010). They are:

1. Bisphenol A (BPA): a chemical used in the production of plastics
2. Oxybenzone: a chemical used to make cosmetics
3. Fluoride: one form of the element fluorine used in tap water
4. Parabens: artificial preservatives used in shaving and hair products
5. Phthalates: chemicals used to make plastic resilient and flexible
6. Butylated hydroxyanisole (BHA): an additive used for preserving fats and oils
7. Perfluorooctanoic acid (PFOA): a material used in Teflon nonstick coatings
8. Perchlorate: a material used in Teflon nonstick coatings
9. Decabromodiphenyl ether (DECA): a flame retardant substance
10. Asbestos: a natural fibrous mineral used in insulation

While federal public agencies review and monitor the impact of these items, government regulations and warnings vary by substance, so it remains important for consumers to be vigilant and informed about the products they use, especially in light of the fact that a lack of quality control in human-made product manufacture can cause environmental hazards. The case of imported drywall is an important example. Residents from more than 40 states, the District of Columbia, American Samoa, and Puerto Rico fear their poor health symptoms and the corrosion of certain metal components in their homes are related to the presence of drywall produced in China. The U.S. Consumer Product Safety Commission (CPSC) has received nearly 4,000 complaints regarding the defective imported drywall.

CPSC experts report that the product was installed in homes built or remodeled from 2001 to 2009. State health departments and the CPSC advise these homeowners to watch for indications of corrosion, including if the home's copper pipes, plumbing fixtures, or uninsulated electrical wires at light switches or receptacles have corroded; if the air conditioner evaporator coils failed early; or if the house has an odor that smells like rotten eggs, matches, or fireworks. When determining whether the drywall is defective, experts suggest that homeowners check the back side of the drywall. Some drywall from China is stamped with

"Made in China." If any corrosion or odor problems are observed, this may indicate that there is defective drywall in the house.

Indoor air tests conducted by the CPSC identified reactive sulfur gases—including hydrogen sulfide and carbonyl sulfide along with emissions of sulfur dioxide—from the drywall. Gas levels are higher in houses containing the imported drywall than those that do not.

The CPSC is coordinating with other federal agencies to address the imported drywall hazard. Consumer groups and builder associations are working with the government and in the courts to find a solution. Extensive investigation into the potential scope of the defective drywall problem and detailed documentation of the drywall's origin is ongoing.

Another environmental health concern related to everyday exposure to toxins is the question of electromagnetic fields. "Danger: mobile phones can 'cook' your brain" screams a news article headline in reference to the alleged danger of consumer cell phone use. Variances in voltage create electric fields; and the higher the voltage, the stronger the resulting field. As electrical current flows, magnetic fields develop; and the stronger the currents, the stronger the field. Static electric fields can exist as charges or voltage differences on the surface of objects.

There are both natural and human-made electromagnetic field sources. Electric charges develop in the atmosphere during thunderstorms, and the Earth's own magnetic field creates a north-south compass needle that birds and fish use for navigation. Increasing demand for electricity, technological advances, and social behavior changes have contributed to the development of additional artificial electromagnetic field sources. People everywhere are exposed to a complicated web of electric and magnetic fields through telecommunications, broadcasting, appliances, and electricity generation and transmission.

To provide protection against the environmental impact from electromagnetic fields, the WHO, in conjunction with the International Commission on Non-Ionizing Radiation Protection and the Institute of Electrical and Electronic Engineers, has developed international exposure guidelines. The WHO also recommends that national authorities adopt international standards to protect residents against adverse levels of electromagnetic fields and establish guidelines restricting access to places where there may be excessive exposure limits.

Responses to stimuli or environmental changes that can be measured in a person are called biological effects and are not usually going to have an adverse effect on individual health. Biological effects occur in a person during routine activities such as playing the piano or riding a bicycle. The human body is naturally able to cope with diverse environmental influences. However, the body does not have the capacity to adjust to all biological effects. Permanent changes that stress the human system over an extended time may represent a health hazard. On the other hand, with an adverse health effect, there is a distinct health problem in an environmentally exposed individual, while a biological effect may or may not have an adverse health effect or hazard. Research continues to determine the identity and impact of this growing list of health hazards.

Contemporary toxicologists adhere to a general standard that originated with 16th-century Swiss physician Theophrastus Philippus Aureolus Bombastus von Hohenheim, the so-called father of toxicology. He was an early pioneer in using chemicals in medicine and believed that "the dose makes the poison." He taught that toxic substances were safe for humans when the amount was below a specific level.

Modern biomonitoring methods allow scientists to detect exposure traces in humans as minute as one part per trillion. These methods are changing the way industries, governments, and medical communities regard human exposure to environmental toxins. The human organ system is comprised of cells and tissue preprogrammed for specific functions. If there is exposure to a hazardous substance, the organ that the substance affects at the lowest dose is referred to as the target organ.

Every person reacts differently when exposed to environmental toxins. Certain groups of people may be more environmentally sensitive, have a predisposition due to their genetic profile, or work in a job that necessitates direct exposure to toxic environmental triggers.

One environmentally linked condition, ideopathic environment illness or intolerance (IEI), has had many different names, including multiple chemical sensitivity (MCS), over time. The public refers to MCS. Physicians refer to IEI. The IEI label reflects the uncertain nature of the condition and its relationship to chemical exposure. The National Institute of Environmental Health Sciences describes it as a "chronic recurring disease caused by a person's inability to tolerate an environmental chemical or class of foreign chemicals." Common among sufferers are complaints of severe sensitivity or allergic reactions to different pollutants, including perfumes or scented products, pesticides, cleaning solvents, new carpets, car exhaust, gasoline and diesel fumes, air pollution, tobacco smoke, plastics, and formaldehyde. Symptoms can involve multiple organ systems and can be severe or debilitating.

The Chemical Sensitivity Foundation estimates that more than 7 million Americans may suffer from IEI (Moore & Roman, 2010). The incidence of the disease is growing, according to the foundation, which points to natural and human-made disasters such as the BP oil spill in 2010 and Hurricane Katrina in 2005. These events caused widespread exposures to chemicals, resulting in immediate and long-term health risks for those exposed.

Some illnesses caused by environmental triggers are clearly defined by their clinical presentation and laboratory test results. For instance, *building-related illness* is a term used when diagnosable illness symptoms are identified and can be related directly to airborne building contaminants. In contrast to IEI sensitivities, these patients experience a limited set of symptoms, which occur only in the affected building.

Many scientists, allergists, and other doctors doubt an IEI diagnosis since there is no known cause for the disease, symptoms vary greatly among patients and are common to other diseases, and there are no specific treatments that work. Clinicians and researchers who believe this is a real medical condition would like to see IEI accepted as an allergic type of illness. They theorize that an unrecognized form of allergy or immunologic hypersensitivity may be the cause.

Of 80,000 chemicals registered in the United States, the Environmental Protection Agency has, under the Toxic Substances Control Act, required the safety testing of only 200.

No longer is it just the coal miner being diagnosed with black lung disease or the firefighter suffering from the residual effects of smoke inhalation. Occupational diseases crosscut all fields, from manufacturing, business services,

---

Household Cleaners

The average U.S. home contains many chemical cleaners and disinfectants. Surprisingly, there are six common household ingredients that will do the job just as well: salt, baking soda, white vinegar, borax, lemon juice, and liquid soap.

Here is a list of products and their substitutes:

Air freshener—To absorb odors, place small bowls of baking soda in the refrigerator and around the house and sprinkle into the bottom of trash cans, or leave small bowls of lemon juice around the house.

Carpet deodorizer—Lightly sprinkle baking soda, cornmeal, or borax on carpets. Let stand 30 minutes, and then vacuum.

Disinfectants—Mix one-quarter cup borax with one-half cup hot water, wipe onto surfaces, and wipe dry.

Drain cleaner—To prevent clogs, pour one-quarter cup salt, one-half cup baking soda, and one-half cup vinegar down the drain and cover it. Allow to stand for several minutes, and then pour boiling water down the drain. To unclog a drain, use a plunger to break up the clog; then flush the drain with the above mixture.

Glass cleaner—Mix five tablespoons white vinegar with one quart warm water, and pour into a spray bottle. Spray onto windows or glass, and wipe with cloth or paper towel.

Scouring powder—Mix equal parts vinegar and salt and scrub with a bristled brush.

Shoe polish—Lightly rub olive oil or nut oil into shoe leather and buff with a soft, clean cloth.

Silver polish—Create a paste with baking soda and water. Rub paste onto the silver; rinse; and polish with a soft, damp cloth.

Wood furniture polish—Mix together two parts vegetable oil and one part lemon juice. Apply a small amount and gently rub into wood with a soft, clean cloth.

Sharon Zoumbaris

agriculture, health care, and transportation to construction and even academics with regard to on-the-job hazards, especially exposure to toxic sources.

Workplace exposures to toxins are thought to cause a wide range of disorders and, in some cases, death, with estimates of hundreds of thousands of illnesses and more than 60,000 disease deaths occurring annually (Public Broadcasting System, 2000). The American Academy of Family Physicians reports musculoskeletal disorders, respiratory diseases, neurological disorders, cancer, heart disease, and stress-related illnesses among the categories of occupational maladies. The academy encourages physicians trying to determine the cause of a particular illness to consider an individual's workplace circumstances and any other environmental hazards.

The research and development of novel substances constantly brings new materials and items into workplaces across the nation. Regulations for usage, safety standards, and monitoring systems are a key concern and the driving force behind the passage by California legislators in 2006 of the nation's first statewide, community-based biomonitoring program. The Department of Health Services and the California Environmental Protection Agency now monitor for chemicals suspected of impacting human health. The data will help officials identify hot spots where exposure to toxins may be harming the health of those populations. For example, volunteers will be tested for the effects of pesticides in the Central Valley or breast cancer in Marin County.

Environmental health is a changing, developing field of study. Still, personal choice continues to dictate use or nonuse of potentially harmful environmental toxins, making education about those toxins increasingly important for Americans. For better or worse, humans and their health status will always be, to some degree, a product of their environment.

Dianne L. Needham

See also Cancer; Cell Phones; Love Canal; World Health Organization (WHO).

References

Agency for Toxic Substances and Disease Registry. "Health Effects of Exposure to Substances and Carcinogens," www.atsdr.cdc.gov/substances/ToxOrganSystems.asp.

American Academy of Allergy, Asthma, and Immunology. "Idiopathic Environmental Intolerances," www.aaaai.org/media/resources/academy_statements/position_statements/ps35.asp.

American Academy of Family Physicians. "Recognizing Occupational Disease," www.aafp.org/afp/980915ap/lax.html.

Carson, Rachel. *Silent Spring.* New York: Houghton Mifflin, 1962.

Centers for Disease Control and Prevention. "CDC's Response to Imported Drywall," www.cdc.gov/nceh/drywall.

Consumer Product Safety Commission. "Drywall Information Center," www.cpsc.gov/info/drywall/index.html.

Kristof, Nicholas D. "Do Toxins Cause Autism?" *New York Times* (February 24, 2010), www.nytimes.com/2010/02/25/opinion/25kristof.html.

Moore, Alicia, and Gerard Roman. "Seminar Explores Multiple Chemical Sensitivities Topic." *Environmental Factor* (December 2010), www.niehs.nih.gov/news/newsletter/2010/december/inside-seminar.cfm.w

Nakazawa, Donna Jackson. *The Autoimmune Epidemic: Bodies Gone Haywire in a World Out of Balance and the Cutting Edge Science That Promises Hope.* New York: Simon & Schuster, 2008.

Ortiz, Deborah. "Governor Signs SB 1379 to Create Nation's First State Biomonitoring Program." *California Progress Report* (September 30, 2006), www.californiaprogressreport.com/site/node/6527.

Park, Alice. "Environmental Toxins: The Hazards Lurking at Home," *Time,* April 1, 2010, www.time.com/time/specials/packages/article/0,28804,1976909_1976895_1976914,00.html.

Pruss-Ustun A., and C. Corvalan. "Preventing Disease through Healthy Environments." World Health Organization (2006), www.who.int/quantifying_ehimpacts/publications/preventingdisease.pdf.

Public Broadcasting System. "Costs of Occupational Illnesses and Injuries." *Frontline* (2000), www.pbs.org/wgbh/pages/frontline/shows/workplace/etc/cost.html.

Society of Toxicology. "What Is Toxicology?" www.toxicology.org/index.asp.

Srinivasan, S., L.R. O'Fallon, and A. Dearry. "Creating Healthy Communities, Healthy Homes, Healthy People: Initiating a Research Agenda on the Built Environment and Public Health. *American Journal of Public Health* 93, no. 9 (September 2003): 1446–50.

United States Environmental Protection Agency. "Indoor Air Facts No. 4 Sick Building Syndrome," www.epa.gov/iaq/pubs/sbs.html.

U.S. Department of Health and Human Services. "Environmental Health." *Healthy People 2020,* www.healthypeople.gov/2020/topicsobjectives2020/overview.aspx?topicid=12.

U.S. Public Health Service Commissioned Corps. "History," www.usphs.gov/aboutus/history.aspx.

Walsh, Bryan. "Environmental Toxins: The Perils of Plastics," *Time,* April 1, 2010, www.time.com/time/specials/packages/article/0,28804,1976909_1976908_1976938,00.html.

Washington State University. "Epigenetic Transgenerational Toxicology Research" (2007), http://skinner.wsu.edu/toxnews/.

World Health Organization. "Electromagnetic Fields" (May 2010), www.who.int/peh-emf/about/WhatisEMF/en/.

ENVIRONMENTAL PROTECTION AGENCY (EPA)

The Environmental Protection Agency (EPA), headquartered in Washington, D.C., is one of the independent agencies of the executive branch, reporting directly to the president of the United States. Because several programs were assigned to different agencies and lacked coordination, Congress created the new agency in 1970 under President Richard M. Nixon to place all of the programs under one umbrella.

The EPA's mission is to protect the environment and, thus, the health of U.S. citizens. It establishes minimum standards, monitors the environment, and enforces regulations. The various programs brought together include the elimination of air pollution and water pollution, controlling noise pollution, and limiting radiation exposure. As toxic waste disposal became more of a problem, the regulation of toxic waste was placed under the purview of the EPA, which now sets standards for its disposal.

The EPA was established as the political reaction to the clamor for a cleanup of the environment, which the government had previously assumed could clean itself. Before the EPA had been created, there was no governmental mechanism for the type of action necessary to take control of the environmental degradation and its deleterious effects on the health and the quality of life of the citizenry.

One of the EPA's programs derives from the Environmental Response, Compensation, and Liability Act of 1980, also called the Superfund. The act was passed to create a framework for the restoration of toxic waste sites. This act requires that those parties who caused the problem—that is, dumped toxic waste—finance the cost of the cleanup. Importantly, the EPA also monitors the activities of other federal agencies and reports on the impact of their activities on the environment. Furthermore, the EPA coordinates and assists state and local governments in their attempts at maintaining a clean environment within their geographic boundaries. The EPA also works with private organizations, working to keep the environment clean.

The EPA employs 17,000 people in Washington, D.C. It has 10 regional offices and laboratories around the country. Employees include the gamut of specialties necessary to run any agency, such as media and computer employees, but it also employs engineers and scientists who specialize in the environment.

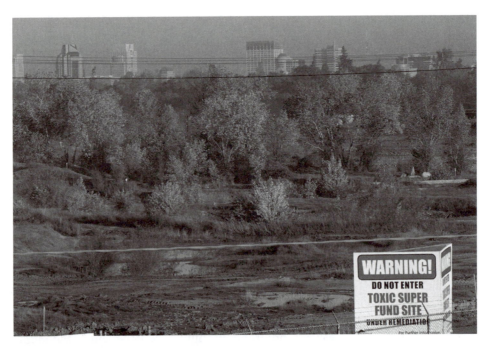

A Superfund site near Sacramento, California. Superfund sites are places where hazardous waste has been identified by the EPA. (Bob Keenan/Dreamstime.com)

The EPA administers all of the environmental laws: the Clean Air Act; the Clean Water Act; the Comprehensive Environmental Response, Compensation, and Liability Act and the Superfund Amendments and Reauthorization Act; the Emergency Planning and Community Right-to-Know Act; the Federal Insecticide, Fungicide, and Rodenticide Act; the Federal Food, Drug, and Cosmetic Act; the National Environmental Policy Act; the Oil Pollution Act of 1990; the Safe Drinking Water Act; the Solid Waste Disposal Act; Resource Conservation and Recovery Act; and the Toxic Substances Control Act.

The EPA conducts many programs (some of which are described in the following discussions) that safeguard the food supply of the United States. The EPA is often criticized by those who say that its regulations stifle business and impede economic growth. Some Republican politicians vow to cut many of its programs as a way to reduce federal spending in difficult economic times.

AgSTAR Program   The AgSTAR program promotes the installation of biogas recovery systems in confined animal feedlots. The goal of the program is to reduce methane emissions.

Pesticide Environmental Stewardship Program   The goal of the Pesticide Environmental Stewardship program is to encourage the stewardship of the soil and the environment by voluntary means and by not merely following the standards but exceeding the standards.

The National Clean Diesel Campaign   The National Clean Diesel Campaign (NCDC) includes these campaigns: Clean Construction USA, Clean Ports USA, Clean School Bus USA, and Diesel Retrofit. The NCDC is part of a plan to make diesel engines cleaner. This effort has been partly regulatory and partly voluntary. This program has the cooperation of national, state, and local agencies, such as school districts, as well as nongovernmental partners.

Coal Combustion Products Partnership   The Coal Combustion Products Partnership (C2P2) is a program that combines the efforts of industry and the government to encourage efficient energy production through the use of coal, reduce the overall consumption of energy, reduce the level of greenhouse gases emitted into the atmosphere, and reduce the amount of solid waste by encouraging the industry to recycle. For example, one goal of the C2P2 program is to replace Portland cement with coal ash in concrete. The goal is to go from the 12.6 million tons used in 2002 to 20 million tons of coal ash in 2010. It was predicted that reaching this goal will result in the reduction of greenhouse gases by at least 6.5 million tons each year and increase the reuse of coal combustion products from 35 percent to more than 45 percent. In 2011, the EPA suspended active participation in this program while they evaluate the program goals.

Combined Heat and Power Partnership   Combined Heat and Power (CHP) is known by another term: cogeneration. The CHP is a methodology that allows for power and thermal energy to be generated from one source. The CHP Partnership (CHPP) operates on a voluntary basis. It is designed to encourage the use of regeneration and thereby reduce the impact of the generation of power on the environment. Each participating facility installs a CHP system. The system is tailored to satisfy both heat and energy requirements of the participating facility.

This retrofitting with CHP makes the facility more efficient—both decreasing the costs of energy generation and production of heat. The CHPP works when members of the cogeneration industry, the EPA, appropriate state and local agencies, energy consumers, citizens, and environmental groups join together to keep making improvements to the systems, let others know about the benefits of cogeneration, and facilitate the joining of the program by new participants, including food industry participants.

Community-Based Childhood Asthma Programs The connection between environmental pollution and the incidence and control of asthma is the motivation behind the creation of the Community-Based Childhood Asthma Program. This voluntary program is conducted in conjunction with public health officials at the federal and local levels in an attempt to reduce the incidence of asthma attacks by reducing environmental triggers. This program identifies best practices and allows families who have children with asthma to help reduce triggers in the home, in schools, day care centers, and other public and private places. Most families have an asthma management plan, and this program is intended to be part of that plan, which also may include medical treatment and drug and other therapies.

EnergyStar The EnergyStar program is designed to help citizens make intelligent choices when purchasing products, such as appliances, that use energy. This program is applicable to both business and private investment in energy-efficient appliances. The program is administered jointly by the EPA and the U.S. Department of Energy. In addition to using less energy, citizens and businesses can save money by using energy-efficient products and promote a cleaner environment.

To make it easier to participate, the EnergyStar program has created a rating system that quantifies the energy efficiency of products. The EPA has worked with producers in all of the sectors of appliance production to support the use of the EnergyStar label on all products. In addition, it encourages producers to create more efficient products to achieve a better rating, create better practices for new construction and retrofitting to achieve higher ratings, and inform consumers in all markets of the benefits of these efficiencies.

Great American Woodstove Changeout Campaign Woodstoves manufactured before 1988 are generally inefficient. To encourage the transition to more efficient models, the EPA and environmental organizations and industry have joined together to form the Great American Woodstove Changeout Campaign. The campaign encourages the installation of more efficient clean-burning stoves that are EPA-certified. One of the goals of the program is to reduce air toxicity both inside and outside, reduce solids in the air, reduce the potential hazards for fire, and improve overall efficiency.

Green Power Partnership More and more sources of green power are being identified. The Green Power Partnership encourages the use of green power sources instead of conventional sources, which may be inefficient and have a great environmental impact. This program is voluntary. Renewable sources of energy, such as solar and wind power, allow commercial and other entities to reduce their environmental impact. The EPA educates, assembles groups, creates resources, and has a program of publicizing partners. Many organic food producers include green production in their practices.

Labs 21 Labs 21 is a joint program of the EPA and the U.S. Department of Energy. It encourages laboratories on a voluntary basis to participate in the reduction of energy and the reduction of pollution by laboratories. Laboratories are high energy users as well as major polluters in all areas—water, air, and soil. The EPA and the U.S. Department of Energy are working together to establish best practices in new construction and retrofitted laboratories to reduce energy costs and diminish environmental damage. The EPA has set a goal to make all EPA laboratories energy self-sufficient so that other laboratories in the country can use their practices as a model.

Outdoor Wood-Fired Hydronic Heaters Program Old outdoor wood-fired hydronic heaters are one more example of inefficient appliances that may still be in use. The Outdoor Wood-Fired Hydronic Heaters program addresses this inefficiency by helping producers create and sell more efficient outdoor hydronic heaters.

Radon Risk Reduction Exposure to radon has been identified as the second leading cause of lung cancer. The Radon Risk Reduction (RRR) program has a goal of eliminating and minimizing this hazard. As real estate changes hands, radon problems in a home can be identified and remediated, if necessary. New home construction is also a part of the program. The RRR program is intended to incorporate radon-reducing features in new home construction.

Responsible Appliance Disposal Partnership Many of the chemicals found in old appliances deplete ozone in the atmosphere. When appliances are not disposed of properly, these chemicals from old freezers, computers, refrigerators, air conditioners, and humidifiers can leach into the environment and do damage. The Responsible Appliance Disposal (RAD) program supports those who recover the ozone-depleting chemicals such as foam insulation and refrigerant from old appliances and see that they are properly disposed of. RAD partners are varied and include universities and utility companies. They ensure that those components (such as metal, plastic, and glass) that can be recycled are recycled. The polychlorinated biphenyls, mercury, and used oil are recovered and properly disposed. The EPA collects and distributes data on the proper collection, disposal, and recycling of the components recovered from disposed appliances. In addition, the EPA collects statistics about disposal and recovery to properly review the program. These benefits, when properly marketed, can help encourage others to participate and help Congress understand the benefit of continuing the program. The RAD partnership also operates an awards program to encourage participation.

SmartWay Transport Partnership The SmartWay Transport Partnership educates consumers to the benefits of choosing truck and rail companies that operate in the most green energy-efficient manner and apply other green practices.

Retailers and other consumers are encouraged either to select an environmentally efficient carrier or to buy products from manufacturers that use efficient carriers.

Greenhill The Greenhill Advanced Refrigeration Partnership is a voluntary program composed of the EPA, the chemical industry that produces refrigerant, refrigeration manufacturers, and the grocery industry. It is designed to encourage the protection of the ozone layer around the Earth by the use of green technologies, environmental support plans, and methodologies. The implementation of the partnership should additionally reduce greenhouse gases and result in significant efficiencies and monetary savings. Because it is a voluntary program, partners do not limit themselves to complying with minimums, but rather pledge to do all that they can to affect the goals of the program. They agree to measure their current impact, including current refrigerant emissions, and then create a plan for the reduction of the emission, complete with target goals and dates. In addition, the partners agree that they will use non-ozone-depleting products and efficient refrigeration techniques as they improve their facilities or build new ones. The EPA hopes that through this program there will be significant improvement in the thinning of the ozone layer.

WasteWise WasteWise is a recycling program of the EPA. It shows the public how recycling and reuse can help save money and be more efficient. It encourages and promotes the use of recycling to reduce the production of waste materials and the purchase of products made of recycled materials. It encourages the manufacture of products with recycled materials. This program has a recognition component to further encourage participation.

The Environmental Protection Agency's budget was $7.8 billion in 2009. Almost half of its budget is used for state-operated programs, which support programs and projects within their respective states.

William C. Smith and Elizabeth M. Williams

See also Asthma; Environmental Health; Love Canal.

References

Environmental Protection Agency, www.epa.gov/.
Lewis, Jack. "The Birth of EPA." *EPA Journal* (November 1985), www.epa.gov/history/topics/epa.15c.htm.

EPHEDRA/EPHEDRINE

Ephedra was banned by the U.S. Food and Drug Administration (FDA) in 2004 based on reports that the weight-loss ingredient increased the risk of heart attacks and strokes. However, ephedra and many other supplements considered risky by the government are still available for purchase according to the watchdog group Consumers Union. Ephedrine is a drug from the plants of the genus *Ephedra,* and is promoted in many herbal diet remedies as a natural weight-loss product. Derived from a Chinese herb called *mahuang,* ephedra is a stimulant used for short-term energy boosts to enhance athletic performance and endurance, to help people exercise longer and feel more alert, to increase metabolism, and to dampen or suppress appetite. Ephedra has been an ingredient in several popular diet supplements, including Metabolife, Diet Pet, and Dexatrim, all part of the multibillion-dollar weight-loss industry.

In 2008 the former chief executive of the dietary supplement company Metabolife International was sentenced to six months in federal prison for lying to the FDA regarding one of the company's ephedra-based weight-loss products. The company had turned over reports to the government in 2002 of some 14,000 ephedra-related events that the company had previously not disclosed. Federal law now requires supplement manufacturers to report serious adverse effects to the FDA, but the government agency still depends on consumers to provide information as well.

Research published as early as December 2000 in the *New England Journal of Medicine* outlined serious complications from dietary supplements containing ephedra, including 10 deaths, 32 heart attacks, 62 cases of cardiac arrhythmia, 91 reports of hypertension, 69 strokes, and 70 seizures. Those figures were compiled between 1993 and 2000. Senator Arlen Specter, chairman of the Senate Subcommittee on Crime and Drugs, criticized the FDA during a hearing in 2009 for the agency's delay in banning ephedra for some 10 years after the FDA issued its first advisory.

Potential problems with ephedrine, according to researchers, is the possibility that the human body may convert ephedra to phenylpropanolamine, an ingredient the FDA banned after it was shown to increase the risk of a kind of stroke in young women. When reports of early problems first were reported, the FDA took no formal action, but by 1997, the agency called for ephedra labeling recommending that daily consumption be held to 24 milligrams. The agency also suggested that users take the supplements no more than seven days in response to studies showing that users who take ephedrine-containing supplements may develop a tolerance to it and must take more of the supplement to achieve the same effect.

The alarm over ephedra use continued to grow after the drug was considered a factor in the death of several high-profile athletes, including Steve Bechler, a 23-year-old minor-league baseball player who collapsed and died while training with the Baltimore Orioles in February 2003. Bechler had been taking a weight-loss supplement containing ephedra at the time of his death. The first statewide ban on ephedra use was signed into law in May 2003 by Illinois governor Rod Blagojevich after the death of a 16-year-old high school football player. The governor urged other states and the federal government to adopt similar bans, and the FDA officially banned ephedra in 2004.

Health organizations, businesses, and professional athletes began to distance themselves from the use of ephedra. Nutritional supplement retailer General Nutrition Centers announced in May 2003 that it would stop selling products containing ephedra. Following Bechler's death, minor-league baseball officials took steps to stop their players from using supplements with ephedra, a restriction already in place for professional and college football players as well as for National Collegiate Athletic Association and Olympic athletes. Ephedra was considered a factor in the deaths of college football players Rashidi Wheeler and Devaughn Darling and Minnesota Viking Korey Stringer. One baseball agent quoted in the March 2003 *Sporting News* estimated that 75 percent of ball players were using ephedrine.

Following Bechler's death, U.S. Department of Health and Human Services Secretary Tommy G. Thompson called for warnings on ephedra labels and for a ban on its use. The American Heart Association was also vocal in its opposition to supplements containing ephedra. On the other hand, dietary supplement industry officials then and now continue to maintain products containing ephedra aimed at U.S. dieters are not a health risk and, when used correctly, can be successful weight-loss aids. The American Generic Labs of Provo, Utah, announced in January 2010 that it had reformulated its popular line of ephedra-based diet pills to again meet FDA regulation changes. Also in 2010, a website was launched to provide information for dieters about the pros and cons of diet pills containing ephedra as a weight-loss aid. According to the website, EphendrineHydrochloride.com is the culmination of scientific research on the facts about ephedra.

Marjolijn Bijlefeld and Sharon Zoumbaris

See also Dieting; Exercise; Metabolism.

References

Brink, Susan, "Diet Drugs: What a Pill." *U.S. News & World Report* (November 20, 2000): 74.

Brody, Jane E. "Potential for Harm in Dietary Supplements." *New York Times* (April 8, 2008): F7.

The Columbia Encyclopedia, 6th ed. New York: Columbia University Press, 2000.

Conlan, Michael F. "Consumer Groups Want FDA to Ban Dietary Supplements with Ephedra." *Drug Topics* 145, no. 18 (September 17, 2001): 18.

Haller, C.A., and N.L. Benowitz. "Adverse Cardiovascular and Central Nervous System Events Associated with Dietary Supplements Containing Ephedra Alkaloids." *New England Journal of Medicine,* 343, no. 25 (December 21, 2000): 1833–38.

"New Blends for Popular Weight Loss Brands: Metabothin, Superdrine and Yellow Devils." *PRWeb Newswire,* www.prweb.com/released/2010/01/prweb3397944.htm.

Rosenthal, Ken. "No More Delays on Drug Testing." *Sporting News* 227, no. 9 (March 3, 2003): 50–52.

Smith, Ian K. "The Trouble with Fat-Burner Pills: Be Suspicious of the Dramatic Weight-Loss Claims of These Supplements." *Time,* August 27, 2001, 66.

EXERCISE

Trying to lose weight without increasing your level of physical activity is like driving a car with no gas in the tank. You may roll forward a little, but you're not really going to get anywhere. One pound equals 3,500 calories. So to lose a pound in, say a week, you'll either have to eat 3,500 calories less or burn off 3,500 calories in exercise, or some combination of the two. Some combination of the two is easier and healthier in the long run.

Exercise burns calories. While the specific rate at which calories are burned depends on individual weight and the intensity of the activity, here are some examples of calorie-burning activities. Walking briskly can burn off about 100 calories per mile. Bicycling for a half hour at nearly 10 miles per hour will burn about 195 calories. Experts recommend at least 30 minutes of vigorous activity five days a week. If you can't find 30 minutes, try two 15-minute intervals, or even three 10-minute intervals. And realize that what's vigorous for a sedentary person is different from a vigorous workout for an athlete. Work at your own pace.

To assist Americans and to encourage daily exercise and personal fitness, the U.S. Department of Health and Human Services (HHS) in 2008 issued a guide, the *Physical Activity Guidelines for Americans,* available at www.health.gov/paguidelines/. The agency created a comprehensive list of recommendations broken into various age categories aimed at helping people include physical activity into their daily schedule. According to the HHS, the guidelines are based on scientific research about health and exercise. A 13-member advisory committee appointed by then HHS secretary Mike Leavitt provided a thorough review of the literature.

Important recommendations from the guidelines for children and adolescents suggest one hour or more of moderate or vigorous aerobic activity each day. Examples of moderate activities are skateboarding, bicycling, and brisk walking. More vigorous activities include sports such as soccer and basketball or jumping rope or running. They also recommended muscle-strengthening activities such as rope climbing or sit-ups three days each week.

Recommendations for adults called for two and a half hours per week of moderate aerobic exercise or one hour and 15 minutes of vigorous activity. Examples of moderate activity include a brisk walk, water aerobics, or yoga. More vigorous activities might include step aerobics, jogging or running, or circuit weight training. The guidelines also suggested that short bouts of physical activity, about 10 minutes, will help many Americans reach their daily physical activity goal. Other suggestions include mixing it up by combining moderate and vigorous physical activities.

The guidelines encourage older adults to follow the guidelines for adults if they have the physical capacity, and those with disabilities should engage in activities that match their abilities in order to avoid inactivity. The American College of Sports Medicine (ACSM) continues to update its physical activity recommendations. Although its basic recommendations remain unchanged from the earlier Physical Activity Pyramid in 1998, the update clarifies exercise duration and intensity. The Physical Activity Pyramid, when introduced, was similar in design to the United States Department of Agriculture's nutritional pyramid, with activities that should be performed the most at the base and less vigorous, less frequent activity at the top.

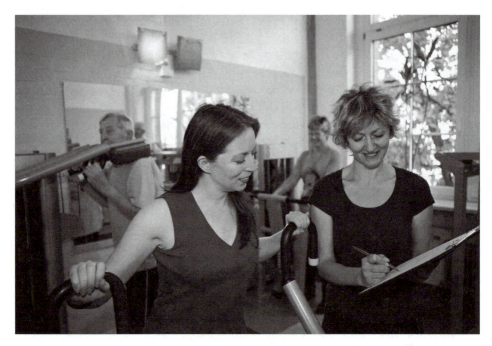

Adults practice circuit training in a gym with a trainer. Circuit training can help develop strength and aerobic endurance along with other health benefits. (Robert Kneschke/ Dreamstime.com)

The ACSM recommendations still call for the bottom level or "everyday activities"—walking, housework or yardwork, outdoor play, walking the dog—to total 30 minutes five days of the week.

The more vigorous activities include active aerobics, sports, and recreation, which should be done at least three times a week for 20 minutes. These vigorous activities, which involve speeding up the heart rate, include basketball, tennis, bicycling, soccer, jumping rope, and hiking. Because these activities elevate the heart rate, three 20-minute intervals per week have about the same health benefits as the activities done every day.

The updated ACSM recommendations also suggest muscle fitness exercises, which should be done two or three times a week. These activities include stretching, light weight lifting, push-ups, curl-ups, and gymnastics. The ACSM recommends that people exercise each major muscle group three to seven days per week and stretch to the point of mild discomfort, but not pain. For strength, the ACSM recommends doing muscle fitness exercises for each major muscle group two or three days a week with a day of rest in between.

The top level of the pyramid is inactivity. In the nutritional pyramid, fats and sugars are at this level—some are required, but they shouldn't be the mainstay of one's diet. Likewise in the activity pyramid, inactivity should be the exception, not the rule. Inactivity should be a small portion of your day—and no more than 30 minutes at a time.

Intensity Levels in Exercise

There are two main categories of intensity levels in physical activity: moderate and vigorous.

Moderate Activity

Walking at a steady pace on a level surface (walking the dog, walking to work or to shop)
Bicycling on a level terrain
Stationary bicycling
Yoga
Ballroom dancing
Water aerobics
Hiking
Doubles tennis
Recreational swimming
Golf
Surfing
Diving
Badminton

Vigorous Activity

Running or jogging
Rock climbing
Bicycling at more than 10 miles per hour or on steep uphill terrain
Jumping rope
Step aerobics (using higher steps and other variables)
Competitive wrestling
Singles tennis
Lap swimming
Cross-country skiing
Competitive sports (football, soccer, rugby, lacrosse, football)
Speed skating
Circuit weight training
Boxing in a ring

Marjolijn Bijlefeld and Sharon Zoumbaris

See also Aerobic Exercise; Anaerobic Exercise; Calories; U.S. Department of Health and Human Services (HHS); Walking; Weight Training.

References

Aaberg, Everett. *Muscle Mechanics*. Champaign, IL: Human Kinetics, 2006.

"Even Moderate Fitness Can Add Years to Your Life," *Healthy Years* 6, no. 10 (October 2009): 2.

Gebel, Erika. "The Science of Sweat: Is Exercise the Best Medicine?" *Diabetes Forecast* 63, no. 7 (July 2010).

Gogerly, Liz. *Exercise*. New York: Crabtree, 2009.

Phillips, Shawn. *Strength for Life: The Fitness Plan for the Best of Your Life*. New York: Ballantine Books, 2008.

Raugh, Randy. *Prime for Life: Functional Fitness for Ageless Living*. Emmaus, PA: Rodale, 2009.

Wadsworth, Andy. *The Complete Practical Encyclopedia of Fitness Training: Body-Shape, Stamina, Power*. London: Lorenz Books, 2009.

"Watch Your Back: Preventing Pain Leads to Happier Life, Career." *States News Service* (June 21, 2010).